OCULAR ANESTHESIA

Scott Greenbaum, M.D., F.A.C.S.

Attending Ophthalmologist
Long Island Jewish Medical Center
Assistant Attending and Former Resident Instructor
Manhattan Eye, Ear, and Throat Hospital
Associate Adjunct and Former Associate Clinical Director
New York Eye and Ear Infirmary
New York, New York

OCULAR ANESTHESIA

W.B. SAUNDERS COMPANY
A Division of Harcourt Brace & Company
Philadelphia London Toronto Montreal Sydney Tokyo

W.B. SAUNDERS COMPANY
A Division of Harcourt Brace & Company

The Curtis Center
Independence Square West
Philadelphia, Pennsylvania 19106

Library of Congress Cataloging-in-Publication Data

Ocular anesthesia / [edited by] Scott Greenbaum

p.   cm.

ISBN 0–7216–5955–1

1. Anesthesia in Ophthalmology.   I. Greenbaum, Scott.
   [DNLM: 1. Eye Diseases—surgery.   2. Anesthesia.   WW 168 019 1997]

RE82.035 1997   617.9′677—dc20

DNLM/DLC   96–22875

Cover illustration by T. C. Hengst

Ocular Anesthesia   ISBN 0–7216–5955–1

Printed in the United States.

Last digit is the print number: 9   8   7   6   5   4   3   2   1

This book is dedicated to
Melissa, Julie, Renee, and Dennis—the loving, caring
foundation upon which my life is built

NOTICE

Medicine is an ever-changing field. Standard safety precautions must be followed, but as new research and clinical experience broaden our knowledge, changes in treatment and drug therapy become necessary or appropriate. Readers are advised to check the product information currently provided by the manufacturer of each drug to be administered to verify the recommended dose, the method and duration of administration, and contraindications. It is the responsibility of the treating physician relying on experience and knowledge of the patient to determine dosages and the best treatment for the patient. Neither the Publisher nor the editor assumes any responsibility for any injury and/or damage to persons or property.

THE PUBLISHER

CONTRIBUTORS

Brian S. Biesman, M.D.
Assistant Professor of Ophthalmology, Tufts University School of Medicine, Boston, Massachusetts
Anesthesia for Oculoplastic Surgery

Sid Borirak-Chanyavat, M.D.
Charles Retina Institute, Memphis, Tennessee
Vitreoretinal Complications of Ocular Anesthesia

Benjamin Chang, M.D.
Assistant Attending, Manhattan Eye, Ear, and Throat Hospital, New York, New York
Anesthesia in Vitreoretinal Surgery

Steve Charles, M.D.
Clinical Professor of Ophthalmology, University of Tennessee College of Medicine, Memphis, Tennessee
Vitreoretinal Complications of Ocular Anesthesia

Eric D. Donnenfeld, M.D.
Assistant Clinical Professor of Ophthalmology, Cornell University Medical College, New York, New York; Department of Ophthalmology, North Shore University Hospital, Manhasset, New York
Anesthesia for Corneal Surgery

Yale L. Fisher, M.D.
Clinical Professor of Ophthalmology, New York Hospital Cornell Medical Center, New York, New York; Surgeon Director/Chief of Retinal Surgery Service, Manhattan Eye, Ear, and Throat Hospital, New York, New York
Anesthesia in Vitreoretinal Surgery

Albert Hornblass, M.D.
Clinical Professor of Ophthalmology, State University of New York Health Science Center, Brooklyn, New York; Surgeon Director, Chief of Ophthalmic Plastic, Lacrimal, Orbital, and Reconstructive Surgery, Manhattan Eye, Ear, and Throat Hospital, New York, New York
Anesthesia for Oculoplastic Surgery

Herbert J. Ingraham, M.D.
Director of Resident Training, Geisinger Medical Center, Danville, Pennsylvania; Clinical Assistant Professor in Ophthalmology, Wills Eye Hospital, Thomas Jefferson University, Philadelphia, Pennsylvania
Anesthesia for Corneal Surgery

Brian H. Jewart, M.D.
Director, Retinal Institute/Associates in Ophthalmology, Pittsburgh, Pennsylvania
Vitreoretinal Complications of Ocular Anesthesia

Craig H. Kliger, M.D.
Fellow, Cornea-External Ocular Disease, Visiting Assistant Professor of Ophthalmology, University of California, Los Angeles, California; Jules Stein Eye Institute, Los Angeles, California
Anesthesia for Refractive Surgery

Jonathan W. Konovitch, M.D.
Attending Anesthesiologist, Director of Anesthesiology, Manhattan Eye, Ear, and Throat Hospital, New York, New York
Anesthesiologist's View of Ocular Anesthesia

Mark J. Kupersmith, M.D.
Professor of Neurology and Ophthalmology, New York University Medical Center, New York, New York; Director of Neuroophthalmology, New York Eye and Ear Infirmary, New York, New York
Neuro-ophthalmologic and Neurologic Complications of Ophthalmic Anesthesia

Jeffrey M. Liebmann, M.D.
Clinical Associate Professor of Ophthalmology, New York Medical College, Valhalla, New York; Assistant Director of Glaucoma Service, New York Eye and Ear Infirmary, New York, New York
Anesthesia for Glaucoma Surgery

Stephen N. Lipsky, M.D.
Pediatric Ophthalmology, Rhode Island Hospital, Brown University, Providence, Rhode Island; Attending Staff, Pediatric Ophthalmology, Kent County Hospital, Warwick, Rhode Island, Landmark Medical Center, Woonsocket, Rhode Island, and Hasbro Children's Hospital, Providence, Rhode Island
Anesthesia for Eye Muscle Surgery

Robert K. Maloney, M.D., M.A. (Oxon.)
Director, Laser Refractive Center, University of California, Jules Stein Eye Institute, Los Angeles, California
Anesthesia for Refractive Surgery

David J. Pinhas, M.D.
Director, Glaucoma Service, Brooklyn Hospital Center, Brooklyn, New York

Anesthesia for Glaucoma Surgery

Renée Richards, M.D., F.A.C.S.
Director, Eye Muscle Department, Manhattan Eye, Ear, and Throat Hospital, New York, New York; Surgeon Director, Manhattan Eye, Ear, and Throat Hospital, New York, New York

Anesthesia for Eye Muscle Surgery

Robert Ritch, M.D.
Professor of Clinical Ophthalmology, New York Medical College, Valhalla, New York; Chief of Glaucoma Service, New York Eye and Ear Infirmary, New York, New York

Anesthesia for Glaucoma Surgery

Floyd Warren, M.D.
Associate Clinical Professor of Ophthalmology, New York University School of Medicine, New York, New York; Director, Neuroophthalmology Service, St. Vincent's Hospital; Attending, Bayley-Seton Hospital, New York, New York

Neuro-ophthalmologic Surgery

FOREWORD

In 1970, when I began demonstrating phacoemulsification to other surgeons, retrobulbar injections were the standard for local ocular anesthesia.

One of the first surgeons to become interested in phacoemulsification was Professor Murry McCaslin from Pittsburgh, who came to observe my surgery. After completing several uneventful cases in the operating room, I took Dr. McCaslin to the patient floor where I wanted to show him some patients who had been operated on the previous day.

The first patient we examined had a beautiful eye. The cornea was clear, there was very little inflammation, and compared to the appearance of the eye after intracapsular extraction, this eye looked almost as if it had never been operated on. I proudly exhibited this patient to Dr. McCaslin, who was duly impressed. We were about to leave when the woman said, "Doctor, when will I see out of this eye?" I told her that as soon as we fitted her for a contact lens or glasses, she would see very well. Her next statement sent a chill through me and Dr. McCaslin.

"But doctor, I don't even see light out of this eye now." Dr. McCaslin and I bumped heads as we both tried to look at her fundus. This patient had had a hemorrhage around the optic nerve, and I remembered that her retrobulbar injection had been somewhat more difficult than usual because she was moving her head.

Obviously it was the retrobulbar injection that had caused the hemorrhage and subsequent destruction of the optic nerve.

That injection in 1970 was the last retrobulbar injection I ever gave. I began looking around for a better way to anesthetize the eye without going back toward the nerve. I quickly discovered that by injecting superiorly through conjunctiva and tendons, the exact same anesthesia could be achieved with absolute safety. This was, I believe, the beginning of peribulbar anesthesia, which I have used successfully and uneventfully in many thousands of cases since.

I am pleased to see Dr. Greenbaum authoring a book on ocular anesthesia.

CHARLES D. KELMAN, M.D.

PREFACE

*The rain descended, and the floods came, and the winds blew,
and beat upon that house; and it fell not: for it was founded upon
a rock [Matthew 7:25].*

In the building project that is every eye surgery, in which the success
of each step is dependent on that of its immediate predecessor, anesthesia is the foundation. If the anesthesia is properly performed, the patient
should be comfortable, confident, and still, and the surgeon should be
able to accomplish the goals of the procedure without distraction. There
should be no lasting adverse sequelae from the administration of anesthesia. When surgical complications arise, the initial anesthesia should
be sufficient in potency and duration to allow the surgeon to manage
them without interruption. This is the goal for which we strive.

Who can better advise us on how to achieve this important goal than
surgeons themselves? A group of experienced surgeons and their current
and former fellows, who write and lecture extensively on their particular
subspecialties, were chosen to share their views on what is optimal
anesthesia for their particular procedures. All areas of eye surgery are
covered, including corneal, refractive, cataract, glaucoma, strabismus,
vitreoretinal, neuro-ophthalmic, and oculoplastic. This joint effort represents the first time such a volume has been written.

In addition, experts who see and manage the complications inherent in
administration of ocular anesthesia, especially vitreoretinal and neuro-
ophthalmic, discuss all aspects of recognizing, managing, and, most
important, avoiding these often devastating events. To this end, the
most modern techniques of ocular anesthesia, including parabulbar,
administration of propofol, and topical, are extensively covered from
many viewpoints. The more standard techniques of general, retrobulbar,
and peribulbar anesthesia are discussed as well, with the goal of maximizing their efficacy for each subspecialty while minimizing their risks.

I hope that this volume will prove useful to those learning to perform
eye surgery and those learning to provide anesthesia for eye surgery as
well as stimulating to those who have been doing so for their entire
careers. I sincerely wish to encourage future interest and innovation in
this most important area in order to help pour the soundest foundation
upon which to build the care of our patients.

SCOTT GREENBAUM, M.D., F.A.C.S.

CONTENTS

CHAPTER 1

ANESTHESIA FOR CATARACT SURGERY

SCOTT GREENBAUM, MD, FACS

HISTORIC PERSPECTIVES

The history of anesthesia for cataract surgery dates back over 2500 years. The earliest authentic writings on the subject were those of Sus'ruta, the ancient Indian surgeon who first described couching, the depression of the cataract into the vitreous, around 600 B.C.[1] He outlined the use of inhalational anesthesia for this method and also described aseptic technique. Later, Egyptian and Assyrian surgeons used carotid compression to produce transient cerebral ischemia, under which couching was performed. Dioscorides, who practiced in the first century A.D., produced a soporific sponge from an extract of mandrake boiled in wine. A Spanish alchemist in the 13th century described a mixture of sulfuric acid and alcohol, which he called "sweet vitriol."[2] In 1730, the substance was renamed ether, and Faraday reported on its accidentally discovered anesthetic effect in 1818. The use of other general anesthetic agents, such as carbonic acid gas, nitrous oxide, and chloroform, was described in the late 18th and 19th centuries.[1(p3117)]

The 18th century was also a time of discovery for more modern techniques of cataract surgery. In 1748, Daviel published an account describing a corneal incision started at the inferior limbus and continued nasally and temporally for approximately 240 degrees. He then performed an anterior capsulotomy and delivered the lens with a curette or spatula, depending on its density. Therefore, this, the first planned cataract extraction, was done in an extracapsular fashion.[3] In 1753, Samuel Sharp described a planned intracapsular extraction using a single knife to make the corneal section. These techniques took more than 100 years to become standard practice, during which time couching procedures continued to be performed using soporific drugs and psychological control of the patient.[2(p236)]

In 1865, Albrecht von Graefe described a scleral incision made with a single passage of a knife followed by the creation of an iridectomy. For this procedure he preferred the use of general anesthetics, especially chloroform.[4] He noted the potential dangers if the patient strained while awakening from anesthesia, and this may have been one of his main incentives for reducing the size of the previously described corneal flap incision of Daviel.

The next great advance in the evolution of anesthesia had its origins in 1855, when Gaedicke isolated the alkaloid of the coca plant. In 1860, Nieman noted its anesthetic effect on his tongue and named it cocaine. Carl Koller further described its use as a local anesthetic, and in 1884 Knapp[5] and Turnbull[6] both reported on the use of cocaine in eye surgery. Knapp described a technique for cataract removal under topical anesthesia using frequent cocaine drops. He also mentioned retrobulbar injection of cocaine for enucleation (the hypodermic needle had been developed in 1853 by Alexander Wood).[7] Turnbull introduced another local anesthetic technique for enucleation, using topical and sub-Tenon's cocaine.

However, an appreciation of the systemic and local toxicity of cocaine soon followed; episodes of syncope, excessive stimulation, hallucinations, and even death made it a less-than-perfect anesthetic. In addition, its corneal epithelial toxicity and drying effect, as well as its prolonged hypoesthesia, led to cases of exposure keratopathy and ulceration.

In 1904, the next step in the advancement of ophthalmic anesthesia began with Einhorn's discovery of procaine hydrochloride, which could be used for infiltration, instillation, and nerve block anesthesia without the toxic effects of cocaine.[2(p240)] Procaine had no inherent vasoconstrictive effects, however; it was absorbed rapidly and had a short duration of action. For this reason, epinephrine was added to slow absorption, thus hastening, intensifying, and lengthening the anesthetic effect. This addition, however, introduced the cardiovascular side effects of sympathetic stimulation in susceptible individuals.

A decade later, van Lint first described a technique for blocking the orbicularis muscle of the eye to prevent blepharospasm during cataract surgery.[8] He injected a combination of procaine and epinephrine near the lateral orbital rim, blocking the terminal branches of the facial nerve and innervating the orbicularis muscle. He advocated waiting 30 to 60 minutes before surgery, thus allowing the block to have its full effect. This block was easy to perform, with a good rate of success. Its localized effect was an advantage; eyelid edema, bruising, and bleeding were its main drawbacks.

O'Brien originated a method for a more proximal facial nerve block in 1929.[9] He injected procaine anterior to the tragus of the ear over the condyloid process of the mandible. He advocated waiting 5 minutes after injecting 2 mL of anesthetic before operating. Although the block was found to be safe, with a reduced risk of bleeding and intravascular injection, the anatomic variability of the zygomatic, mandibular, and buccal branches of the facial nerve reduced the certainty of a complete block.

In 1943, Lofgren and Lundquist synthesized lidocaine, and 3 years later Lofgren reported on its anesthetic properties.[10] It was found to have a more rapid onset, better diffusion, and longer duration than procaine. In addition, its early proponents believed that lidocaine was less toxic.[11] However, more toxicity was observed in higher concentrations. Circulatory depression was also associated with lidocaine, whereas respiratory depression was noted with procaine.[12]

The next major advance came in 1949, when Atkinson reported on the use of hyaluronidase in an attempt to increase the diffusion of procaine.[13] His method originated in the observation that aqueous testicular extract increased the spread of vaccinia virus.[14] This extract was later identified as hyaluronidase.[15] Atkinson found that the addition of 6 turbidity-reducing units per milliliter to a solution of 2% procaine with epinephrine provided more profound anesthesia and akinesia in both retrobulbar and facial nerve blocks without reducing the duration of action.

In 1953, Atkinson proposed another approach to blocking the facial nerve, introducing his needle through an intradermal wheal at the inferior edge of the zygomatic bone "a little posterior to the lateral margin of the orbit."[16] He then infiltrated anesthetic along the zygomatic arch, which he believed was the ideal site to block the upper branches of the facial nerve, while sparing those innervating the lips and lower facial muscles. The benefits of this method included the avoidance of lid edema as well as injection into major vessels and nerves. As with O'Brien's technique, however, its main drawback was the unpredictability of its effect because of the anatomic variability of the facial nerve's branches.

Ten years later, Nadbath and Rehman introduced the most proximal variation on the facial nerve block.[17] They injected anesthetic behind the mandibular ramus to block the main trunk of the facial nerve, exiting the stylomastoid foramen. Although this approach was the least subject to anatomic variation, its site was a veritable minefield of major blood vessels and cranial nerves. In addition, access to the dura surrounding the spinal cord was reported when this method was used in certain frail patients, with resultant respiratory depression and actual paralysis.[18] More commonly, hoarseness, pooling of secretions, and dysphagia were noted when the glossopharyngeal, vagus, and spinal accessory nerves were blocked along with the facial nerve.[19]

The literature of the next two decades is replete with case reports and complications of retrobulbar anesthesia, the most serious being blindness and death.[20–32] Alternatives to standard intraconal retrobulbar anesthesia were used as well. In 1985 and again the following year, Davis reported on the use of peribulbar anesthesia.[33, 34] He credited Kelman for its introduction in the mid-1970s. Davis's technique involved three injections, two given anteriorly, into and just beneath the orbicularis muscle of the upper and lower lids and one posteriorly along the floor of the orbit near the equator of the globe. Although Davis cited 1600 cases without complication,[34] it took only a year from the date of his publication for the first reports of globe penetration to be published.[35, 36]

Transconjunctival retrobulbar anesthesia was another technique to be introduced in the mid-1980s.[37] Gills advocated this method to reduce the potential for globe perforation and to avoid the need for a separate facial nerve block. The details of this and other anesthesia techniques for cataract surgery are discussed in greater detail later in this chapter.

In 1990, Hansen, Mein, and Mazzoli described a modification of Turnbull's sub-Tenon technique.[38] Although sub-Tenon's anesthesia had not been forgotten in the intervening 106 years, it had been relegated to a largely ancillary position. Atkinson advocated the technique as a supplement to retrobulbar anesthesia in patients with preoperative inflammation.[10(p50)] The author observed Dr. Arnold Turtz at the Manhattan Eye, Ear, and Throat Hospital perform sub-Tenon's technique with a blunt metal cannula to improve the anesthetic effect of a retrobulbar block or to provide postoperative anesthesia to patients who had received general anesthesia as their primary block.

In 1950, Kirby had reported his abandonment of retrobulbar anesthesia in favor of sub-Tenon's technique because of the all-too-frequent complications of retrobulbar hemorrhage and proptosis with the former technique. He routinely used a needle to inject a combination of procaine, tetracaine (Pontocaine), and potassium sulfate before surgery.[2(p245)] Forty years later, Yanoff described an ocular perforation with the anterior sub-Tenon's injection.[39] In 1992, the author reported on the elimination of the needle in sub-Tenon's anesthesia through the use of a flexible, blunt polyethylene cannula.[40] In the same year, Stevens described the use of a blunt metal cannula in delivering sub-Tenon's anesthesia without a needle.[41]

The 1990s also heralded the resurgence of another noninjection technique: topical anesthesia. Although Koller had introduced topical cocaine in 1884, its toxicity limited its popularity. In 1956, Atkinson had reported using tetracaine for topical ocular anesthesia.[42] In 1966, Thorson,

Jampolsky, and Scott had described a topical proparacaine anesthetic in strabismus surgery.[43] In 1986, Shimizu had demonstrated the use of topical cocaine (3%) in performing clear corneal cataract surgery.[44] Finally, in 1992, Fichman presented a method for performing topical anesthesia with tetracaine and began popularizing its use in the United States.[45]

Many surgeons who write and lecture on topical anesthetic techniques use the term "vocal local" to underline the importance of constant communication with the patient during the procedure. In his discussion of papers presented at the 16th annual session of the American Academy of Ophthalmology and Otolaryngology at Chicago in 1955, Sadove remarked, "I want to emphasize that a few carefully chosen words are as potent as any sedation . . . vocal is about as good as local."[46]

In summary, it can be seen that rediscovery and modification of previously described techniques have been the driving forces in the evolution of ocular anesthesia since 1884.

ANATOMIC PERSPECTIVES

Understanding how to provide the most effective ocular anesthesia in the safest manner requires an anatomic knowledge of the nerves, blood vessels, muscles, and bony landmarks of the orbit, face, and globe. Although this anatomy is unique to any given patient, some basic rules apply that can be of great help.

The first consideration in providing anesthesia for cataract surgery or any other purpose is understanding the goals of the block. Which parts of the eye does one intend to leave without sensation? Which muscles does one wish to paralyze? Once these questions are addressed, the next task at hand is to understand the cranial neuroanatomy.

The trigeminal nerve carries the sensory innervation of the eye and adnexa in three divisions: ophthalmic, maxillary, and mandibular. Except for a portion of the sensory input from the lower lid that is carried by the maxillary division, the sensory fibers of the eye and adnexa are found in the ophthalmic division. This division in turn has three components: frontal, lacrimal, and nasociliary. The frontal nerve usually branches into two more divisions: the supraorbital, which carries sensation from the conjunctiva and skin of the central two thirds of the upper lid, and the supratrochlear, which carries sensory fibers from the medial third of the upper lid. The lacrimal nerve carries sensory input from the skin and conjunctiva of the lateral aspect of the upper lid.[47] The nasociliary nerve carries sensory fibers from the cornea, iris, ciliary body, perilimbal bulbar conjunctiva, and optic nerve sheath; these fibers proceed through its long ciliary branches and sensory root to the ciliary ganglion. The infratrochlear branch of the nasociliary nerve carries sensory input from the medial canthus, medial portion of lower lid skin and conjunctiva, caruncle, lacrimal sac, and canaliculi.

Once it is known which branches are responsible for carrying sensory input from which structures, an approach can be planned that has a reasonable chance of blocking the targeted area. Because, for example, the nasociliary nerve carries fibers that pass through the intraconal space, a standard intraconal retrobulbar block may provide excellent intraocular and partial surface anesthesia. It could not be expected, however, to block the conjunctiva of the upper or lower lids or the lateral aspect of the globe effectively. Because the frontal and lacrimal branches enter the orbit through the superior fissure, above the annulus of Zinn, and the maxillary division enters the orbit through the infraorbital foramen, below the annulus, an intraconal approach will probably not block the structures that these branches innervate effectively. If an intraconal retrobulbar block is the only one administered before surgery, patients can be expected to feel irrigating solutions being dropped on the conjunctiva, away from the limbus; they will also be aware of the lid speculum and any manipulation of the lateral surface of the globe. They will probably attempt to close the eye in response to these stimuli. This is the basis for the traditional facial-retrobulbar block combination.

As has been mentioned, a litany of facial blocks have been devised to prevent patients from squeezing the eye shut during surgery. None of these blocks keeps patients from wanting to close the eye; they only keep the patients from succeeding. Because the facial block also involves added discomfort, many anesthesiologists and surgeons provide intravenous sedation along with it. Thus, limiting the initial block to the intraconal retrobulbar space also limits its potential benefits, requiring two supplemental procedures. Anatomy determines effect. Figure 1–1 shows the branches of the ophthalmic division of the trigeminal nerve, and Figure 1–2 depicts the relationship between the muscle cone and the sensory nerves.

The more anterior blocks—peribulbar, parabulbar-sub-Tenon's, and topical—reduce or eliminate the need for a separate facial block by providing better surface anesthesia than the retrobulbar. Although the

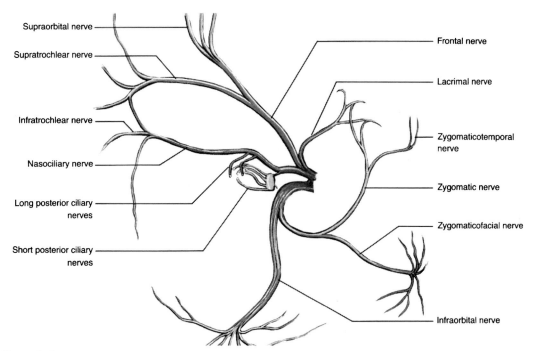

Figure 1–1. Sensory nerves, frontal view. (From Dutton JJ. Atlas of clinical and surgical orbital anatomy. p 52. Philadelphia: WB Saunders, 1994, p 52. Used with permission.)

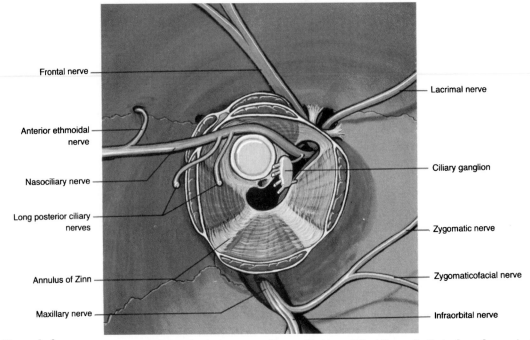

Frontal nerve

Anterior ethmoidal
nerve

Nasociliary nerve

Long posterior ciliary
nerves

Annulus of Zinn

Maxillary nerve

Lacrimal nerve

Ciliary ganglion

Zygomatic nerve

Zygomaticofacial nerve

Infraorbital nerve

Figure 1–2. Sensory nerves, frontal view, apex. (From Dutton JJ. Atlas of clinical and surgical orbital anatomy. Philadelphia: WB Saunders, 1994, p 52. Used with permission.)

first two also provide intraocular anesthesia through their effect on the nasociliary branch, topical blocks provide only surface anesthesia, so that intraocular sensations, such as stretching of the zonulae, during filling of the anterior chamber may be felt throughout surgery. Some authors advocate the addition of a subconjunctival injection to add more anesthetic effect to a topical block.[48(pp 182, 183)]

The motor supply of the superior, medial, and inferior rectus muscles, the inferior oblique muscle, and the levator palpebrae superioris muscle is carried by the oculomotor nerve (Figs. 1–3, 1–4). It also carries proprioceptive input from these muscles and parasympathetic fibers to the ciliary ganglion. As the oculomotor nerve enters the orbit through the supra orbital fissure, it splits into two divisions: superior and inferior. The superior division is smaller, courses forward within the superolateral portion of the intraconal space, and then turns medially toward the lateral aspect of the superior rectus muscle, where it divides into a network of small branches.[49] The innervation of all extraocular muscles is multifocal, with nerve fibers extending distally and proximally between the muscle fibers, before ending at myoneural junctions.[47(p38)] Some branches innervate the superior rectus muscle, whereas others pass through it to enter the levator muscle through its inferior surface.

The inferior division of the oculomotor nerve splits into at least three trunks within the intraconal space, and these in turn divide into 8 to 10 branches as they course forward, lateral to the optic nerve. The medial rectus is innervated by branches that run from beneath the optic nerve into the muscle, beginning at its posterior third. The inferior rectus muscle is similarly penetrated at its posterior conal surface by branches of the inferior division of the oculomotor nerve. The inferior oblique

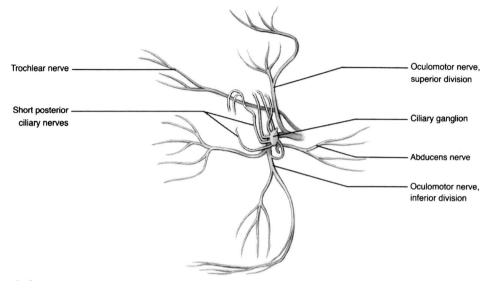

Figure 1–3. Motor nerves, frontal view. (From Dutton JJ. Atlas of clinical and surgical orbital anatomy. Philadelphia: WB Saunders, 1994, p 50. Used with permission.)

muscle is innervated by a branch that initially contains parasympathetic fibers; these fibers originate in the Edinger-Westphal nucleus and enter the ciliary ganglion inferolateral to the optic nerve. The remainder of this branch then breaks up into smaller fascicles, which penetrate the inferior oblique at its posterolateral aspect.[47(p38)]

The trochlear nerve supplies motor fibers to the superior oblique muscle. It enters the orbit through the superior oblique fissure above

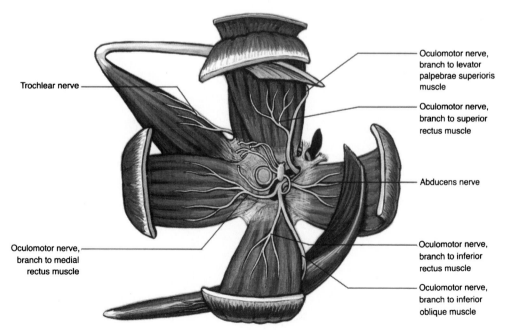

Figure 1–4. Motor nerves, frontal view with extraocular muscles. (From Dutton JJ. Atlas of clinical and surgical orbital anatomy. Philadelphia: WB Saunders, 1994, p 50. Used with permission.)

the annulus of Zinn, along with the frontal and lacrimal branches of the ophthalmic division of the trigeminal nerve. It crosses the superior rectus origin above the levator and enters the superolateral surface of the superior oblique muscle.[47(p40)]

The abducens nerve enters the orbit through the superior orbital fissure, along with the oculomotor nerve. They are sometimes divided by a dense septum connecting the superior rectus origin to the superior rectus sheath.[47(p38)] The abducens nerve enters the lateral rectus sheath just anterior to the annulus of Zinn and first enters the lateral rectus muscle at the medial aspect of the junction of its posterior and medial thirds.[47(p41), 50]

The ciliary ganglion is an irregular structure measuring 1×2 mm and lying just temporal to the optic nerve (see Figs. 1–3, 1–4) 7 to 10 mm from the orbital apex.[47(p39), 51] In it the presynaptic parasympathetic fibers from the Edinger-Westphal nucleus synapse with the postsynaptic fibers that form the short ciliary nerves. All but 3 to 5% of these fibers innervate the ciliary muscle; the remainder supply the iris sphincter. The ganglion also contains sensory branches of the nasociliary nerve and sympathetic fibers en route to the choroidal vasculature.

When attempting to provide akinesia, it should be kept in mind that the motor nerves enter the rectus muscles at the junction of their posterior and medial thirds or more anteriorly.[52] It is also important to remember that these fibers run both distally and proximally between the muscle fibers before they end at the myoneural junctions. A motor block may, therefore, be achieved at many points along their path. The oculomotor divisions may be blocked in the posterior orbit before their insertion into the rectus muscles, but it is necessary to keep in mind the proximity of the optic nerve, the ophthalmic vein, and the anterior muscular branches to the oculomotor branches in this region (Figs. 1–5, 1–6). Because the nerve and artery supplying the inferior oblique muscle

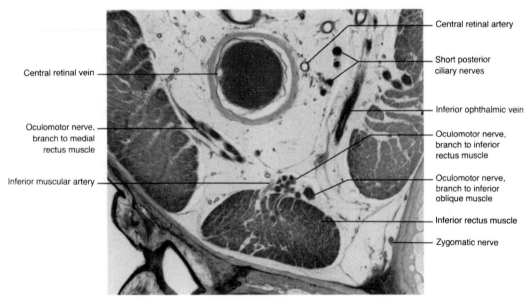

Figure 1–5. Inferior rectus muscle in posterior orbit at the entrance of the oculomotor nerve rootlets. (From Dutton JJ. Atlas of clinical and surgical orbital anatomy. Philadelphia: WB Saunders, 1994, p 168. Used with permission.)

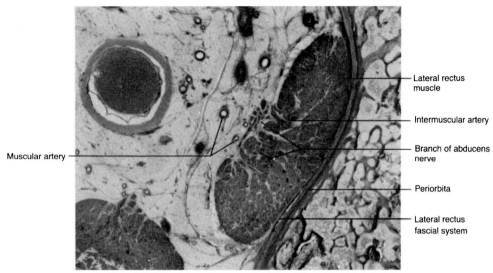

Figure 1–6. Lateral rectus muscle at the entrance of the abducens nerve rootlets. (From Dutton JJ. Atlas of clinical and surgical orbital anatomy. Philadelphia: WB Saunders, 1994, p 175. Used with permission.)

insert more anteriorly (Fig. 1–7), they are more vulnerable to needle trauma from peribulbar or retrobulbar blocks delivered along the floor of the orbit.[48(p53)] The superior oblique muscle is innervated and receives its blood supply in the posterior orbit (Fig. 1–8). Because it is relatively immobile in the superotemporal orbit, it is possible to injure this muscle with blocks in this area.

Local blocks delivered in the mid- or anterior orbit depend on diffusion

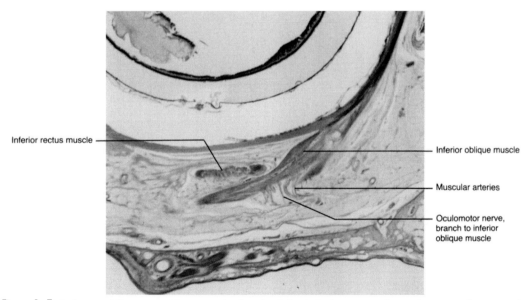

Figure 1–7. Inferior oblique muscle near the level of the inferior rectus insertion onto the posterior globe. (From Dutton JJ. Atlas of clinical and surgical orbital anatomy. Philadelphia: WB Saunders, 1994, p 176. Used with permission.)

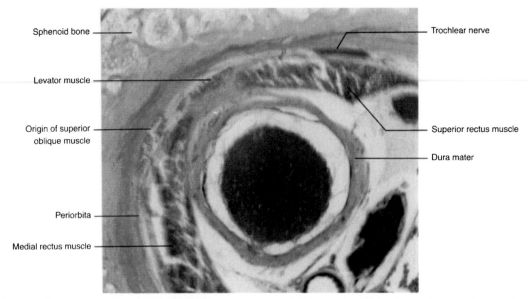

Sphenoid bone

Levator muscle

Origin of superior oblique muscle

Periorbita

Medial rectus muscle

Trochlear nerve

Superior rectus muscle

Dura mater

Figure 1–8. Origin of the superior oblique muscle in the orbital apex just above the annulus of Zinn. (From Dutton JJ. Atlas of clinical and surgical orbital anatomy. Philadelphia: WB Saunders, 1994, p 178. Used with permission.)

of the anesthetic agent into either the posterior orbit to the origin of the nerve branches or the muscles themselves at the point where distal branches insert into myoneural junctions. The first process is dependent on the anatomy of the connective tissue planes that subdivide the orbit into compartments (Figs. 1–9, 1–10). This architecture is variable between patients. The classic teaching of a single intermuscular septum that connects the rectus muscles and divides the orbit into an intraconal space and an extraconal space is overly simplified. Histologic examina-

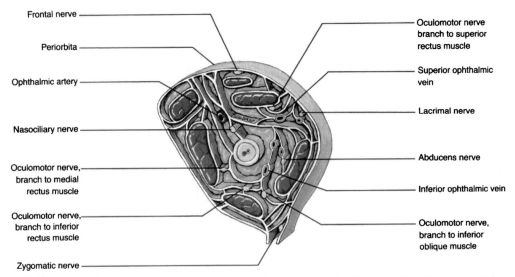

Frontal nerve

Periorbita

Ophthalmic artery

Nasociliary nerve

Oculomotor nerve, branch to medial rectus muscle

Oculomotor nerve, branch to inferior rectus muscle

Zygomatic nerve

Oculomotor nerve branch to superior rectus muscle

Superior ophthalmic vein

Lacrimal nerve

Abducens nerve

Inferior ophthalmic vein

Oculomotor nerve, branch to inferior oblique muscle

Figure 1–9. Orbital fascial system, frontal view, posterior midorbit. (From Dutton JJ. Atlas of clinical and surgical orbital anatomy. Philadelphia: WB Saunders, 1994, p 103. Used with permission.)

tion of the orbit reveals an arrangement of roughly parallel and partially broken septa of various thicknesses with and without fenestrations.[48(p97)] This anatomic variability, therefore, accounts for the variability in akinesia seen with orbital blocks.

Atkinson discussed supplementing incomplete akinesia by injecting 0.5 to 1.0 mL of anesthetic solution 3 cm back along a rectus muscle if it was still active after retrobulbar block. He grasped a horizontal rectus muscle with forceps and rotated the eye away from the needle or placed a muscle hook under the eyelid and separated it from a vertical rectus muscle before injection.[10(p45)] Because the rectus muscles measure 40 to 42 mm in length without their tendons, which in turn may vary from 3.7 mm for the medial rectus to 8.8 mm for the lateral, Atkinson's injection was administered 14 to 21 mm anterior to the origin of the muscle. This would place it anterior to the insertion of the oculomotor branch innervating the muscle. Because akinesia can be achieved with this technique, the anesthetic must be diffusing within the muscle, blocking distal branches of the oculomotor divisions at their most distal myoneural junctions. However, this technique may produce myotoxicity with prolonged paresis of the muscle.[53, 54]

Because permanent extraocular muscle damage is more a product of the actual intramuscular or intraneural injection than of the concentration of anesthetic injected,[48(p194), 55] a less traumatic delivery of anesthetic could be used around the extraocular muscles to achieve akinesia without risking either myotoxicity or needle trauma to the adjacent structures such as the optic nerve and the orbital vessels. Using the sub-Tenon's space for this delivery allows for such nontraumatic akinesia.

Tenon's capsule is the anterior extension of the visceral dura.[48(p52)]

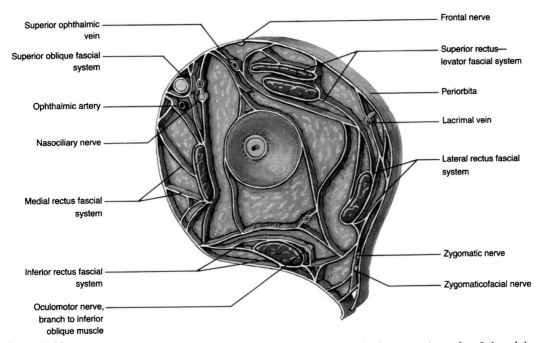

Figure 1–10. Orbital fascial system, frontal view, midorbit through the posterior pole of the globe. (From Dutton JJ. Atlas of clinical and surgical orbital anatomy. Philadelphia: WB Saunders, 1994, p 104. Used with permission.)

Because it invests the anterior portions of the extraocular muscles, and the intermuscular septa fuse with Tenon's capsule posteriorly, anesthetic injected within the sub-Tenon's space will have direct communication with the muscles themselves and with the distal nerve fibers innervating them (Fig. 1–11). Even the lateral rectus muscle, which has the longest tendinous insertion of 8.8 mm,[47(p18)] has actual muscle fibers and, therefore, distal myoneural junctions overlying the globe just posterior to the equator, where they can be bathed in and blocked by sub-Tenon's anesthesia. In fact, the tendon ends and the muscle fibers begin approximately 15.7 mm from the limbus (the lateral rectus insertion is generally found 6.9 mm from the limbus), less than 4 mm posterior to the equator of the average sized eye.[56] Here these muscle fibers and myoneural junctions can be readily blocked. The three other rectus muscles have significantly shorter tendons[47(p18)] (medial, 3.7 mm; inferior, 5.5 mm; superior, 5.8 mm), so that actual muscle fibers and their junctions with distal twigs of the oculomotor branches overlie the equator, which is the site of anesthetic infusion in parabulbar anesthesia. This is the mechanism of akinesia in sub-Tenon's or parabulbar anesthesia.[40, 41]

For safe akinesia with retrobulbar injections, it is important to know how far to advance the needle before injecting. Needle length, angle of insertion, and orbital dimensions all determine safety. Although injections in the orbital apex may be highly effective, the density of vital structures in this region raises the risk-benefit ratio of this approach above that of more anterior techniques. As a guide for avoiding needle trauma to the optic nerve, Katsev, Drews, and Rose measured the dis-

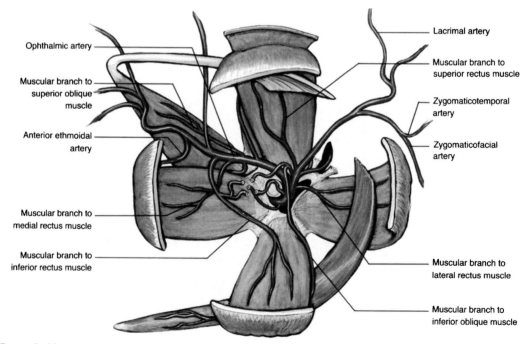

Figure 1–11. Orbital arteries, frontal view with extraocular muscles. (From Dutton JJ. Atlas of clinical and surgical orbital anatomy. Philadelphia: WB Saunders, 1994, p 74. Used with permission.)

tance from the junction of the middle and lateral thirds of the infraorbital rim to the supranasal aspect of the foramen.[51] In studying 120 orbits of 60 subjects, they found the distance averaged 48 mm (range, 42–54 mm). Because the optic nerve is fixed in place as it enters the optic foramen, and it has an average diameter of 3.5 mm, needles 38 mm or longer carry a significant risk of perforating this nerve anterior to the foramen. Others have estimated the distance to be even shorter,[57] not taking into account the path the needle would take when used for retrobulbar and posterior peribulbar anesthesia. In any case, the risk of damage to the optical structures obviously diminishes with shorter needles. Because it is impossible to know the exact orbital dimensions of a given patient, Katsev et al. recommended a needle length of 31.5 mm (1.25 in).

Even short needles, however, can penetrate orbital arteries and veins; it is estimated that 1 to 3% of retrobulbar injections result in hemorrhage. Therefore, a knowledge of the vascular anatomy of the orbit may be helpful in reducing this relatively common occurrence (Fig. 1–12). The ophthalmic artery carries the main orbital blood supply in 96% of the population, with the middle meningeal artery sharing equally in 3% and solely supplying 1%.[58] The ophthalmic artery can be divided into four portions.[59] The first is the main trunk, which enters the orbit inferotemporal to the optic nerve in 70% and inferonasal or directly inferior to the nerve in 30% of individuals. The second portion approaches above or below the nerve, coursing medially. The third portion crosses over the nerve in 81% and below in 19%.[60] Finally, the fourth and longest portion begins as the artery courses forward, in the supero-

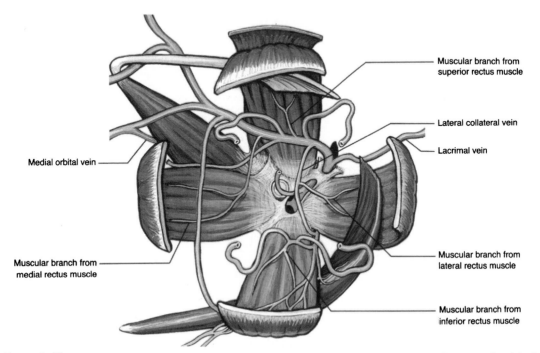

Muscular branch from
superior rectus muscle

Lateral collateral vein

Lacrimal vein

Medial orbital vein

Muscular branch from
lateral rectus muscle

Muscular branch from
medial rectus muscle

Muscular branch from
inferior rectus muscle

Figure 1–12. Orbital veins, frontal view. (From Dutton JJ. Atlas of clinical and surgical orbital anatomy. Philadelphia: WB Saunders, 1994, p 86. Used with permission.)

medial orbit, between the superior oblique muscle and the optic nerve, exiting the muscle cone just posterior to the junction of the nerve and the sclera. In 80% of the population, it runs between the medial rectus and superior oblique muscles and continues anteriorly near the medial orbital wall. The branching of the ophthalmic artery is extremely variable, with no one standard pattern.[47(p69)]

Orbital veins vary even more than the arteries, except for major trunks.[47(p82)] Unlike arteries, veins travel within the septal layers of the orbital fascial system.[61, 62] Except for the lacrimal and ethmoidal veins, there is no parallel course running between corresponding arteries and veins.[63] Although the orbital arteries are centrally arranged in the posterior orbit, the veins are mainly peripheral.[64] They usually form two main trunks: the superior and inferior ophthalmic veins (Fig. 1–13). The superior vessel leaves the orbit through the supraorbital fissure and passes above the annulus of Zinn, near the lateral rectus, along the lateral edge of the superior rectus muscle. The inferior vessel begins as a plexus between the globe and the inferior rectus muscle, running posteriorly along its lateral border and then usually below the annulus of Zinn. Some 40% of individuals possess a medial ophthalmic vein.[47(p83)] This vessel arises from branches of the superior ophthalmic and angular veins, running in the extraconal space, along the medial orbital wall. Additionally, 20% of the population possess another trunk, the "veine ophthalmologique moyenne" of Henry.[63, 65] It starts as a muscular branch of the medial rectus, extending backward above the inferior ophthalmic vein, and exits the orbit lateral to the muscle cone. Because the venous system is so variable, the best way to avoid it is to stay away from any orbital septa. Injections into the spaces between the four rectus muscles and nasal to the medial rectus, the adipose tissue compartments,[48(p31)] may provide the best possibility of avoiding the orbital vessels, nerves, and muscles. Individual techniques for doing this are discussed later in the chapter, but suffice it to say none is foolproof. The greater the knowledge of orbital anatomy, the greater is the respect gained for the risks of injection anesthesia.

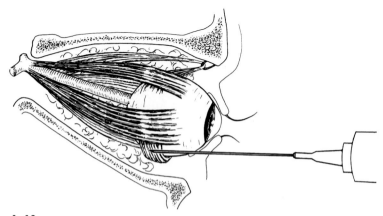

Figure 1–13. Inferotemporal injection with the lateral portions of the right eye removed. The needle does not enter the muscle cone. (From McGoldrick KE. Anesthesia for ophthalmic and otolaryngologic surgery. Philadelphia: WB Saunders, 1992, p 246. Used with permission.)

GENERAL ANESTHESIA

Although the specific techniques for induction of general anesthesia are discussed in another chapter, it is important to consider as well the indications, contraindications, ophthalmic effects, and complications of this procedure. In 1955, Atkinson wrote that the indications for general anesthesia in eye surgery included operations on young children, on adults undergoing extensive orbital surgery, and on those who objected to local anesthesia.[10(p78)] Although only the first and third of these apply to cataract surgery, general anesthesia may also be considered in patients who are unable to cooperate, such as the mentally retarded or those with general movement disorders, nystagmus, an inability to lie flat, excessive anxiety, or claustrophobia.

Inability to communicate with the patient may contribute to a decision to choose general anesthesia, but an interpreter can often be used to instruct a patient preoperatively or even intraoperatively, thus facilitating surgery under local anesthesia. It is also advisable for the surgeon to learn a few crucial phrases in the patient's language. It can be very helpful to have an interpreter write down translations of "look up," "look down," "don't move," "open the eye," and "close the eye" and affix them to the wall of the operating room or to the microscope. Patients with hearing impairment should be encouraged to wear their hearing aids.

Bleeding disorders have in the past been considered a relative indication for general over local anesthesia; however, newer techniques such as sub-Tenon's–parabulbar and topical anesthesia avoid the risks of retrobulbar hemorrhage and thus eliminate the advantage of general anesthesia in these cases.

In the 1950s, when intracapsular cataract surgery was the state of the art, general anesthesia was believed to be helpful in the prevention of vitreous loss through "relief of abnormal muscle tone due to fear of pain."[2(p559)] Studies of the era compared a 7% loss of vitreous under local anesthesia with a 3% loss under general anesthesia.[66] Constant stress was placed on the importance of a stay suture to close the eye quickly should the patient lighten under general anesthesia and put a strain on the endotracheal tube. Cataract surgery today is executed in a more controlled manner within a closed system. The occasional intracapsular extraction is still performed, of course, as in the case of a subluxed lens with a large zonular dehiscence. In these cases, the lessons of the past should not be forgotten.

In 1980, Backer, Tinker, and Robertson published a study demonstrating that elderly patients with a history of myocardial infarction were at a significantly higher risk for a second infarction with general than with local anesthesia.[67] However, a study done 3 years later by Lang at the Massachusetts Eye and Ear Infirmary demonstrated a low rate of morbidity and mortality with both general and local anesthesia in ophthalmic surgery.[68] In reviewing nearly 15,000 cases between 1977 and 1979, Lang found that they were evenly divided between the two types of anesthesia and that there were only two postoperative deaths, also equally divided between the two groups. The only two myocardial infarctions occurred in the local group, both in patients who had a history of infarction more than 6 months before surgery. In comparing the two groups, however, it must be kept in mind that these were not randomly selected and that the local anesthesia patients had a significantly higher average age. What this study does highlight is the overall safety of eye surgery in general when the appropriate anesthetic technique is chosen for a given patient. Again, this choice should be based on factors other than the type of surgery being performed. As early as 1974, Lynch, Wolf, and Berlin compared the rate of vitreous loss in iris prolapse during cataract extractions performed under local and general anesthesia, and they found no significant difference.[69]

The broad range of contraindications to general anesthesia are discussed in another chapter, but there are some that apply to specific patients, and these are mentioned here. In up to 90% of myotonic dystrophy cases, for example, cataracts develop in the early years.[70] The myotonia and muscular dystrophy seen in these patients increase the risk of general anesthesia.[71] In these patients significant bradycardia may develop with a prolonged PR interval that can be unresponsive to atropine. The patients may also suffer respiratory complications as a result of their decreased vital and maximum breathing capacities, resulting in prolonged postoperative respiratory depression. In addition, they experience an increased risk of aspiration because of delayed gastric emptying and abnormal swallowing. All of these factors make local anesthesia the preferred method in these patients.

Care must also be taken when considering general anesthesia in patients with Marfan's syndrome. They often have cardiovascular abnormalities such as incompetent or prolapsed valves, arrhythmias, and aortic aneurysms, which may dissect with an elevation in blood pressure.[72] In addition, pulmonary anomalies such as bronchogenic cysts, abnormal lobulations, and emphysematous changes can lead to spontaneous pneumothorax. The risk of tension pneumothorax increases during controlled breathing.[73] For all these reasons, local anesthesia may again be safer for such individuals.

In considering whether to use general anesthesia, total physical condition must be taken into account, as must any medications the patient may be taking that could interact with the anesthetic. If possible, smoking should be discontinued. A history of prostatic enlargement should be followed up by a urologic consultation before surgery. Patients who are difficult to intubate, such as those with cervical spondylosis, should be identified and carefully evaluated. Prior reactions to general anesthesia should be investigated as should a family history of unexplained perioperative death or malignant hyperthermia.

Although the incidence of malignant hyperthermia is considered to be 1 per 15,000 anesthetic events in children and 1 per 50,000 in adults,[74] the true incidence varies with the definition of the condition and the anesthesia used. A study done in Denmark estimated an incidence of 1 per 5000 if episodes of fever, unexplained tachycardia, and masseter muscle rigidity were included in cases in which succinylcholine and an inhalation agent were used.[75] The specific diagnosis and treatment of malignant hyperthermia are beyond the scope of this chapter, but it is important to remember that with current treatment the mortality rate is approximately 10%. Therefore, in adult patients who may be susceptible to this condition, local anesthesia is obviously preferable to general anesthesia.

When general anesthesia is required in pediatric cases, a history of malignant hyperthermia susceptibility triggers a cascade of precautionary steps. These include intravenous dantrolene, continuous body temperature monitoring, and the use of agents considered to be relatively safe for this population, such as narcotics, benzodiazepines, barbiturates, and nondepolarizing muscle relaxants. Finally, careful monitoring should be continued for at least 8 hours postoperatively.

A thorough review of all medications the patient is taking must be made before cataract surgery, especially when it is to be performed under general anesthesia. Guidelines for preanesthetic management include the cessation of diuretics, which could cause urinary retention in patients with unsuspected prostatic enlargement, and the discontinuation of those psychotropic agents that might interact with general anesthesia, such as monoamine oxidase inhibitors, which intensify and prolong the anesthetic effect. However, vasodilators and antiarrhythmic agents should be continued through the day of surgery. Their elimination could lead to rebound hypertension and tachycardia, conditions that, along with congestive heart failure and unexplained anemia, represent the major cardiovascular contraindications to general anesthesia.

Because diabetics have a greater incidence of cataracts than the general population, the perioperative management of insulin and oral hypoglycemics deserves special attention here. General anesthesia and surgery represent a major disruption of the day-to-day existence of the diabetic patient, and the treatment regimen must be altered accordingly. Type I diabetics tend to be more affected by changes in therapy than non–insulin-dependent Type II diabetics, so that these patients with juvenile-onset disease should have their surgery scheduled as early in the day as is feasible.[74(p224)] Both groups should be given one third to one half of their standard morning dose of intermediate or long-acting insulin. The blood glucose level should be checked before insulin administration and at hourly intervals throughout the perioperative period, and any hyperglycemia should be treated with small amounts of short-acting insulin. Hypoglycemia should be treated with a continuous intravenous infusion of 5% dextrose, the rate of administration to be guided by blood sugar levels.

Patients taking oral hypoglycemics should have the medication discontinued on the day of surgery. They too should have a fasting blood sugar level in the morning and a continuous intravenous infusion of dextrose, as guided by blood sugar levels, monitored frequently. Once the patient is able to resume a regular diet, which in the case of cataract extraction should be relatively soon after surgery, the normal insulin or oral therapy is resumed.

In diabetic patients, the type of anesthesia used does not determine the morbidity and mortality of the surgery. Rather, the pre-existing status of the diabetes, specifically the presence or absence of retinopathy, nephropathy, neuropathy, as well as peripheral vascular and cardiovascular disease, is predictive of the surgical risk. In a study of diabetics undergoing nonocular procedures, the overall risk of complications was 15%.[76] The greatest incidence was 35%, in those with peripheral vascular disease, whereas patients with none of these conditions had a complication risk of approximately 5%.

Some of the ophthalmic medications used in the treatment and preparation of patients undergoing cataract surgery may also interact with general anesthetic agents. Epinephrine, for example, may be used on a long-term basis by glaucoma patients for the reduction of intraocular pressure. It may also be used intraoperatively in cataract surgery for its mydriatic effect; in patients who are inadequately dilated, an infusion of epinephrine into the anterior chamber can be helpful in dilating the pupil enough so that surgery can be performed without the aid of iridectomy, sphincterotomy, or iris hooks. Epinephrine is also routinely added to the fluid used for intraocular irrigation during cataract surgery.

However, what are the implications of its use, and how much is safe? The major concern is the interaction between epinephrine and halogenated hydrocarbon anesthetics, which can potentiate ventricular fibrillation. This effect may be especially dramatic with epinephrine and cyclopropane, and this combination should definitely be avoided. On the other hand, epinephrine can be safely used with halothane; the maximal safe dose has been reported as 68 µg/kg infused into the anterior chamber.[77]

The rate of administration plays a role as well. It has been estimated that 10 mL of a 1:100,000 solution of epinephrine may be safely administered in 10 minutes in the presence of halothane, or up to 30 mL per hour in a healthy 70-kg patient.[78] Lesser complications such as hypertension, syncope, headache, diaphoresis, tachycardia, and extra systoles have been reported in patients using topical epinephrine.[79, 80] Because as little as 0.5 mg of it may trigger these effects, and one drop of a 2% solution contains this amount, it may be advisable to substitute another glaucoma treatment for epinephrine in patients scheduled for general anesthesia.

Another glaucoma treatment that is less commonly used but that may be seen in the setting of aphakia is echothiophate, a long-acting anticholinesterase. If a patient has received this drug in the 4 weeks before surgery, anesthetic agents that are metabolized by plasma pseudocholinesterase should be avoided or at least significantly restricted.[81] These include succinylcholine, cocaine, procaine, and chloroprocaine. Overdosage of succinylcholine in this setting can lead to prolonged apnea. Because echothiophate can itself cause cataracts as well as vomiting, hypotension, and abdominal pain, it is more likely to be used by a patient undergoing secondary implant surgery than one having a cataract extraction.

Acetazolamide is a carbonic anhydrase inhibitor used in the long-term treatment of glaucoma and in the short-term treatment and prophylaxis of postoperative intraocular pressure elevation. Both ocular and renal carbonic anhydrase activity is inhibited, so that bicarbonate, water, sodium, and potassium are wasted with its use. Patients on continuous acetazolamide therapy are often hypokalemic and hyponatremic, a combination that can potentiate significant arrhythmias under general anesthesia. Because these electrolyte imbalances are worsened by hepatic or renal failure, acetazolamide should be avoided in such cases. It should also be avoided in patients with chronic obstructive pulmonary disease because they have a tendency to retain carbon dioxide and, therefore, to become acidotic. Short-term treatment of intraocular pressure with intravenous acetazolamide has become a popular technique. The drug begins to have an effect in 5 minutes and peaks by 30 minutes. It should be noted that this is a sulfonamide derivative and thus carries a risk, however rare, of anaphylaxis, Stevens-Johnson syndrome, erythema multiforme, and aplastic anemia.

General anesthesia is more likely to cause significant adverse systemic effects than local or ocular complications. In addition, those ocular problems that do occur are usually not serious. They include corneal abrasion, chemical keratitis, hemorrhagic retinopathy, and, rarely, retinal ischemia.

The incidence of corneal abrasion under general anesthesia has been reported to be as high as 44%.[82] However, simple precautions, such as instilling a bland ointment or taping closed the lids of the unoperative eye, may prevent surface trauma produced by the surgical drape, anesthetic mask, or simply exposure. Decreased tear production under general anesthesia, proptosis, and poor Bell's phenomenon may worsen corneal exposure, requiring eyelid suturing in some susceptible patients. Other potential dangers to the cornea are the inadvertent trauma by the anesthesiologist during induction[83] or by an ill-fitting anesthetic mask.

Reusable masks may also cause chemical injury to the cornea because of the liquid disinfectants used on them.[84] Disposable masks or those that can be autoclaved are simple solutions to this problem.

Postoperative vomiting, difficult extubation, and straining on the endotracheal tube may lead to the formation of retinal hemorrhages, a condition dubbed Valsalva retinopathy.[85] This is usually benign because its source is the venous circulation and the location is intraretinal. These hemorrhages clear without interrupting vision unless they are located in the macula.

Retinal ischemia is by far the most serious adverse effect of general anesthesia. It may be caused by an oversized anesthetic mask, by inadvertent pressure exerted by an assistant, or by the surgeon's leaning on the unoperative eye. In the case of posterior segment surgery, it can also result from expansion of intraocular gases in the presence of high concentrations of nitrous oxide.[86] Fortunately, this condition is rare and can be readily prevented if kept in mind during surgery.

RETROBULBAR ANESTHESIA

In 1985, 76% of the members of the American Society of Cataract and Refractive Surgeons (ASCRS) who responded to an annual survey indicated that they preferred retrobulbar anesthesia with a facial nerve block for cataract surgery.[87] Another 16% preferred retrobulbar anesthesia without the facial block. Thus, 92% of these surgeons were performing retrobulbar blocks as their procedure of choice a little over a decade ago. The latest survey published in 1993 listed 40% as preferring retrobulbar anesthesia plus facial block and 19% as choosing retrobulbar anesthesia alone, a decline from 92 to 59%.

The technique that the majority of respondents still preferred varies from Atkinson's classic description published in 1955 but not substantially. He wrote,

Good results will be obtained and orbital hemorrhage rarely occurs if the following directions are observed: An intradermal wheal is made. A 3.5 cm 23 gauge needle with a rounded point is introduced through this wheal at the inferior temporal margin of the orbit and the skin is moved upward with the needle until the point just clears the orbital margin. About 0.5 cc of the anesthesia solution is now injected so that pain will not be experienced when the orbital septum is pierced. Incidentally, the septum can be pierced more easily close to the orbital margin and is pierced more easily if the needle is rotated producing a boring effect. A pause of a few moments allows the anesthesia to work during which time the patient is directed to look upward and away from the site of injection. This is done to move the inferior oblique muscle and fascia between the lateral and inferior rectus muscles forward and upward, out of the way. The needle is directed straight back close to the floor of the orbit, until the point is beyond the globe and fascia before directing it upward toward the apex of the orbit for a depth of 2.5 to 3.5 cm depending on the size of the orbit. When the needle has reached the proper depth, one should aspirate before injecting the anesthetic solution in order to determine whether or not the needle has entered a vessel. However, in this location, it would be most unlikely unless there is an abnormally large vessel. The anesthetic solution is then slowly injected, the amount depending upon the size of the orbit, the operation that is to be done and whether or not hyaluronidase has been added to the anesthetic solution. When hyaluronidase is not used, 1.5 ml [of anesthetic] is considered a safe amount for intraocular operations. At least 5 minutes should elapse before the operation is begun ... more effective results are obtained for cataract extractions and larger injections may be given if hyaluronidase is added to the anesthetic solution. It may be safely injected until there is a noticeable proptosis, which usually occurs after injecting 2 to 3 cc in the average orbit. The hyaluronidase causes the solution to diffuse rapidly and the proptosis quickly subsides. Pressure over the eye, combined with moving it in the orbit for at least 5 minutes, produces still greater diffusion of the anesthetic solution, enhances anesthesia and akinesia, and increases hypotony. Each is an important defense against vitreous loss and other complications.[10(p43)]

The major change in this technique as used today is the direction of gaze the patient is asked to assume during the block. This came about because of a 1981 study by Unsold and associates, in which computed tomographic (CT) images of retrobulbar needle placement in a cadaver were studied with two different techniques.[88] In one side of the cadaver, the eye was sutured into the position described by Atkinson mentioned previously. Then a 3.5-cm 25-gauge needle was introduced just above the orbital rim and was directed superomedially toward the optic canal. In the other side, the eye was sutured into a position of inferotemporal gaze, and the needle was directed in a more inferior direction. In the first case, CT scanning demonstrated that the needle tip was extremely close to the optic nerve, having crossed underneath it and stopped medially in front of the optic canal. By having the patient look upward and inward, the anesthesiologist would have caused the optic nerve to rotate downward and outward into or at least very close to the path of the needle.

In addition, these scans revealed the close proximity of the ophthalmic artery and superior ophthalmic vein to the needle. Even the inferior oblique muscle, which Atkinson made a point of describing as being moved away from the injection by the upward and inward direction of gaze, was found to be displaced anteriorly, temporally, and inferiorly. This brought it into the path of the needle, which was at its lateral border. Interestingly, the first report of inferior oblique trauma in three patients who underwent retrobulbar anesthesia and in one who underwent peribulbar was published in 1995.[55]

In the second set of scans, done with the eye directed downward and outward, the needle was found to lie above the inferior rectus muscle anterior to the inferior aspect of the supraorbital fissure. It was within the muscle cone but away from the optic nerve, the superior ophthalmic vein, and the ophthalmic artery. The inferior oblique muscle was found to rotate posteriorly, medially, and superiorly away from the needle path.

Unsöld and colleagues concluded that most of the complications of the traditional retrobulbar technique could be explained by direct trauma to the optic nerve or the orbital vessels. He also postulated that, in the traditional position, the dural sheath of the optic nerve was on stretch and was, therefore, more readily penetrated, allowing easier access to the subarachnoid space, the central retinal artery, and the nerve itself. Similarly, the contraction of the inferior oblique muscle with an upward and inward gaze made it a target more susceptible to puncture. Unsold and associates' observations provided an impetus for many surgeons and anesthesiologists to change their technique, so that more and more retrobulbar blocks are now performed with the patient in primary gaze.

In 1987, Nicoll and coworkers reported a study evaluating standard retrobulbar anesthesia performed with both an upward and an inward gaze and straight-ahead or "minimally upward" gaze.[89] Of 6000 patients who received retrobulbar anesthesia, 16 experienced symptoms suggestive of central nervous system spread: blindness of the contralateral eye, drowsiness, abnormal shivering, vomiting, respiratory depression, hemiplegia, aphasia, convulsions, unconsciousness, and cardiac arrest. The combined incidence of these symptoms in both groups was 1 in 375. The incidence in the 2000 patients who looked upward and inward was 1 in 333, whereas in the group who looked straight ahead or slightly upward, it was 1 in 400. This difference is not statistically significant.

Unsold and colleagues' observations were, after all, based on the study of a single cadaver and might have overemphasized the importance of gaze direction. One eye was directed "downward and outward" and a 35-mm needle was introduced in a direction described as "slightly more" inferior to the "traditional technique." In Nicoll and associates' study, one group of patients was looking straight ahead or slightly upward while a 38-mm needle was introduced via "a standard inferotemporal approach." The difference in needle length and angle of introduction may explain the difference between the theoretical advantage of Unsold and colleagues' findings and in the disappointing reality of those by Nicoll and associates.

Katsev and colleagues' study may explain the disagreement.[51] In 120 human orbits, they measured the distance between the retrobulbar needle site (the junction between the middle and lateral thirds of the intraorbital rim) and the optic foramen. They found that 11% of optic nerves could be perforated by a 38-mm needle, the length used in Nicoll and colleagues' study. This may have been so long that it overcame the advantage of rotating the optic nerve toward or away from the point. Unsold and others did not report the size of the orbit they studied, and in any case no two skulls or orbits are identical. In comparing the Unsold findings with the Katsev findings, it could be concluded that in any individual the shorter the needle and the more it is rotated away from the area of the optic nerve, the less likely is a complication. Katsev and colleagues suggested using a needle of 31 mm. Unsöld and associates' rotation of the eye downward and outward toward the injection site might not be objectionable to a cadaver but certainly might be to a patient. Having the patient assume the primary position of gaze and using a 31-mm needle may, therefore, represent the safest combination for retrobulbar anesthesia.

These studies have led to alternative retrobulbar approaches. In 1983 Gills and Loyd reported on a modified retrobulbar block performed transconjunctivally with a 31-mm needle and the patient looking "slightly" upward.[37] The site of injection was 5 mm from the lateral canthus, and the technique involved a combination of three or four injections. The first was made 1 minute after proparacaine was instilled; 1.5 mL of 1% lidocaine without epinephrine was injected "down to the level of the muscle cone." Then 5 mL of 0.75% bupivacaine was injected with the needle inserted to a depth of 25 mm "plus." A third injection of 2 to 3 mL more bupivacaine was made into the retrobulbar space if akinesia was not present after 10 minutes. Finally, another injection was made through the lower lid 5 mm from the lateral canthus to a depth of 2 to 5 mm to block the facial nerve, in effect a modified van Lint block.

In a later report on their technique, Gills and Loyd advised a medial "periconal" (peribulbar) injection of 2 to 4 mL of 2% mepivacaine (Carbocaine) in cases with persistent medial or superior rectus function.[48(p128)] The authors warned against using 0.75% bupivacaine for this periconal block because of the possibility of myotoxicity, with subsequent medial rectus fibrosis or ptosis. They reported a total absence of optic nerve or globe perforations with this technique. Only one case of apnea was noted, but the rate of retrobulbar hemorrhage or diplopia was not mentioned. These complications might well be expected to increase as a result of the multiple injections involved. The risk of retrobulbar hemorrhage with retrobulbar blocks has been estimated at 1 to 3%.[31] Some areas of the orbit have been shown to be relatively less vascular than others. However, as was pointed out in the section on orbital anatomy, the highly variable pattern of arterial and especially of venous branching makes it desirable to minimize the number of injections given.

In an effort to avoid the globe and the optic nerve, however, many experts on injection anesthesia have advocated multineedle techniques. The type of needle preferred by most is a sharp disposable one that can be introduced with less patient discomfort, thus requiring less intravenous sedation. It is considered no more likely to produce scleral, optic nerve, or blood vessel perforation than a blunt needle.[90]

Hustead's multi-injection technique includes an inferotemporal injection of 0.5 mL of a mixture of two parts 0.75% bupivacaine and one part 2% mepivacaine, with epinephrine and hyaluronidase. It is administered with a 2.5-cm (1 inch) 30-gauge needle introduced to a depth of 20 mm. The same needle is partially withdrawn and redirected toward the intraorbital foramen. Then 1.25 mL of anesthetic is injected anterior to the orbital septum to prepare for the lid block. The needle is withdrawn completely. After 30 seconds a .625-cm (¼ inch) 27-gauge needle is introduced along the same inferotemporal route beneath the lateral rectus muscle to a point ⅝ mm behind the globe (presumably the anesthesiologist checks the axial length before injecting). The 4 mL of anesthetic is slowly injected. The needle is again partially withdrawn and introduced into the preseptal space near the infraorbital foramen to serve as a partial lid block. Ocular compression is performed, and ocular mobility is checked after 5 minutes. A medial periconal injection is then performed with a 30-gauge needle directed superiorly or inferiorly, depending on which muscles are predominantly mobile. In 5% of cases, a fifth injection is done superotemporally to yield complete akinesia. Hustead reported no incidence of hemorrhage in his last 6000 cases.[48(p145)]

Hamilton also begins with a 30-gauge needle.[48(p138)] He introduces it transconjunctivally in the inferotemporal position after administering topical anesthetic. Then 1 mL of 0.2% mepivacaine with epinephrine and hyaluronidase is injected behind the inferior tarsal plate 10 mm from the conjunctival surface. This injection is given to anesthetize the path of the next one, which is done with a 27-gauge needle previously bent to an angle of 10 degrees for half of its 31-mm length. The bevel of the needle is on the concave side. This needle is introduced transconjunctivally with the patient in primary gaze. The site is the farthest lateral extension of the inferior fornix, just behind the inferior tarsal plate. The target site is the sagittal plane of the lateral limbus, as in the Gills-Loyd retrobulbar block, which requires a medial tilt of the needle pathway. The 10-degree bend mimics the rise in the orbital floor. Once the needle has been inserted to a depth of 25 to 31 mm, some 3 to 4 mL of 2.0% mepivacaine with epinephrine and hyaluronidase is injected over 2 minutes. Ocular compression of 10 minutes follows this injection, and if any motility remains, a medial periconal injection is performed using a 30-gauge needle as in Hustead's technique.

Two other modifications in the retrobulbar technique have been made by Thornton and Straus. Both have changed the design of the needle to avoid globe perforation.

The 25-gauge Thornton retrobulbar needle was designed without cutting edges; it has a sharp, smooth point and a 15-degree bevel.[48(p155)] Although its design is intended to "run truer through tissue," it has been reported to cause undesirable globe rotation in about a third of cases because of septal adherence to the needle shaft.[48(p159)]

Straus designed a curved retrobulbar needle with a 20-mm radius, a 25-mm chord length, and a 10-mm straight distal portion, creating a 30-degree angle in reference to the needle hub.[91] This radius of curvature was designed to exceed that of the average globe. The angle of the distal segment was intended to parallel that of the optic nerve and the globe. Although Straus reported no globe or optic nerve trauma in 10,000 patients and only one retrobulbar hemorrhage, similarly curved needles have failed to eliminate these complications entirely in the past.[48(p154)]

The popularity of retrobulbar anesthesia has declined in the past decade, but it is still the most frequently used technique. It is actually not one technique at all but rather a family of single or multiple injections ending up somewhere behind the eye. Many different alterations have been proposed that are designed to reduce the incidence of complications. This proliferation of modifications in the technique Atkinson described more than 40 years ago, and the continued reports of maloccurrence, suggest that the ideal retrobulbar method is still in evolution.

PERIBULBAR ANESTHESIA

In 1986 Davis and Mandel reported on their use of peribulbar anesthesia.[92] According to their article, the technique was actually introduced by Kelman in the mid-1970s but not published at that time. Davis and Mandel make one injection, a finger's width medial to the lateral canthus, through the lower lid just above the inferior orbital rim. There 0.5 mL of lidocaine is injected subcutaneously, and a second 0.5 mL is injected into the orbicularis muscle. Then 1 mL of anesthetic is introduced beneath the orbicularis muscle "into the anterior orbit" and 2 mL through the upper lid in the same manner, beginning just below the supraorbital notch. This is followed by 1 minute of ocular compression. In their original article, the authors did not describe the needle used for the first two injections, but in a later report[48(p122)] they mentioned the use of a 1.25-cm (½ inch) 27-gauge needle.

A more posterior injection is then made using a 23-gauge 3.125-cm (1¼ inch) blunt retrobulbar needle; 4 mL of 0.75% bupivacaine mixed with 4 mL of 1% lidocaine and hyaluronidase is administered. An inferior injection is given 15 mm medial to the lateral canthus just above the inferior orbital rim, and 1 mL of anesthetic is injected just beneath the orbicularis muscle. "The needle is then advanced along the inferior orbit to the equator of the globe."[92] (This is evidently an assumed depth because the authors do not mention measuring or adjusting for the patient's axial length before injecting.) Then 1 mL of anesthetic mixture is delivered in this region (Figs. 1–13, 1–14). "The barrel of the syringe is angled over the malar eminence, and the needle is advanced in a superior and medial direction to the full depth of the needle." Another 1 to 2 mL are injected. These steps are repeated beneath the supraorbital notch anteriorly and "at the superonasal equator of the globe." The third stage of this superoposterior injection is then delivered "to the superior orbital fissure" where another 1 mL of anesthetic is injected. (Because the distance from the superior orbital rim to the supraorbital fissure is actually 4.5 to 5 cm,[47(p3)] the 31-mm (1¼ inch) needle is in reality falling far short of this target.)

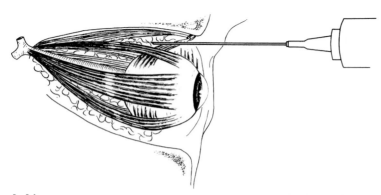

Figure 1–14. Supranasal injection as seen from above with the roof of the orbit removed. The needle is inserted medial to the supraorbital notch (not shown) and just beyond the equator of the globe. (From McGoldrick KE. Anesthesia for ophthalmic and otolaryngologic surgery. Philadelphia: WB Saunders, 1992, p 246. Used with permission.)

The authors always aspirate before injecting, and they describe the volumes delivered as approximate and dependent on the dimensions of the eye and orbit. After a total volume of 12 to 14 mL of anesthetic mixture is given through the four injections described, the eyelids may be tense as a result of the filling of the orbital volume. Then 8 minutes of ocular compression ensue, and the completeness of the block is evaluated. The authors describe achieving complete akinesia in 90% of cases with practice. In the remaining 10%, an additional 3 to 4 mL are injected at a site determined by the muscles not completely blocked. The onset of anesthetic effect is described as 10 to 12 minutes from the time of injection. No further facial block is required, most likely because of the multiple injections into and just below the orbicularis muscle, which are in themselves distal facial nerve blocks. Davis and Mandel described an excellent safety record in their first 1600 patients. They concluded that this technique "eliminates the need for standard retrobulbar injections." However, it is possible to wonder how much the two most posterior injections they describe differ from "standard" retrobulbar injections. Although the peribulbar injection is not intended to enter the muscle cone, the delivery of anesthetic through a needle introduced 31 mm deep into the orbit, starting at the infraorbital rim and advancing superomedially, more than casually resembles the retrobulbar anesthetic technique, as does the superior injection made anterior to the supraorbital fissure. Davis and Mandel later modified their technique[48(p122)] using a blunt 2.19-cm (⅞ inch) 23- or 25-gauge needle instead of the 3.125-cm (1¼ inch) needle previously described. The later report also substitutes an anesthetic mixture of two-thirds 0.75% bupivacaine and one-third 1% lidocaine without epinephrine but with hyaluronidase. This represents a longer acting mixture than the original, which contained half lidocaine and half bupivacaine.

The shortening of the needle for more anterior delivery of anesthetic was a response by the authors to reports of optic nerve trauma, globe perforation, and respiratory depression after peribulbar anesthesia. This was another resemblance to the retrobulbar technique. Indeed, the site of injection chosen by Davis and Mandel was nearly identical to the one Braun described in 1918[93] and Pitkin and colleagues later abandoned because of similar adverse effects.[94] Specific complications of these techniques are discussed later in the chapter, but it is clear that deep orbital injections carry with them vision and life-threatening risks no matter what their direction.

A study comparing the efficacy of retrobulbar and peribulbar or periocular injections for cataract surgery by Weiss and Deichman in 1989 demonstrated that, like their complications, the therapeutic effects of the techniques were similar.[95] Although only 79 patients were included in the study, it was performed in a randomized, masked, prospective fashion. In both groups, 5 mL of a half and half mixture of 2% lidocaine and 0.75% bupivacaine with epinephrine and hyaluronidase were used. A single injection was performed with the patient in primary gaze. Interestingly, the only difference in technique between the two groups was the length of the needle used.

In the retrobulbar group, a 38-mm (1½ inch) 25-gauge needle was inserted "almost to the hub," starting at the juncture of the lateral third and medial two thirds of the infraorbital rim and "aiming toward an imaginary posterior extension of the visual axis." In the periocular group, the identical site and angle of administration were used, with a 16-mm 25-gauge needle. No facial block was given to either group, but 10 minutes of ocular compression was administered in both. At this point, the surgeon evaluated lid and globe akinesia as well as the depth of anesthesia. If the globe was not totally akinetic or anesthetized, a supplemental block of 0.5 mL of anesthetic was injected in the supra-trochlear region. No intravenous sedation was administered.

There was no significant difference between the two groups in the degree of lid or globe akinesia, anesthesia, or patient-reported comfort. There was also no significant difference between the two groups in the number of patients who required a supplemental block; 21% of the retrobulbar and 28% of the periocular patients received one. The only significant difference between the two groups was the greater degree of chemosis seen with the periocular patients.

Weiss and Deichman speculated that a reduction in the needle length and volume of anesthetic made their particular technique safer and no less efficacious than the standard retrobulbar method or the multi-injection peribulbar procedure (actually, in 28% of cases their periocular technique did include more than one injection). However, their sample size was too small to come to this conclusion with any reliability. Certainly, shortening the needle at least changes the type of complications seen after injection anesthesia.

Another "anterior" peribulbar technique was described by Bloomberg in 1986[96] and reviewed 5 years later.[97] An 18- to 24-mm 27-gauge needle is used to inject 8 to 10 mL of a half and half mixture of 2% mepivacaine and 0.75% bupivacaine to which hyaluronidase and sodium bicarbonate (0.2 mL/10 mL of solution) are added. It is possible that the pH adjustment of the anesthetic speeds the onset of akinesia.[98, 99] If the longer needle is used, it is advanced only for three quarters of its length. The site of injection is the standard juncture of the lateral third and medial two thirds of the infraorbital rim, and the needle is directed toward the floor of the orbit, away from the globe. Ocular compression is an important adjunct to this technique; Bloomberg advocated 12 to 20 minutes using a Honan balloon set at 30 to 40 mm Hg.

Bloomberg reported a rate of supplemental blocks for residual move-ment of 10 to 50%. These blocks are made with an 18-mm needle in the quadrant of the still-active muscle. The needle is placed tangential to the globe and is directed approximately 10 degrees toward the optical axis, unlike the original injection.

Another anterior peribulbar technique for the creation of anesthesia with incomplete akinesia was described by Pannu.[48(p146)] Like Weiss and Deichman, he uses a 16-mm 25- or 27-gauge needle, having had two episodes of respiratory depression in the first approximately 200 cases he performed using a 24-mm needle. He injects 4 to 5 mL of 1 or 2% lidocaine. The site of injection is identical to the previous techniques described, and Pannu makes it a point to touch the orbital floor as he directs the needle downward and away from the globe. He does not use ocular compression, nor does he perform supplemental injections, be-cause movement is tolerated during his surgery.

In their latest study of peribulbar anesthesia,[100] Davis and Mandel evaluated a number of prospectively collected peribulbar blocks performed mostly for cataract surgery at 12 different facilities between 1988 and 1992. A total of 16,224 cases were studied. These blocks were performed in at least 12 different ways by ophthalmologists, anesthesiologists, and nurse anesthetists. Most included intravenous sedation. All involved 10 to 60 minutes of ocular compression and an inferotemporal injection site. Two of the 12 centers performed two primary injections, whereas 10 performed only the inferotemporal injection, with a supplemental one given if necessary.

Davis and Mandel's technique has apparently evolved since their first publication. Their current block begins with a 2-mL injection of warmed (98°F) 1% lidocaine that has been diluted in a 4:1 to 9:1 mixture with a balanced salt solution. This injection is given with a 12-mm 27-gauge needle into and through the orbicularis muscle and into the anterior orbit inferotemporally. Its purpose, according to the authors, is to anesthetize the lids in preparation for the second injection. This is given with a 18- to 24-mm 23- to 26-gauge needle in the same inferotemporal location. A 10-mL syringe is filled with 6 mL of 0.75% bupivacaine, 3 mL of 1% lidocaine, and 1 mL of hyaluronidase. Between 4 and 10 mL are injected, presumably in the manner previously described, with the eye in primary position. Intravenous sedation with 6 to 10 mL of midazolam is delivered "as needed."

Then ocular compression for 10 to 25 minutes is applied. After 8 to 10 minutes, akinesia is checked and a superonasal or inferonasal injection of the same mixture is given as needed. In 9% of the 1200 cases using this technique, a supplemental block was required. In another 2%, an "additional nerve block," presumably facial, was required.

Davis and Mandel reported that almost all of their patients had nearly complete akinesia and that even when it was incomplete no positive vitreous pressure was noted. The amount of movement remaining did not interfere with surgery. Approximately 75% of their cases were performed by phacoemulsification and 25% by extracapsular extraction.

The other centers included in this study reported similar results. The highest rate of supplemental blocks reported was 11% by a center that already began with two blocks. Despite these multiple injections, however, the rates of orbital hemorrhage, globe perforation, and central nervous system involvement were low. The study did not evaluate the incidence of extraocular muscle trauma or ptosis, nor was there a protocol for examining patients postoperatively. For example, it is unclear how many patients were dilated for postoperative retinal evaluation.

Another drawback of this study was that it did not evaluate the degree of anesthesia patients experienced except in a small subgroup of 200 subjects. Of these patients, 140 remembered having the injection. The authors did not mention how many of the 200 had intravenous sedative or why they waited until the day after surgery to question their patients. Of those who remembered the block, one third had mild to severe discomfort, but two thirds had no discomfort. If it is assumed that the discomfort mentioned was due to the block (which would explain why the 60 patients who did not remember the injection were excluded from evaluation) and not the surgery, there is no mention of the effectiveness of the peribulbar technique in providing anesthesia in this study.

Although Davis and Mandel conceded that peribulbar anesthesia is not "one hundred percent safe," they do demonstrate that it can be given relatively safely and effectively in large numbers by a variety of providers. It is mainly due to their work that the percentage of cataract operations done by members of the ASCRS under peribulbar anesthetic continues to grow. In 1985 4% of surgeons who responded to the ASCRS survey used peribulbar, whereas in 1993 35% did so.[87] The popularity of peribulbar anesthesia for cataract surgery is not in question, but as more surgeons, anesthesiologists, and nurse anesthetists use shorter needles directed away from the globe, it is still unclear which if any complications will increase in incidence. This point is addressed later in the chapter.

PARABULBAR (SUB-TENON'S) ANESTHESIA

Orbital dissections have revealed that Tenon's capsule is the anterior extension of the visceral layer of dura investing the optic nerve.[48(p52)] Therefore, the sub-Tenon's space is continuous with the subdural space and is, in effect, an anatomic pathway from the limbus to the retrobulbar space. Within this space lie the sensory and motor nerves of the globe as well as the four rectus muscles themselves; they penetrate Tenon's capsule behind the equator of the globe. These muscles are invested posteriorly with an extensive network of connective tissue septa that fuse with Tenon's capsule approximately 2 mm from the corneal limbus.[47(p94)] Because conjunctiva fuses with Tenon's capsule in this same area, the sub-Tenon's space can be easily accessed through a snip of the scissors made 2 to 3 mm behind the limbus. From this site, therefore, anesthetic, antibiotic, anti-inflammatory, antiangiogenesis, or other solutions can be delivered along the globe, around the rectus muscles, to the nerves innervating them and into the retrobulbar space around the optic nerve. Figure 1–15A to D demonstrates the passage of 2 mL of anesthetic from the limbus around the lateral rectus muscle to the optic nerve sheath. (This demonstration can be easily repeated by performing a magnetic resonance imaging scan immediately after parabulbar anesthesia; because any liquid will light up on the T2-weighted scan, no contrast material is required.)

Credit for the anatomic appreciation of the sub-Tenon's space goes to O'Ferrall and Bonnet.[101] Credit for using it to deliver anesthetic should go to Turnbull, who dropped 4% cocaine into a cut made through conjunctiva and Tenon's capsule before an enucleation.[6] Credit for bringing the technique back to the attention of the ophthalmic community belongs to Mein, Woodcock, and Hansen, who published two articles in 1990 demonstrating that vitreoretinal and cataract surgery could be performed successfully under sub-Tenon's anesthesia.[38, 102] Their work and that of Smith[103] and Redmond[104] in Great Britain and Furata and associates in Japan[105] have led to three methods of sub-Tenon's anesthesia.

Parabulbar anesthesia[40] is the method by which a sub-Tenon's infusion of anesthetic mixture is administered from the site previously described, 2 to 3 mm posterior to the limbus, through a specially designed flexible cannula. The site was chosen for its anatomic advantages. A single cut is all that is required to access bare sclera and the sub-Tenon's space. Cauterizing the space before making an incision, as suggested by Hugh

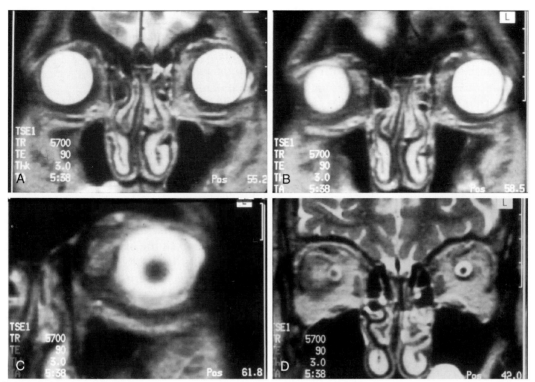

Figure 1–15. Magnetic resonance imaging study immediately after administration of parabulbar anesthesia to a patient about to undergo cataract surgery in the left eye. The anesthetic is highlighted in the T2-weighted image. *A,* Bolus of anesthetic is evident near the site of administration just posterior to the equator. *B,* Spread of anesthetic is demonstrated around the globe more posteriorally. *C,* Anesthetic surrounding the junction of the globe and optic nerve is evident. *D,* Anesthetic surrounds the optic nerve; note the difference between the intensity of the right and left optic nerve signals.

Williams subsequent to publication of this technique (personal communication, 1993), has been extremely helpful in limiting both subconjunctival hemorrhage and the unintended extension of the incision. This cautery has also improved the ease of accessing the sub-Tenon's space, because the gentle application of the bipolar cautery, barely touching but not pressing down on the conjunctival surface, causes the fusion of Tenon's capsule and conjunctiva, lifting Tenon's capsule away from the sclera.

Although the incision can be done anywhere along the globe, more posterior placement requires dissection through three separate layers of tissue; conjunctiva, Tenon's capsule, and intermuscular septum. This procedure is not unduly difficult for the practiced ophthalmic surgeon, but it is not one that an anesthesiologist or nurse anesthetist would find as easy to learn as the single snip involved in the anterior method. Once the sub-Tenon's space is identified, a polyethylene cannula with a flat bottom, expanded proximal hub, and distal opening along its bottom surface (the Greenbaum anesthesia cannula) is introduced through the incision so that the cauterized opening in conjunctiva and Tenon's capsule fits snugly over its hub. This requires that the opening be approximately 0.5 mm in diameter. It is a simple matter to create such an incision using either a Vannas or sharp Westcott scissors under a drop of topical anesthetic. The larger Westcott scissors should not be opened more than halfway, however, in creating this incision.

The infusion is not begun until there is a tight seal between the cannula hub and the fused conjunctiva-Tenon's-intermuscular septum. If the original incision is too large to allow this seal, the tissue is folded tautly over the cannula with a fine-toothed forceps. From 1.0 to 2.0 mL of anesthetic solution is then infused quickly to create a pressure head through the distal opening of the cannula of sufficient force to dissect hydraulically along the globe, around the rectus muscles, past the ciliary ganglion, and finally to the optic nerve itself. Because the cannula is 10 mm in length from hub to tip and is inserted 2 to 3 mm posterior to the limbus, the opening in the bottom of the cannula sits posterior to the equator of the globe. Fluid tracks along the path of least resistance. By sealing the opening created for its passage and conforming to the sclera and sealing the tunnel in Tenon's capsule created by its passage, the cannula discourages anterior extension of the infused fluid and encourages posterior dissection to the only unblocked opening in Tenon's capsule, the one surrounding the optic nerve. Although some fluid does in fact extend anteriorly around the cannula, Figure 1–15 demonstrates the posterior excursion of anesthetic fluid to the junction of the optic nerve and the globe.

The speed of infusion must be brisk. The intended effect is a gush of fluid, not the slowly expanding puddle that would be created by a needle or by a conventional metal cannula. The opening in the 15-gauge half-round Greenbaum anesthesia cannula is "D" shaped and approximately 2 mm in diameter. Because of the flat bottom and half-round shape, the flow characteristics are those of an 18-gauge cannula. Rate of flow is determined by the pressure head and the facility of flow. Therefore, the equation is $F = (P_1 - P_2) C$, where F is the rate of flow, $P_1 - P_2$ is the pressure head created by the syringe, and C is the facility of flow.[106] Because the facility of a tube is proportional to its diameter, the cannula and its opening were designed to be of maximal size while still being clinically useful and not excessively bulky.

The amount of anesthetic infused was chosen by gradually reducing the volume from an initial 5 mL and observing the amount of akinesia and anesthesia obtained. Reduction to the current volume of 1.0 to 2.0 mL has not led to a diminution of clinical effect. A 3-mL syringe is used to infuse the anesthetic because it is easy to handle in a sterile fashion under the surgical microscope, where the block is most often delivered at the beginning of surgery. Filling the syringe with 3 mL of anesthetic mixture leaves an additional 1.0 to 2.0 mL of solution ready should additional anesthetic be required. However, we have not required a second injection in our last 2 years of experience with this technique. The amount of force that can be generated by quickly depressing the plunger is approximately 400 mm Hg.[48(p58)] The volume of anesthetic infused has, therefore, been minimized so as to allow this pressure head to dissect back hydraulically to the retrobulbar space without creating a tight orbit.

The particular mixture we use is 1.5 mL each of 0.75% bupivacaine and 2 or 4% lidocaine, depending on the maximum percentage available at the time. No significant reduction in effect has been noted with the use of 2% lidocaine. However, given the small amount used and the high margin of safety, it seems desirable to maximize potency so as to ensure the greatest patient comfort as well as adequate akinesia. Other surgeons and anesthetists have successfully used lidocaine alone in various percentages as well as etidocaine. The use of bupivacaine is intended to increase the duration of anesthesia. Indeed, we use the parabulbar technique at the end of pediatric cataract surgery under general anesthesia to infuse 1.5 mL of 0.75% bupivacaine alone. This practice has led to a high degree of comfort and satisfaction by children and their parents during the night and day after surgery.

For those surgeons who desire to leave the patient unpatched and able to see after surgery, an infusion of 1 to 1.5 mL of 1 to 2% lidocaine alone is suggested. This technique has also been successfully used to perform panretinal photocoagulation: the patient is able to see throughout and at the end of the procedure is extremely comfortable even when deeper penetrating wavelengths like that for krypton are used. With our anesthetic mixture and volume, a significant reduction in optic nerve function is noted in all cases. This is desirable in that patients are protected from the discomfort often seen under topical anesthetic resulting from the strong light from the operating microscope.

In 1994, Griffiths, Pillai, and Lustbader studied the effect of optic nerve blockade under retrobulbar anesthesia.[107] The authors enrolled 50 patients undergoing anterior segment surgery. They injected a mixture of 2% lidocaine and 0.75% bupivacaine with hyaluronidase in a retrobulbar fashion. Only 10% of their patients had no light perception after injection, whereas 8% had light perception vision. Also, 42% had hand motion vision and 40% had finger-counting vision. The degree of visual effect did not correlate with the degree of akinesia. These values are not significantly different from those seen with parabulbar anesthesia, clinically confirming the retrobulbar spread of anesthetic seen in Figure 1–15.

The effect of parabulbar anesthesia is immediate. There is no need to pause before operating. The technique can be performed either in a holding area or in the operating room under the microscope. Unlike retrobulbar or peribulbar techniques, which require varying degrees of ocular compression to reduce orbital pressure, parabulbar anesthesia has no such association and has immediate efficacy, making it the most efficient of the anesthetic methods for eye surgery. A 1993 prospective study comparing retrobulbar, peribulbar, and sub-Tenon's anesthesia found no significant rise in intraocular pressures with sub-Tenon's or retrobulbar anesthesia but a significant (5 mm Hg) rise after peribulbar anesthesia.[108] This study supports the safe elimination of ocular compression after parabulbar anesthesia.

As opposed to its immediate anesthesia, the akinetic effect of parabulbar anesthesia takes 4 to 5 minutes to develop. This discrepancy is probably due to the larger caliber and myelination of the motor axons. The mechanism of akinesia is probably on a local muscular level. The four rectus muscles penetrate the posterior Tenon's capsule behind the equator of the globe.[47(p94)] They are innervated on their scleral side by branches of the third and sixth cranial nerves. Therefore, these muscles and the distal twigs innervating them are individually bathed in anesthetic mixture in the same way that Atkinson supplemented the akinesia of his retrobulbar blocks by injecting anesthetic directly into muscle that was still active. By infusing anesthetic around the muscle from its scleral side, the parabulbar technique provides akinesia in the only way possible without using a needle. By the time the surgeon enters the eye, the akinesia will be adequate for intraoperative manipulation, such as capsulorrhexis, phacoemulsification, and cortical aspiration.

If a small amount of movement exists after an adequate period of time, an inferior traction suture is suggested to stabilize the eye. This suture is placed tangential to the 6 o'clock limbus through clear cornea at one-half corneal depth, using a 6-0 silk suture on a corneal needle. For cases performed from the temporal position, this suture is placed at the 3 or 9 o'clock limbus and is clamped over a drape retractor nasally. This suture is left long, and when it is clamped to a drape retractor, it can be used to direct the eye away from the site of incision, facilitating dissection. We strongly prefer this technique to superior rectus suturing because it is associated with far less postoperative ptosis. No superior suture is necessary for any additional degree of infraduction because this one can be tightened, loosened, or reclamped as needed. When used, it is usually released immediately after scleral dissection before capsulorrhexis. It is helpful to have patients cooperate in moving the eye during placement of the lid speculum, having them look away from the limb of the speculum so as to avoid corneal epithelial trauma.

While this technique is being learned, additional anesthesia can be safely infused through the same opening created for the initial block or through a newly created one to supplement the akinetic or anesthetic effects of this parabulbar anesthesia. Unique to sub-Tenon's anesthesia is that the original block and any supplementation can be performed without the additional risk of globe or optic nerve perforation, retrobulbar hemorrhage, extraocular muscle trauma, respiratory depression, or corneal epithelial toxicity, which can interfere with the surgeon's view of the posterior capsule. That adequate levels of akinesia can be obtained without these risks and in most cases without supplementation is also unique to this technique. The increased margin of safety provided by akinesia and by patients' increased level of comfort, over that seen with other anesthetic techniques, is a further desirable result of parabulbar anesthesia.

As Turnbull discovered more than a century ago, sub-Tenon's anesthesia provides a greater level of sensory block than even retrobulbar anesthesia because of the blockage of the sensory origins of all three branches of the ophthalmic division of the trigeminal nerve. Retrobulbar anesthesia blocks the nasociliary branch, providing excellent intraocular and corneal anesthesia, yet it misses the bulbar and palpebral conjunctiva. Topical anesthesia provides excellent surface anesthesia but does not block intraocular sensation like that felt during iris manipulation or stretching of the zonulae when the anterior chamber is filled. By infusing anesthetic directly beneath Tenon's capsule and the conjunctiva and posteriorly to the ciliary ganglion, parabulbar anesthesia provides the greatest amount of sensory block. For this reason, we do not advise using a facial block. Patients do not feel the surgery and are not bothered by the operating microscope light; therefore, they do not want to squeeze the eye closed. Facial blocks are given with other techniques to prevent patients from squeezing in response to noxious stimuli. Presumably, they can still feel the stimuli but are prevented from responding. With parabulbar anesthesia, there is no response because there are no perceived stimuli.

After surgery, sub-Tenon's infusions of any steroids or antibiotics the surgeon chooses can be safely performed with the same cannula and the same opening. This avoids the risk of intraocular injection and resulting retinal toxicity. Anesthetic can also be added in the same way for postoperative analgesia, a practice especially advisable in pediatric cases done under general anesthesia. Because the pharmacokinetics of anesthetic agents do not change whether they are injected through a sharp needle or infused through a blunt cannula, the use of bupivacaine in this setting will allow for long-acting postoperative analgesia.

It is important to make the initial incision in a quadrant of the globe away from the rectus muscles to avoid toxicity from infusion of these agents as well as from the anesthetic. Any quadrant can be chosen: inferotemporal, inferonasal, superotemporal, or superonasal. The inferior quadrants are ergonomically easier to access when operating superiorly, whereas the superior ones may be more accessible from the temporal approach. We generally suggest crossing over the cornea with the dominant hand to create the opening. If cosmesis is of primary importance, the opening in Tenon's capsule should be done superiorly, where it can be hidden by the upper lid. More than 40,000 cases have now been done with this parabulbar technique, with no report of vision-threatening complications to date.

In 1992, almost simultaneously with the publication of the parabulbar technique came a report on another sub-Tenon's block by Stevens.[41] In this technique, a curved metal cannula is inserted through an incision created approximately 5 mm from the limbus. At this location, three levels of dissection are required to access the sub-Tenon's space. Three to 3.5 mL of a mixture of 2% lignocaine and 0.5% bupivacaine are infused. The first 1 mL is delivered just posterior to the equator, whereas the remainder is administered after moving the cannula 15 to 20 mm back. Stevens chose the inferonasal quadrant to avoid damage to the temporal vortex vein with his metal cannula. A waiting period of 15 minutes is then allowed for the anesthetic to take effect. In about half the cases reported, a facial block was administered and less than "complete" akinesia was noted. In 16% of patients, a supplemental infusion of 1.5 mL of anesthetic was given, with an additional 5-minute waiting period.

Over the past few years, a third sub-Tenon's anesthetic technique has been developed in Japan by Fukasaku.[109] The first of his "pinpoint" methods involved the injection of 1.5 mL of 2% lidocaine beneath Tenon's capsule with a 27-gauge needle after instillation of 4% lidocaine drops. The second involved the placement of a sponge saturated with 4% lidocaine in the superior fornix. Both of these methods were abandoned by the author because of an "unacceptable incidence of pain." The third technique involves the placement of a curved metal cannula through an incision in conjunctiva, Tenon's capsule, and the intramuscular septum 8 to 12 mm posterior to the limbus in the superotemporal quadrant. The cannula was advanced approximately 20 mm, and 1 mL of 2% lidocaine was injected. Fukasaku reported rapid, complete anesthesia with no akinesia. He compared the comfort level of patients who were blocked with retrobulbar, sub-Tenon's, or topical anesthesia and found that those who received the cannula-delivered sub-Tenon's block were the most comfortable. The lack of akinesia with this technique serves as further clinical confirmation that the mechanism of motor blockade with parabulbar anesthesia is on the local level because individual muscles are blocked just posterior to the equator as they penetrate Tenon's capsule, a site missed by Fukasaku's long cannula.

Some anesthesiologists seem hesitant to adopt the sub-Tenon's technique because it requires an incision in conjunctiva, Tenon's capsule, and the intermuscular septum. On the other hand, those same individuals do not hesitate to place a needle blindly behind or beside the eye into an orbit filled with nerves, blood vessels, and muscles. To compound this problem, the globe itself is not of uniform size or shape. Highly myopic globes are not just longer than average but wider as well. Anterior and posterior staphylomas provide unexpected obstacles, with an increased risk of needle trauma because of their increased dimensions.

A single snip through a fused, cauterized layer of connective tissue just posterior to the limbus for the delivery of a parabulbar block is clearly far safer. Indeed, two vitreoretinal surgeons writing on the complications of cataract surgery noted that "the major advantage of this technique is its safety."[110] They recommended that surgeons using retrobulbar or peribulbar anesthesia "consider changing to this simple and safe technique."

TOPICAL ANESTHESIA

Although topical anesthesia for cataract surgery is not a new technique, it is undergoing a resurgence with the increasing popularity of clear corneal phacoemulsification followed by insertion of foldable intraocular lenses. A 1994 survey of members of the ASCRS reported that only 4% of respondents use this technique,[87] but it appears that a much larger percentage of lecturers giving talks on cataract surgery do so. It is clearly a technique with both real advantages and real drawbacks. In 1986, Shimizu reported on his use of topical 3% cocaine for clear corneal cataract surgery. In 1992, Fichman presented his experience with cataract surgery under topical anesthesia at the annual symposium of the ASCRS. Many variations have been described by others since then.

Fichman's technique begins immediately before the surgical scrub. He uses 0.5% tetracaine drops, which he does not give in the preoperative period to avoid epithelial toxicity.[111] After draping of the patient and placement of a lid speculum, two additional drops of tetracaine are administered. Fichman then waits for 30 seconds and assesses the anesthetic effect by questioning the patient while manipulating the conjunctiva. Additional drops are given until complete topical anesthetic effect is obtained. Fichman and all other authors writing on this subject emphasize the importance of constant verbal communication with the patient before, during, and after surgery. Every sensation the patient is likely to experience is explained before performing the step that will elicit it. Paul Arnold, in a lecture on peribulbar anesthesia given in 1994, reported that during his experience with topical anesthesia he was "exhausted by the amount of psychotherapy" he was performing. Fichman refers to this as "constant coaching."

Fichman does not use a bridle suture but depends on the patient's ability to fixate on the operating microscope light and to look away from the incision site when he is beginning the operation. He noted that it is important to "release the patient from any previous instructions"[111] to avoid operating on a confused patient with a moving eye.

Fichman reported that, although patients may initially be photophobic, they will eventually be able to tolerate the intensity of the operating microscope light, which he sets to the lowest illumination at the beginning of the case (he provided no guidelines for increasing the intensity throughout surgery, however). He also stated that only one patient was unable to stand the light.

Fichman reported frequent complaints during phacoemulsification when the eye is inflated. When patients do complain, he releases the foot pedal immediately and lowers the bottle "so that the globe is barely inflated with the foot pedal still in position one (irrigating only)." He then gradually elevates the bottle to its desired height (he again provided no guidelines for this). He repeats this step each time he enters the eye for these patients. He also advises that "a small dose of IV sedation a minute prior to lens injection may be advisable so as to lessen ciliary-body irritation." He has even gone so far as to inject "a small amount of topical anesthetic directly into the anterior chamber," noting that his "preferred anesthetic" is nonpreserved tetracaine. This is a technique currently being investigated by Gills and others, using nonpreserved lidocaine as well.

For cases lasting longer than 15 to 20 minutes, Fichman adds an additional one to two drops of tetracaine (presumably on an open eye). He reported that this additional dose has worked well in cases lasting up to 45 minutes.

To avoid the pain of ciliary spasm experienced by patients who undergo phacoemulsification under topical anesthesia, Fichman has abandoned the use of intraocular miotics. Instead, he has reduced the amount of epinephrine he uses in the irrigating solution (presumably lessening mydriasis during surgery) and instills carbachol drops postoperatively to avoid the risk of vasovagal response seen with miotics. In cases in which he believes an intraocular miotic is necessary, he provides additional intravenous sedation.

Fichman avoids subconjunctival injections at the end of the operation to prevent discomfort and "cosmetic deformity." Instead, he places on the eye a collagen shield that has been presoaked in an antibiotic-steroid combination. He also prescribes a narcotic analgesic but has reported that "most" patients fail to take it. He cited the elimination of needle trauma, plus the improved cosmesis and better vision in the first 24 hours after surgery, as his reasons for using topical anesthesia.

Although there is no arguing with the first justification, the latter two demand further comment. In exchange for an extremely short-term (1 day) improvement in the patient's "quality of life," the surgeons performing phacoemulsification under topical anesthesia must modify and perhaps compromise their surgical technique. They must reduce the intensity of microscope light and, presumably, the clarity of their view at the beginning of the procedure. They must lower the irrigating bottle and adjust it repeatedly, reducing and changing the depth of the anterior chamber, and hence the room to operate, as well as the distance between the corneal endothelium and the phacoemulsification probe. They reduce the quantity of epinephrine in the irrigating solution and in turn the amount of mydriasis during surgery. They use intraocular topical anesthetics, subjecting the eye to the potential risk of permanent corneal endothelial damage (see section on complications). In other words, they must be willing to put the iris, posterior capsule, and corneal endothelium at increased risk, with all the long-term ramifications of this potential trauma. All this to provide most patients with a whiter eye without a patch for one additional day of their lives. What is the purpose? Is it purely psychological and patient motivated? Is it intended to speed up operating time for the benefit of the elderly patient and society as a whole (by potentially reducing the cost of surgery)? Is it part of the intent, perhaps, to improve surgeons' ability to market their services? These are questions still requiring answers.

The use of other agents for topical anesthesia in phacoemulsification has also been reported. Williamson uses lidocaine, touting its reduced corneal epithelial toxicity, increased duration of action, and improved depth of anesthetic effect in comparison with tetracaine.[111, 112] He begins with tetracaine preoperatively before instilling the dilating drops. He cautions the nursing staff to advise patients about keeping their eyes closed before surgery, thus avoiding exposure and drying of the cornea. The preoperative dose of lidocaine administered is two sets of four drops of topical 4% lidocaine 8.5 to 10 minutes before entering the operating room. Williamson recommended "rigid patient selection" for these procedures and suggested that patients be well dilated to avoid the pain inherent in iris manipulation.[111]

Before operating, he administers four more drops of lidocaine, allowing additional time for dilation of the pupil if required. Alternatively, he adds a subconjunctival injection of 1% lidocaine to his topical regimen in these cases. Williamson stated that peribulbar needles and anesthetic, as well as intravenous sedation, should be available in the operating room if needed. He cautioned that oversedation must be avoided in patients undergoing topical anesthesia because their cooperation is required and recommended "mild sedation" for the pain experienced with filling of the anterior chamber or iris manipulation, advice similar to that given by Fichman for tetracaine-blocked patients. According to Williamson, subconjunctival anesthesia should be added if extracapsular cataract surgery is performed or if a superior rectus suture is used when a scleral tunnel is dissected. He uses a disposable contact lens and antibiotic-steroid drops postoperatively, taping the eye closed for 30 minutes after surgery.

Williamson has written that the threat to reimbursement for anesthesia services during cataract surgery makes the use of topical anesthesia "almost imperative."[111] Several questions remain, however: Who is to administer intravenous sedation during filling of the anterior chamber, for chafing of the iris, or in the odd case in which a peribulbar block is used to supplement the topical anesthesia? Who is to monitor the patient after its administration? More important, is Williamson aware of the other anesthetic techniques that have eliminated the risks inherent in the use of needles without increasing the use of intravenous sedation?

He, too, cited the value of "instantaneous visual rehabilitation" (although he does reduce the extra day of vision by half an hour).

In his description of topical lidocaine use for phacoemulsification, Grabow cautioned that patients lose clear view of the operating microscope light during the procedure and that two instruments can be used for stabilizing the eye and providing fixation.[111] He also advised 10-mg doses of intravenous propofol (Diprivan) for patients who are uncomfortable during the procedure. He noted that topically blocked patients require more intraoperative intravenous support than those who are needle blocked, again calling into question Williamson's use of topical anesthesia without an anesthesiologist. Grabow cautioned against topical anesthesia in patients who are hard of hearing, who are dysphasic, who speak a language foreign to the surgeon, and who cannot be relied on to follow the surgeon's commands. He also cautioned against using this technique with those who cannot fixate well, specifically those with strabismus, nystagmus, macular scars, or very dense cataracts.

Despite all the limitations, warnings, and possible supplemental blocks inherent in the use of topical anesthesia, as raised by even its greatest proponents, there is no question that, in the best of circumstances, cataract surgery can be successfully performed with this technique. There is no shortage of early cataracts in patients who dilate well, speak the surgeon's native tongue, are able to comprehend and follow directions, and have a high threshold of discomfort and anxiety. However, even in these cases, things go wrong.

Someone once said that the only way to avoid complications is not to operate; even in a perfect situation, unforeseen and unforeseeable problems do occur. Because experts in topical anesthesia warn against its use as the only block for extracapsular extraction or for cases that run longer than 45 minutes, there is a question about their protocol for dealing with intraocular complications. Broken capsules, dislocating nuclei, prolapsing vitreous, and edematous corneas are to some small degree risks of phacoemulsification that can never be totally eliminated; the challenge of managing them while simultaneously providing additional anesthesia is a daunting one. Operating under a level of anesthesia that is sufficient for the quick, perfect phacoemulsification but inadequate for a longer, more complicated case, the surgeon must, at the very moment when attention is most needed to manage an evolving problem in the eye, turn attention away from the often downwardly cascading series of events to the provision of additional anesthesia.

If the surgeon chooses to provide additional anesthesia by dropping more topical anesthetic in an open eye or, as Fichman advised, by infusing inside the eye a topical anesthetic that is neither formulated nor approved for intraocular use, the patient is being exposed to potential intraocular toxicity (see Complications of Ocular Anesthesia section). The surgeon may opt to close the eye or to remove the instruments and allow a self-sealing incision to seal and then administer peribulbar or retrobulbar anesthesia. However, this subjects the patient to the inherent risks associated with use of a needle that topical anesthesia was meant to avoid and to an increase in orbital pressure when the eye may be most vulnerable to it.

When Williamson uses the peribulbar needles that he advises be kept available in the operating room during topical anesthesia, the question arises as to how much additional intravenous sedation he asks his anesthesiologist to provide and how he decompresses the eye to avoid further complicating a situation in which a nucleus may be subluxating or vitreous may be prolapsing. These circumstances are rare, but physicians must anticipate rare circumstances and plan for them. The first rule of ethics taught in medical school is "Primum no nocere," or "First do no harm." Although the intention of avoiding needle trauma is admirable, doing so in a way that provides "the daily minimum requirement" of anesthesia may be trading one possible complication for another possibly worse one. This practice would obviously be more palatable if there were no alternative to it.

Experts on topical anesthesia advise the use of "subconjunctival" injections of anesthetic when a superior bridle suture is required, extracapsular cataract extraction is to be performed, a scleral tunnel is to be dissected, or the pupil is poorly dilated. However, it is difficult to see why patients should be subjected to the risk of anterior eye wall perforation, as was reported by Yanoff and Redovan in 1990,[39] if the intention is completely eliminating the risk of needle trauma. Why not completely eliminate needles while providing a level of anesthesia more than adequate for performing all forms of cataract surgery with or without complications, namely parabulbar or sub-Tenon's anesthesia?

In deciding whether or not to use topical anesthesia, surgeons might first investigate their intent and then honestly evaluate their surgical history. If the intent is complete elimination of needle trauma or intravenous sedation, another technique should obviously be used. Surgeons having a significant rate of complications or conversion to extracapsular cataract extraction should likewise consider using more complete anesthesia.

If, however, the sole motivation is to speed up operating time, to improve cosmesis, or to eliminate postoperative patching for the first 18 to 24 hours, surgeons might do well to ponder whether these goals are worth the added risk, however large or small. Parabulbar or sub-Tenon's anesthesia takes the same or less time. It may not be quite as appealing cosmetically, but perhaps our concern should be for how our patients see rather than how they look.

FACIAL NERVE BLOCKS

Although facial nerve blocks are discussed in other chapters, specifically "Anesthesia for Corneal Surgery," their use in cataract surgery is somewhat different. Their history has already been covered; what remains is a detailed discussion of how, when, and whether to use each block.

Van Lint's was the first description of the facial block[8]: "Introduce the needle 1 cm back of the intersection of a horizontal line extending from the lowest part of the inferior margin of the orbit and a vertical line from the most temporal part of the lateral margin of the orbit, about the center of the zygoma" (Fig. 1–16). "The needle is introduced as far as the bone, and directed inward and slightly downward into the deep tissues just below the orbital margin. The injection is given as the needle is withdrawn. Through the same opening in the skin, the needle is again inserted as far as the bone, and directed upward and inward near the

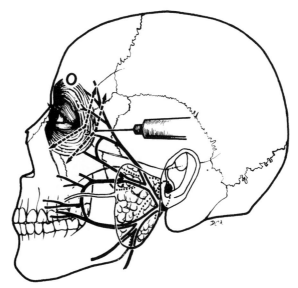

Figure 1–16. Van Lint block. In the classic block, the initial injection site begins near the lateral orbital rim. After a skin wheal, the needle is directed perpendicular to contact the periosteum. It is then redirected deep to the lower orbicularis oculi. Anesthetic is injected upon withdrawal of the needle. The needle is redirected cephalad to complete a "V." In the modified van Lint block, the first injection is made approximately 1 cm lateral to the orbital rim. The needle is made to contact the periosteum, and 1 mL of anesthetic is injected. The needle is directed cephalad and caudad in a "V" over the periosteum. Anesthetic may be injected as the needle is advanced or withdrawn. (O = orbicularis ocularis muscle.) (From Zahl K. Blockade of the orbicularis oculi. Ophthalmol Clin North Am 1990;3:94. Used with permission.)

orbital margin close to the bone." In 1914 van Lint recognized that he could inject anesthetic at the trunk of the facial nerve, but he believed that blocking other branches of the nerve was undesirable.

O'Brien's description of a more proximal facial nerve block was published 15 years later (Figs. 1–17 to 1–19). He wrote, "The point of injection is just anterior to the tragus of the ear, below the posterior portion of the zygomatic process, and directly over the condyloid process

Figure 1–17. O'Brien block. The relationship of the mandibular ramus to the posterior zygomatic process and external auditory meatus is shown. (From Zahl K. Blockade of the orbicularis oculi. Ophthalmol Clin North Am 1990;3:94. Used with permission.)

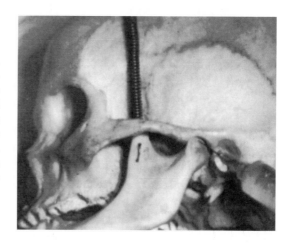

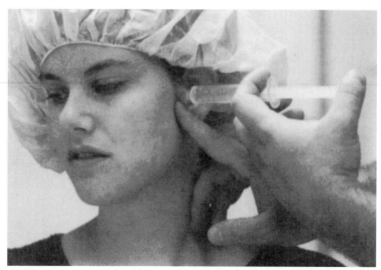

Figure 1–18. O'Brien block. This demonstrates palpation of the condyle of the temporomandibular joint with the index finger anterior to the tragus. The initial injection is given over the posterior zygomatic process and not in the joint capsule. Spaeth recommends redirection of the needle toward the lateral canthus and infiltration of further anesthetic to block lower communicating branches of the seventh nerve. (From Zahl K. Blockade of the orbicularis oculi. Ophthalmol Clin North Am 1990;3:95. Used with permission.)

of the mandible. Going straight inward with a short needle, one strikes the bony condyloid process at a depth of about 1 cm. As soon as this bone is felt with the needle, I begin injecting the 2% solution of procaine hydrochloride and, gradually withdrawing, inject about 2 [mL] of the solution."[9] Spaeth recommended increasing the volume to 7 mL, with an

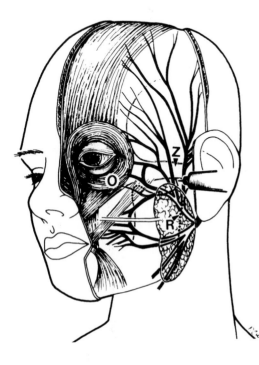

Figure 1–19. O'Brien block. The bony features and course of the facial nerve over the mandibular ramus in relation to the face are shown. (O = orbicularis ocularis; Z = zygomatic process; R = mandibular ramus.) (From Zahl K. Blockade of the orbicularis oculi. Ophthalmol Clin North Am 1990; 3:95. Used with permission.)

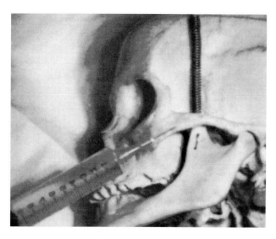

Figure 1–20. Atkinson block. The relationship of the zygomatic arch to the orbit is shown. The needle is positioned in the direction of the injection. (From Zahl K. Blockade of the orbicularis oculi. Ophthalmol Clin North Am 1990;3:96. Used with permission.)

additional 5 mL injected after redirecting the needle toward the lateral canthus, putting his technique somewhere between the O'Brien and van Lint blocks.[113] However, facial paralysis has been reported with this method.

Atkinson described a block that was more proximal than van Lint's but more distal than O'Brien's (Figs. 1–20, 1–21): "a different site for injection has been chosen. It is along the inferior edge of the zygomatic bone and upward across the zygomatic arch toward the top of the ear. A 23 gauge 3.5 cm needle with rounded point, the same needle as is used

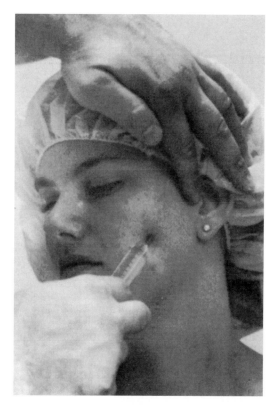

Figure 1–21. Atkinson block. The initial injection site for the Atkinson block is demonstrated. The needle is inserted at the inferior portion of the zygomatic arch (usually below the lateral margin of the orbital rim). Anesthetic is injected (5–10 mL) along the arch as the needle is advanced. (From Zahl K. Blockade of the orbicularis oculi. Ophthalmol Clin North Am 1990;3:96. Used with permission.)

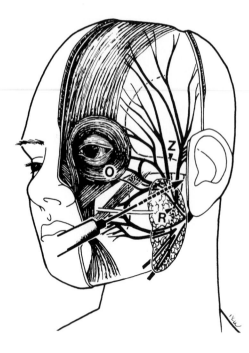

Figure 1–22. Atkinson block. The landmarks of the zygomatic arch and orbit, branches of the facial nerve in relation to the face, are shown. (O = orbicularis ocularis; Z = zygomatic process; R = mandibular ramus.) (From Zahl K. Blockade of the orbicularis oculi. Ophthalmol Clin North Am 1990; 3:97. Used with permission.)

for retrobulbar injections, may be used. It is introduced through an intradermal wheal at the interior edge of the zygomatic bone, a little posterior to a vertical line drawn from the lateral margin of the orbit. The injection is made close to the bone and the anesthetic solution is injected as the needle advances. The index finger of the free hand is placed over the arch of the zygoma just anterior to the ear and over the superficial temporal vessels. This is done to prevent the vessels [Fig. 1–22] from being pierced by the needle and to indicate the direction the needle should follow. About 3 mL of the anesthetic solution are injected. Firm pressure exerted over the site of injection will provide a more rapid and complete block."[16]

Nadbath's proximal facial nerve block, described in 1963,[17] results in total hemifacial akinesia (Figs. 1–23 to 1–25) by blocking the main trunk of the nerve as it exits the stylomastoid foramen. The needle is inserted behind the posterior border of the ramus of the mandible in front of the mastoid process. It is helpful to have patients open the mouth widely to palpate this space before injection. The injection should be given with a short 25-gauge disposable needle, advancing it in an anterocephalad direction. It is crucial to aspirate before injecting 3 to 5 mL of anesthetic to avoid intravascular injection into one of the many blood vessels in this region.

The main disadvantage all facial blocks have in common is pain. They usually require pretreatment with a short-acting intravenous sedative such as methohexital (Brevital). This is, in effect, a block for a block. The need for a facial block is greatest with retrobulbar anesthesia, moderate with peribulbar anesthesia, and nonexistent with parabulbar or sub-Tenon's anesthesia. This is due to the combination of excellent surface as well as intraocular anesthesia with the latter two techniques

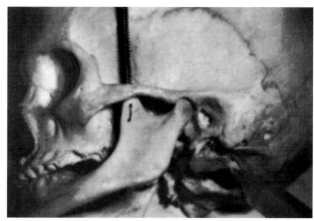

Figure 1–23. Nadbath-Rehman block. The relationship of the stylomastoid foramen (located between the mastoid process and stylus) and the external auditory meatus is shown. The needle is positioned in an anterocephalad direction to avoid penetration of the jugular foramen. (From Zahl K. Blockade of the orbicularis oculi. Ophthalmol Clin North Am 1990;3:97. Used with permission.)

and the lack of adequate surface anesthesia with the first two. By providing both surface and intraocular anesthesia through the parabulbar block, the surgeon or anesthesiologist is eliminating the patient's desire to squeeze the eyes closed. A facial block only eliminates the ability to do so.

The number of surgeons using retrobulbar anesthesia with a facial block has decreased from 76% in 1985 to 40% in 1993.[87] Although most of these converts have switched to peribulbar blocks, some have chosen to continue using retrobulbar anesthesia without the facial counterpart. Cataract surgery is most often performed in the elderly, who are more likely to have concurrent medical problems as well as other medications on board. Thus, the attempt to reduce or eliminate the use of facial blocks with their required intravenous sedation is highly desirable.

Figure 1–24. Nadbath-Rehman block. The injection technique is demonstrated. The index finger rests on the mastoid process, and the needle is inserted between the mastoid process and the posterior border of the mandibular ramus. The needle is advanced in an anterocephalad direction. (From Zahl K. Blockade of the orbicularis oculi. Ophthalmol Clin North Am 1990;3:98. Used with permission.)

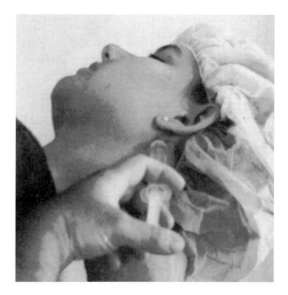

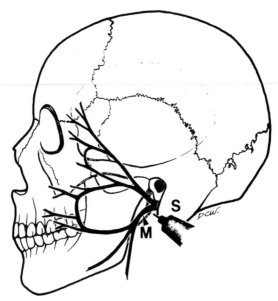

Figure 1–25. Nadbath-Rehman block. The exit of the facial nerve from the stylo-mastoid foramen posterior to the ear is shown. (M = mandibular ramus; S = styloid process.) (From Zahl K. Blockade of the orbicularis oculi. Ophthalmol Clin North Am 1990;3:88. Used with permission.)

Many ophthalmic surgeons clearly agree with this and are changing their anesthetic method of choice accordingly. Williamson's prediction of a future without anesthetic support for cataract surgery may prove to be true; witness the decreasing numbers of assistant surgeons today as well as an attempt in Wisconsin to eliminate reimbursement for anesthetic personnel at most routine cataract operations. If so, methods that require no facial block or intravenous sedation will be the most desirable. This might prove to be a motivation for those who have not yet considered sub-Tenon's techniques. Because Grabow reported an increased use of intraoperative intravenous sedation with his conversion to topical anesthesia,[111] elimination of intravenous sedation should not be a motivation for adopting that technique.

Some forms of cataract surgery clearly require more lid akinesia than others. The more the eye is opened, the greater is the risk of expulsive choroidal hemorrhage, iris prolapse, vitreous loss, and posterior capsular rupture from increased vitreous pressure.[110] In performing intracapsular surgery under retrobulbar anesthesia, the need for excellent lid akinesia is crucial because patients will want to squeeze the eye whenever they feel manipulation of the conjunctiva away from the limbus as a result of the incomplete sensory block inherent with retrobulbar anesthesia. Because intracapsular surgery involves the use of many sutures for closure, this conjunctival stimulation is extremely significant. An incomplete block should be supplemented before beginning the operation. However, if intracapsular surgery is performed under parabulbar anesthesia, it is our experience that no facial block is required because the patient feels no surface sensation and has no stimulus to squeeze the eye. Intracapsular surgery done under peribulbar block should be evaluated on a case-by-case basis as to the need for supplemental facial blocks. However, in this case, the need for prolonged and complete orbital decompression is paramount. No author has advised performing intracapsular surgery (or, in fact, anything but phacoemulsification) under topical anesthesia.

Extracapsular cataract surgery is a wastebasket term for many techniques. Some surgeons maintain a relatively closed system during the procedure, with many sutures preplaced and tied after nucleus expression. Some place a couple of sutures and begin irrigating and aspirating the cortex with a large probe, keeping the incision relatively open. The nucleus can be prolapsed with the pressure of a muscle hook or with an irrigating vectus, needle, or lens spoon. The same guidelines that apply to intracapsular surgery are obviously more applicable to extracapsular techniques performed in a less controlled system and less applicable to those done in a more controlled, closed manner. Certainly, retrobulbar or peribulbar blocks can be successfully used without additional facial anesthesia in most of these cases. Parabulbar blocks have been used extensively by expert and novice surgeons alike without a problem. In a 1993 report on topical anesthesia, the addition of a subconjunctival (sub-Tenon's?) injection when extracapsular surgery is attempted with this technique is advised.[111]

Perhaps the most important benefit of phacoemulsification is that it can be performed in an almost completely closed and controlled environment. To some degree, this fact turns the existence of positive vitreous pressure into an asset rather than a detriment. A moderate amount of pressure helps to prolapse nuclear quadrants after the nucleus is divided in the nuclear cracking or chopping process. In the original three-step nuclear prolapsing method popularized by Maloney, vitreous pressure was almost required. That technique was actually more difficult in the rare patient who had previously undergone trans–pars plana vitrectomy. The need for lid akinesia is clearly less pressing in phacoemulsification, and any of the four techniques of ocular anesthesia can be successfully used with it.

Guidelines for ocular decompression parallel those for facial blocks. Large-volume peribulbar blocks require the most complete decompression; smaller volume blocks are less dependent on it. Parabulbar anesthesia produces a film of anesthetic surrounding the globe and extraocular muscles. This sub-Tenon's distribution does nothing to increase the orbital pressure. If a large volume of anesthetic is used, as has previously been described with older sub-Tenon's techniques,[102] ocular compression might perhaps be used, but such a practice is not advised. By providing akinesia, parabulbar anesthesia further prevents a rise in ocular pressure by lessening the increase seen with muscle contraction. It is this last point that limits the use of topical anesthesia to phacoemulsification, because this procedure is not hindered by the rise in pressure inherent in extraocular muscle contraction, which is associated with topical anesthesia. A preoperative attempt could be made to decompress the eye undergoing surgery under topical anesthesia, but the pressure in the decompression device should be kept low (20–25 mm Hg) to avoid vagal stimulation.[48(p117)] This same technique can be used after administration of parabulbar anesthesia to reduce any anterior chemosis if the surgeon feels the need for it (my colleagues and I do not).

COMPLICATIONS OF OCULAR ANESTHESIA

With all of the advances made in cataract surgery over the past two decades, it might be supposed that the patient's and surgeon's tolerance for anesthetic-related complications would be diminished. Yet only a veritable handful of surgeons today can offer their patients a 100% guarantee that there will be no risk of needle-related trauma. There are manifold dangers inherent in any use of a needle, whether it be directed behind, around, in front of, or alongside the eye: globe perforation, optic nerve trauma, extraocular muscle trauma, retrobulbar hemorrhage with possible subsequent retinal vein or arterial occlusion, and intrathecal anesthesia with possible respiratory depression and death. Whether the needle is blunt or sharp and whether its length is short, medium, or long, the risk of these events can be completely eliminated only by using parabulbar-sub-Tenon's (with a blunt cannula) or purely topical (not topical plus subconjunctival injection) anesthesia. For this reason, Stewart and Lambrou recommended "that surgeons using retrobulbar or peribulbar anesthesia consider changing to this simple and safe technique (parabulbar or posterior sub-Tenon's anesthesia)."[110(p63)]

The literature is filled with reports of adverse effects experienced with retrobulbar, peribulbar, and subconjunctival needle-delivered anesthesia. The risk of globe perforation has been estimated at anywhere from 1:1000[114] to 1:4200.[36] The first estimate was of patients undergoing retinal detachment surgery, and the second involved those undergoing cataract surgery, given peribulbar injections from a single anesthesiologist (presumably a very experienced one). If the average value falls somewhere in between, and if approximately 1.5 million patients undergo needle-delivered anesthesia in the United States each year, then about 750 Americans a year, or 2 a day, are potentially blinded as part of their elective, presumably vision-enhancing, surgery.

If a patient is unfortunate enough to have an eye that is 26 mm or longer, it has been estimated that the risk of globe perforation with retrobulbar or peribulbar anesthesia increases to 1:140.[32] This makes sense because longer eyes are also wider and more prone to anterior and posterior staphylomas, increasing the likelihood of perforation. In fact, this complication has been reported with anterior subconjunctival injections as well,[39] perhaps for this reason. In a 1995 ultrasound study of retrobulbar blocks, 14 of 25 needles were found to be indenting the globe; none of them were farther than 3.3 mm from it.[115] It seems surprising that more eyes are not perforated. It may be that some cases go unreported or are subclinical and not noted postoperatively.

There is a small but real risk of retinal detachment after any form of cataract surgery, even with an intact posterior capsule. Although much of this may be due to vitreous detachment stemming from increased hydration, some may perhaps be due to unsuspected peripheral retinal tears stemming from globe perforation. This is made more plausible by the fact that all the surgeons in the previously noted ultrasound study erroneously thought their needle was at least 5 mm from the globe.

The risks of optic nerve trauma and subdural anesthetic injections are anatomically intertwined. In a study of 6000 consecutive patients undergoing ophthalmic surgery under retrobulbar anesthesia, the risk of central nervous system spread was 1:375.[89] Although some of the subsequent effects were minor, such as shivering or drowsiness, half were life threatening, including apnea, respiratory depression, convulsions, and cardiopulmonary arrest. Other unpleasant complications included blindness of the contralateral eye, hemiplegia, and unconsciousness. It is entirely possible that many cases of "postsurgical optic atrophy" are actually related to unrecognized needle trauma. If there is any doubt that respiratory arrest after retrobulbar injection can be due to a direct spread of anesthetic intrathecally, it should be allayed by a report demonstrating recovery of anesthetic from the cerebrospinal fluid after such an event.[116] Likewise, surgeons should certainly be alerting their patients during informed consent that they may be undergoing risk of life-threatening complications as a result of retrobulbar anesthesia.

The risk of retrobulbar hemorrhage from needle-delivered anesthesia before surgery is reported as being anywhere from 1:1000 to 1:60.[117] This complication has been reported both with retrobulbar and peribulbar anesthesia.[118] Most of these hemorrhages are not vision threatening, although blindness has been reported from one after a peribulbar block.[117] However, many require postponement of surgery, and all are disconcerting to patient and surgeon alike.

Extraocular muscle trauma, with subsequent diplopia, is being increasingly recognized as resulting from local anesthetic needles. Inferior rectus trauma with subsequent paresis or contracture has been reported after both retrobulbar and peribulbar anesthesia.[119–124] This complication may have become more common because of the increased popularity of peribulbar blocks. In an effort to avoid the globe, surgeons may be more likely to hit the muscles surrounding it. A 1995 report of inferior oblique muscle trauma in four patients who underwent retrobulbar or peribulbar blocks noted a contracture of the muscle in three and paresis in one.[55] It should be noted that the authors of this report advised adopting sub-Tenon's anesthesia as a way of avoiding diplopia. Again, surgeons should certainly mention diplopia as a possible risk while providing informed consent before needle-delivered anesthesia.

Drug-related complications may also be seen with both needle-delivered and topical anesthesia. One case of hyaluronidase allergy after retrobulbar anesthesia was found to simulate expulsive choroidal hemorrhage. The patient required a second procedure for intraocular lens implantation because of a rapid increase in orbital pressure.[125] Because hyaluronidase is not used with parabulbar anesthesia, this is not a concern of surgeons using this technique. This is a rare complication, but the use of an agent that is both expensive and potentially dangerous should be of concern to all those using hyaluronidase to improve the effectiveness of retrobulbar and peribulbar blocks. Millions of dollars are spent each year on this substance. Adopting parabulbar or another form of sub-Tenon's infusion, or using topical anesthesia, would eliminate both the potential risk and the very real expense of this enzyme.

Topical anesthesia may, however, subject the patient to other drug-related risks. As previously noted, Fichman advocated the use of intraocular tetracaine[111] during topical anesthesia for periods when the patient becomes uncomfortable. Even when a topical agent is not delivered directly into the eye, many cases of unintended intraocular anesthesia are probably caused by surgeons dropping additional topical agents on the eye. There is one report of inadvertent anterior chamber tetracaine injection causing a semidilated, atonic pupil and bullous keratopathy that did not resolve.[126] Perhaps the dilution was different from the one Fichman uses.

In any case, it would be very hard to live with a complication directly caused by topical anesthesia, a method intended to increase safety. It would probably be at least as hard to defend the intentional intraocular use of an agent not intended for intraocular use, leading to a vision-threatening complication. A corroborating report on the complications of intraocular lidocaine injection found similarly dilated, atonic pupils as well as retinal toxicity; one patient experienced a permanent visual field defect.[127] A recent study presented by Kim and coworkers at the 1996 American Academy of Ophthalmology (unpublished) demonstrated transient endothelial edema caused by intraocular lidocaine. These articles definitely call into question the safety of intraocular anesthesia as a supplement to topical anesthesia. More study is clearly required before this procedure can be safely advised.

In his editorial, "Avoiding Complications from Local Anesthesia," Lichter speculated on ways "to avoid iatrogenic injury that can turn a hoped-for happy visual result into a nightmare."[128] As we have seen, there is such a way. In the entire literature, there has been just one report of a real complication with sub-Tenon's anesthesia. This was the creation of a tight orbit with a 6-mL infusion.[102] This problem is unique. Our experience with parabulbar anesthesia has been totally devoid of complications. As Stewart and Lambrou postulated, this may in part be due to the reduction of anesthesia infused to 1.5 mL.[110] Thus far, more than 40,000 parabulbar blocks have been given worldwide. Not every one can be expected to have worked perfectly, but no complications have been reported other than subconjunctival hemorrhage or chemosis. This, then, appears to be the method for which Lichter was searching.

WHICH BLOCK FOR WHICH METHOD?

Although phacoemulsification is fast becoming the method by which most surgeons perform cataract surgery, there will probably never be only one way for all surgeons to perform all operations on all patients. In a perfect future, we may perhaps be able to inject an enzyme through the capsule, dissolving the lens. It could be aspirated through a pipette, followed by the injection of a liquid intraocular lens that would harden to a semisoft consistency, retaining the ability to change shape during accommodation. Even so, a number of cases will probably always require phacoemulsification, irrigational aspiration, and even intracapsular surgery. In choosing anesthesia for today and tomorrow, two variables must be kept in mind. First, the larger the incision (in other words, the more open the surgical environment) and the earlier the technique is on a particular surgeon's "learning curve," the more desirable is akinesia. Second, on the other hand, anesthesia and analgesia are desirable regardless of the technique or the surgeon's experience.

To provide akinesia for an intracapsular extraction, therefore, it might be better to use general anesthesia or a larger volume of parabulbar anesthetic (2–3 mL at one or two sites). These added precautions would certainly not be advisable for phacoemulsification. Although millions of intracapsular procedures have been successfully performed under retrobulbar and peribulbar anesthesia, the many complications of these techniques are only now being fully appreciated. We strongly believe that the continued use of such methods will only add to the number of patients left with unanticipated, undesirable secondary effects of anesthesia. If one cataract patient in the next million suffers intractable diplopia because of the use of a needle, when there are currently available at least three techniques that provide more than adequate anesthesia in a much safer manner, that one is too many. A 1995 prospective study of parabulbar anesthesia, presented at the 1995 meeting of the Association of Research in Vision and Ophthalmology, demonstrated the excellent safety and more than adequate efficacy of a surgeon's early experience with parabulbar anesthesia in 53 consecutive anterior segment cases.[129]

With the future promising better and less traumatic techniques for extracting the lens and rehabilitating vision, better and less traumatic ways of providing anesthesia to assist in accomplishing this important task in the safest and most comfortable manner must be developed. Parabulbar anesthesia, although currently "the road less traveled,"[130] is the route that we should continue to follow in the coming years.

REFERENCES

1. Duke-Elder WS. Textbook of ophthalmology, vol 3. London: Kimpton, 1940, p 3115.
2. Kirby DB. Surgery of cataract. Philadelphia: JB Lippincott, 1950.
3. Hubbell A. Jacques Daviel and the beginning of the modern operation of extraction of cataract. JAMA 1902; July 26.
4. Von Graefe A. On linear extraction. BMJ 1867;1:379.
5. Knapp H. On cocaine and its use in ophthalmic surgery. Arch Ophthalmol 1884;13:402.
6. Turnbull CS. Editorial. Med Surg Rep 1884;29:628.
7. Traquair HM. Anesthesia in ophthalmic surgery. Trans Ophthalmol Soc UK 1938;58:697.
8. Van Lint A. Paralysie palpebrae temporaire provoquee dans l'operation de la cataracte. Ann Ocul (Paris) 1914;151:420.
9. O'Brien CS. Akinesis during catact extraction. Arch Ophthalmol 1929;1:447.
10. Atkinson WS. Anesthesia in ophthalmology. Springfield, IL: Charles C Thomas, 1955.
11. Adriani J. Local and regional anesthesia for minor surgery. Surg Clin North Am 1951;31:1507.
12. DeJong RH. Local anesthetics. Springfield, IL: Charles C Thomas, 1977.
13. Atkinson WS. Use of hyaluronidase with local anesthesia in ophthalmology: a preliminary report. Arch Ophthalmol 1940;42:628.
14. Duran Reynals F. The effect of extracts of certain organs from normal and immunized animals on the infecting power of the vaccine virus. J Exp Med 1929;50:327.
15. Chain E, Duthie ES. Identity of hyaluronidase and spreading factor. Br J Exp Pathol 1940;21:324.
16. Atkinson WS. Akinesia of the orbicularis. Am J Ophthalmol 1953;36:1255.
17. Nadbath RP, Rehman I. Facial nerve block. Am J Ophthalmol 1963;55:143.
18. Cofer HF. Cord paralysis after Nadbath facial nerve block. Arch Ophthalmol 1986;104:337.
19. Wilson CA, Ruiz RS. Respiratory obstruction following the Nadbath facial nerve block. Arch Ophthalmol 1985;103:1454.
20. Ramsay RC, Knobloch WH. Ocular perforation following retrobulbar anesthesia for retinal detachment surgery. Am J Ophthalmol 1978;86:61.
21. Kraushar MF, Seelenfreund MH, Freilich DB. Central retinal artery closure during orbital hemorrhage from retrobulbar injection. Trans Am Acad Ophthalmol Otolaryngol 1974;78:OP65.
22. Meyers EF, Ramirez RC, Boniuk I. Grand mal seizures after retrobulbar block. Arch Ophthalmol 1978;96:847.

23. Beltranena HP, Vega MJ, Garcia JJ, Blankenship G: Complications of retrobulbar marcaine injection. J Clin Neuroophthalmol 1982;2:159.

24. Sullivan KL, Brown GC, Forman AR, et al. Retrobulbar anesthesia and retinal vascular obstruction. Ophthalmology 1983;90:373.

25. Brookshire GL, Gleitsmann KY, Schenk EC: Life-threatening complication of retrobulbar block: a hypothesis. Ophthalmology 1986;93:1476.

26. Antoszyk AN, Buckley EG. Contralateral decreased visual acuity and extraocular muscle palsies following retrobulbar anesthesia. Ophthalmology 1986;93:462.

27. Friedberg HL, Kline OR Jr. Contralateral amaurosis after retrobulbar injection. Am J Ophthalmol 1986;101:688.

28. Paulter SE, Grizzard WS, et al. Blindness from retrobulbar injection into the optic nerve. Ophthalmic Surg 1986;17:334.

29. Javitt JC, Addiego R, et al. Brainstem anesthesia after retrobulbar block. Ophthalmology 1987;94:718.

30. Wittpenn JR, Rapoza P, et al. Respiratory arrest following retrobulbar anesthesia. Ophthalmology 1986;93:867.

31. Morgan CM, Schatz H, Vine AK, et al. Ocular complications associated with retrobulbar injections. Ophthalmology 1988;95:660.

32. Duker JS, Belmont JB, Benson WE, et al. Inadvertent globe perforation during retrobulbar and peribulbar anesthesia. Ophthalmology 1991;98:519.

33. Davis DB II. Retrobulbar and facial nerve block ? no; peribulbar ? yes (letter). Ophthalmic Surg 16:604, 1985.

34. Davis DB II, Mandel MR. Posterior peribulbar anesthesia: an alternative to retrobulbar anesthesia. J Cataract Refract Surg 1986;12:182.

35. Berg P, Kroll P, Kuchie HJ. Iatrogenic perforations in peri- and retrobulbar injections. Klin Monatsbl Augenheilkd 1986;189:170.

36. Kimble JA, Morris RE, Witherspoon CD, Feist RM. Globe perforation from peribulbar injection. Arch Ophthalmol 1987;105:749.

37. Gills JP, Loyd TL. A technique of retrobulbar block with paralysis of the orbicularis oculi. Am Intra-ocular Implant Soc J 1983;9:339.

38. Hansen EA, Mein CE, Mazzoli R. Ocular anesthesia for cataract surgery: a direct sub-Tenon's approach. Ophthalmic Surg 1990;21:696.

39. Yanoff M, Redovan EG. Anterior eyewall perforation during subconjunctival cataract block. Ophthalmic Surg 1990;21:262.

40. Greenbaum S. Parabulbar anesthesia. Am J Ophthalmol 1992;114:776.

41. Stevens JD. A new local anaesthesia technique for cataract extraction by one quadrant sub-Tenon's infiltration. Br J Ophthalmol 1992;76:670.

42. Atkinson WS. Observations on anesthesia for ocular surgery. Trans Am Acad Ophthalmol Otol 1956;60:377.

43. Thorson J, Jampolsky A, Scott A. Topical anesthesia for strabismus surgery. Trans Am Acad Ophthalmol Otol 1966;70:968.

44. Shimizu K. Surgery from Japan. Audiovis J Cat Implant Surg 1986;2.

45. Fichman RA, Hoffman J. Anesthesia for cataract surgery and its complications. Curr Opin Ophthalmol 1994;5:21.

46. Sadove MS. Discussions of papers on ocular anesthesia. Trans Am Acad Ophthalmol Otol 1956;60:396.

47. Dutton JJ. Atlas of clinical and surgical orbital anatomy. Philadelphia: WB Saunders, 1994.

48. Gills JP, Hustead RF, Sanders DR, eds. Ophthalmic anesthesia. Thorofare, NJ: Slack, 1993.

49. Sacks JG. Peripheral innervation of extraocular muscles. Am J Ophthalmol 1983;95:520.

50. Nathan H, Ouaknine G, Kosary IZ. The abducens nerve: anatomical variations in its course. J Neurosurg 1979;41:561.

51. Katsev DA, Drews RC, Rose BT. An anatomic study of retrobulbar needle path length. Ophthalmology 1989;96:1221.

52. Von Nordon GK. Burian-von Nordon's binocular vision and ocular motility: theory and management of strabismus. St. Louis, MO: CV Mosby, 1985.

53. Carlson BM, Emerick S, Komorowski TE, Rainin EA. Extraocular muscle regeneration in primates: local anesthesia-induced lesions. Ophthalmology 1992;99:582.

54. Rainin EA, Carlson BM. Postoperative diplopia and ptosis: a clinical hypothesis on the myotoxicity of local anesthetics. Arch Ophthalmol 1985;103:1337.

55. Hunter DG, Lam GC, Guyton DL. Inferior oblique muscle injury from local anesthesia for cataract surgery. Ophthalmology 1995;102:501.

56. Scheie HG, Albert DM. Textbook of ophthalmology. Philadelphia: WB Saunders, 1977.

57. Galindo A, Keilson LR, Mondshine RB, Sawelson HI. Retro-peribulbar anesthesia. In: Zahl K, Meltzer MA, eds. Regional Anesthesia for Intraocular Surgery. Ophthalmol Clin North Am 1990;3:74.

58. Hayreh SS, Dass R. The ophthalmic artery: I. Origin and intracranial and intra-canalicular course. Br J Ophthalmol 1962;46:65.
59. Hayreh SS, Dass R. The ophthalmic artery: II. Intra-orbital course. Br J Ophthalmol 1962;46:165.
60. DeSantis M, Anderson KJ, King DW, Nielsen J. Variability in relationships of arteries and nerves in the human orbit. Anat Anz 1984;157:227.
61. Bergin MP. Relationships between arteries and veins and the connective tissue system in the human orbit: I. The retrobulbar part of the orbit: apical region. Acta Morphol Neerl Scand 1982;20:1.
62. Bergin MP. Relationships between arteries and veins and the connective tissue system in the human orbit: II. The retrobulbar part of the orbit: septal complex region. Acta Morphol Neerl Scand 1982;20:17.
63. Brismar J. Orbital phlebography: III. Topography of the orbital veins. Acta Radiol (Diagn) (Stockh) 1974;15:577.
64. Bergin MP. Some histologic aspects of the structure of the connective tissue system and its relationships with the blood vessels in the human orbit. Acta Morphol Neerl Scand 1982;20:293.
65. Henry JGM. Contribution a l'etude de l'anatomie des vaisseaux de l'orbite et de la loge caverneuse-pas injection de matieres plastiques du tendon de Zinn et de la capsule de Tenon. These de Paris, 1959. Cited in Bergin MP: Vascular architecture in the human orbit. Lisse, Netherlands: Suets and Zeitlinger, BV, 1982.
66. Birge HL, Zimmerman LW, Tovell RM, et al. Intraocular surgery under general anesthesia: a study of the problems from 1950 to 1954. Trans Am Acad Ophthalmol Otolaryngol 1956;54:381.
67. Backer CL, Tinker JH, Robertson DM. Myocardial reinfarction following local anesthesia for ophthalmic surgery. Anesth Analg 1980;59:257.
68. Lang DW. Morbidity and mortality in ophthalmology. In: Bruce RA, McGoldrick KE, Oppenheimer P, eds. Anesthesia for ophthalmology. Birmingham, AL: Aesculapius Publishing, 1982, p 195.
69. Lynch S, Wolf GL, Berlin I. General anesthesia for cataract surgery: a comparative review of 2217 consecutive cases. Anesth Analg 1974;53:909.
70. Luntz MH. Clinical types of cataracts. In: Duane TD, ed. Clinical ophthalmology. Philadelphia: JB Lippincott, 1988, p 14.
71. Aldridge LM. Anaesthetic problems in myotonic dystrophy: a case report and review of the Aberdeen experience comprising 48 general anaesthetics in a further 16 patients. Br J Anaesth 1985;57:1119.
72. Wells DG, Podolakin W. Anesthesia and Marfan's syndrome: case report. Can J Anesth 1987;34:311.
73. Mostafa SM. Anaesthesia for ophthalmic surgery. Oxford: Oxford University Press, 1991, p 165.
74. McGoldrick KE. Anesthesia for ophthalmic and otolaryngologic surgery. Philadelphia: WB Saunders, 1992.
75. Ording H. Incidence of malignant hyperthermia in Denmark. Anesth Analg 1985;64:700.
76. MacKenzie CR, Charlson ME. Assessment of perioperative risk in the patient with diabetes mellitus. Surg Gynecol Obstet 1988;167:293.
77. Smith RB, Douglas H, Retruscak J. Safety of intraocular adrenaline with halothane anaesthesia. Br J Anaesth 1972;44:1314.
78. Ritchie JM, Greene NM. Local anesthetics. In: Gilman AG, Goodman LS, Gilman A, eds. The pharmacologic basis of therapeutics. New York: Macmillan, 1980, p 312.
79. Ballin N, Becker B, Goldman ML. Systemic effects of epinephrine applied topically to the eye. Invest Ophthalmol 1966;5:125.
80. Lansche RK. Systemic reactions to topical epinephrine and phenylephrine. Am J Ophthalmol 1966;49:95.
81. DeRoeth A, Dettbar WD, Rosenberg P. Effect of phospholine iodide on blood cholinesterase levels. Am J Ophthalmol 1963;59:586.
82. Batra YK, Bali M. Corneal abrasions during general anesthesia. Anesth Analg 1977;56:363.
83. Watson WJ, Moran RL. Corneal abrasion during induction. Anesthesiology 1987;66:440.
84. Durkan W, Fleming N. Potential eye damage from reusable masks. Anesthesiology 1987;67:444.
85. DeVoe AG, Norton EWD, Kearns TP, et al. Valsalva hemorrhagic retinopathy: discussion. Trans Am Ophthalmol Soc 1972;70:307.
86. Stinson TW, Donlan JV. Interaction of SF6 and air with nitrous oxide. Anesthesiology 1979;51:S16.
87. Leaming DV. Practice styles and preferences of ASCRS members-1993 survey. J Cataract Refract Surg 1994;20:459.

88. Unsöld R, Stanley J, DeGroot J. The CT-topography of retrobulbar anesthesia. Arch Klin Ophthalmol 1981;217:125.

89. Nicoll JMV, Acharya PA, Ahlen Kjell, et al. Central nervous system complications after 6000 retrobulbar blocks. Anesth Analg 1987;66:1298.

90. Grizzard WS, Kirk N, Pavan PR, et al. Perforating ocular injuries caused by anesthesia personnel. Ophthalmology 1991;98:1011.

91. Straus JG. A new retrobulbar needle and injection technique. Ophthalmol Surg 1988;19:134.

92. Davis DB, Mandel MR. Posterior peribulbar anesthesia: an alternative to retrobulbar anesthesia. J Cataract Refract Surg 1986;12:182.

93. Braun H, Harris ML, ed. Local anesthesia. Philadelphia: Lea & Febiger, 1924, p 218.

94. Pitkin GP, Southworth JL, Hingson RA, ed. Conduction anesthesia. Philadelphia: JB Lippincott, 1946, p 336.

95. Weiss JL, Deichman CB. A comparison of retrobulbar and periocular anesthesia for cataract surgery. Arch Ophthalmol 1989;107:96.

96. Bloomberg L. Administration of periocular anesthesia. J Cataract Refract Surg 1986;12:677.

97. Bloomberg L. Anterior peribulbar anesthesia: five years experience. J Cataract Refract Surg 1991;17:508.

98. Galindo A. pH adjusted local anesthetics: clinical experience. Reg Anesth 1983;8:35.

99. Zahl K, Jordan A, McGroaty J, et al. The use of pH-adjusted bupivicaine/hyaluronidase for peribulbar anesthesia. Anesthesiology 1990;72:230.

100. Davis DB, Mandel MR. Efficacy and complication rate of 16,224 consecutive peribulbar blocks. J Cataract Refract Surg 1994;20:327.

101. Snyder C. An operation designated "the extirpation of the eye." Arch Ophthalmol 1965;74:429.

102. Mein CE, Woodcock MG. Local anesthesia for vitreoretinal surgery. Retina 1990;10:47.

103. Smith R. Cataract extraction without retrobulbar anaesthetic injection. Br J Ophthalmol 1990;74:205.

104. Redmond RM, Dallas NL. Extracapsular cataract extraction under local anaesthesia without retrobulbar injection. Br J Ophthalmol 1990;74:203.

105. Furata M, Toriumi T, Kashiwagi K, Satoh S. Limbal anesthesia for cataract surgery. Ophthalmic Surg 1990;21:22.

106. Moses RA. Adler's physiology of the eye: clinical application. St. Louis, MO: CV Mosby, 1981, p 228.

107. Griffiths JD, Pillai S, Lustbader JM. The effect of retrobulbar anesthesia on optic nerve function (abstract). Invest Ophthalmol Vis Sci 1994;35:1544.

108. Stevens J, Giubilei M, Lanigan L, Hykin P. Sub-Tenon, retrobulbar and peribulbar local anaesthesia: the effect upon intraocular pressure. Eur J Implant Refract Surg 1993;5:25.

109. Fukasaku H, Marron JA. Pinpoint anesthesia: a new approach to local ocular anesthesia. J Cataract Refract Surg 1994;20:468.

110. Stewart M, Lambrou F. The management of preoperative, intraoperative, and postoperative complications of cataract surgery from the perspective of vitreoretinal surgeons. Adv Clin Ophthalmol 1994;1:63.

111. Fine IH, Fichman RA, Grabow HR. Clear-corneal cataract surgery and topical anesthesia. Thorofare, NJ: Slack, 1993.

112. Marr WG, Wood R, Senterfit L, et al. Effect of topical anesthesia on regeneration of corneal epithelium. Am J Ophthalmol 1957;43:606.

113. Spaeth GL. A new method to achieve complete akinesia of the facial muscles of the eyelids. Ophthalmic Surg 1976;7:105.

114. Cibis PA. General discussion: opening remarks. In: Shepens CL, Regan CDJ, eds. Controversial aspects of the management of retinal detachments. Boston: Little, Brown, 1965, p 222.

115. Birch AA, Evans M, Redembo E. The ultrasonic localization of retrobulbar needles during retrobulbar block. Ophthalmology 1995;102:824.

116. Kobet KA. Cerebral spinal fluid recovery of lidocaine and bupivacaine following respiratory arrest subsequent to retrobulbar block. Ophthalmic Surg 1987;18:11.

117. Peterson WC, Yanoff M. Complications of local ocular anesthesia. Int Ophthalmol Clin 1992;32:23.

118. Puustjarvi T, Purhonen S. Permanent blindness following retrobulbar hemorrhage after peribulbar anesthesia for cataract surgery. Ophthalmic Surg 1992;23:450.

119. de Faber J-THN, von Noorden GK. Inferior rectus muscle palsy after retrobulbar anesthesia for cataract surgery. Am J Ophthalmol 1991;112:209.

120. Grimmett MR, Lambert SR. Superior rectus muscle overaction after cataract extraction. Am J Ophthalmol 1992;114:72.

121. Esswein MB, von Noorden GK. Paresis of a vertical rectus muscle after cataract extraction. Am J Ophthalmol 1993;116:424.

122. Ong-Tone L, Pearce WG. Inferior rectus muscle restriction after retrobulbar anesthesia for cataract extraction. Can J Ophthalmol 1989;24:162.
123. Hamed LM, Mancuso A. Inferior rectus muscle contracture syndrome after retrobulbar anesthesia. Ophthalmology 1991;98:1506.
124. Hamilton SM, Elsas FJ, Dawson TL. A cluster of patients with inferior rectus restriction following local anesthesia for cataract surgery. J Pediatr Ophthalmol Strabismus 1993;30:288.
125. Minning CA. Hyaluronidase allergy simulating expulsive choroidal hemorrhage (report). Arch Ophthalmol 1994;112:585.
126. Fraunfelder FT. Drug-induced ocular side effects and drug interactions. Philadelphia: Lea & Febiger, 1982, p 486.
127. Lincoff H, Zweifach P, Brodie S, et al. Intraocular injection of lidocaine. Ophthalmology 1985;92:1587.
128. Lichter PR. Avoiding complications from local anesthesia (editorial). Ophthalmology 1988;95:565.
129. Markoff DD. Parabulbar anesthesia for cataract surgery (abstract). Invest Ophthalmol Vis Sci 1995;36:S809.
130. Frost R. The road not taken. In: Lathem EC, ed. The poetry of Robert Frost. New York: Henry Holt, 1979, p 105.

CHAPTER 2

ANESTHESIA FOR CORNEAL SURGERY

HERBERT J. INGRAHAM, MD
ERIC D. DONNENFELD, MD

INTRODUCTION

GOALS OF ANESTHESIA FOR CORNEAL SURGERY

Impressive advances in surgery of the anterior segment and cornea have occurred over the past 25 years, and similar progress has been made in the fields of general and regional anesthesia. Anesthesia is a critical component of surgery, and from the patient's perspective it is perhaps the most important aspect. With good communication and cooperation between the ophthalmologist and anesthetist, the operative experience can be relatively safe, pleasant, and pain free while providing an easy transition to the postoperative period.

No matter which type of anesthesia is chosen for a given corneal procedure, the goals remain the same. The patient should be free of pain, and anxiety should be controlled. Good akinesia of the extraocular muscles and eyelid is critical in intraocular surgery unless there is a self-sealing wound. Intraocular pressure must be maintained within a narrow range to avoid serious vision-threatening complications and is particularly important in the setting of an open globe. Anesthesia should be safe and effective, minimizing the risk of ocular and systemic morbidity. Finally, the systemic effects of surgery, including alterations in the respiratory, cardiovascular, and endocrine systems, must be monitored and controlled. Each of these issues is discussed further because each one impacts on the appropriate selection of anesthetic approach for specific procedures in a variety of clinical settings.

BRIEF HISTORY OF OPHTHALMIC ANESTHESIA

Until the description of the anesthetic properties of nitrous oxide in 1800 by Davy,[1] little was available to ease the suffering of patients undergoing surgery. Unfortunately, this technique did not gain widespread popularity, and it was not until Morton[1] demonstrated the use of ether for general anesthesia in 1846 that an agent was widely used. The discovery of cocaine a decade later heralded the beginning of the era of regional anesthesia, and in 1884 Koller[2] first reported the use of topical cocaine for ocular surgery. Knapp[3] described the use of retrobulbar cocaine for an enucleation the same year. Systemic toxicity limited the use of retrobulbar cocaine for most ophthalmic procedures, and it was not until van Lint[4] popularized the use of procaine in 1914 for a facial nerve block that the procedure was more widely accepted. A number of techniques to obtain akinesia of the orbicularis followed and are discussed in more detail later.

In 1936 Atkinson described his technique of retrobulbar injection for ocular surgery using procaine.[5] The author advocated the use of a blunt-tip needle to avoid the intraorbital structures while injecting inside the muscle cone followed by ocular massage to soften the eye. Although he was not the first to describe the technique, he is credited with its subsequent popularity and dominance of ocular anesthesia. It was not until 1986, when Davis and Mandel[6] described the peribulbar approach developed by Kelman and others, that a significant improvement was made on Atkinson's technique of 50 years previously. The injection of anesthetic outside the muscle cone with reduced risks of ocular trauma and systemic effects provided yet another tool in the armamentarium of ocular anesthesia.

SELECTION OF APPROPRIATE ANESTHESIA

PREOPERATIVE EVALUATION

The selection of appropriate anesthesia for any procedure in a given clinical setting requires cooperation and communication among the patient, ophthalmologist, and anesthesiologist. Although some procedures can certainly be performed under local anesthesia without the assistance of anesthesia personnel (particularly in the office or minor procedure room setting), there is general consensus that patient care is improved if a trained anesthetist is available to monitor the patient.[7] The preoperative interview, ideally performed on a day before the surgery, is an important part of this process. During this interview, a patient's medical history, medications, drug allergies, previous adverse anesthetic reactions, or other special circumstances can be examined and a treatment plan devised. In ophthalmic patients, this is particularly important; a 1985 study of 100 cataract patients found the average age to be 75 years; 84% of patients had one or more serious systemic conditions.[8]

PREOPERATIVE TESTING

As a general rule, preoperative testing should be determined by the patient's medical history and the plan of anesthesia care rather than a routine battery of tests. A hematocrit is indicated,[9] except in the young, healthy patient, whereas complete blood cell count with coagulation profile is of limited use except in oncology patients and in those taking anticoagulants. An electrolyte panel is advised for patients with renal disease, with diabetes, or who are taking diuretics. Electrocardiogram (ECG) and chest x-ray films should be reserved for those with a cardiac history or respiratory condition, respectively. Urinalysis, once a routine test, probably has little value, except in the presence of referable symptoms or renal compromise. Liver enzymes may be indicated if general anesthesia is anticipated. This common-sense approach allows the delivery of cost-effective, high-quality care and is tailored to the individual patient.

DRUG INTERACTIONS

A number of medications taken regularly by patients have the potential to cause anesthetic complications, particularly in the setting of general anesthesia. Patients taking cholinesterase inhibitors, including topical phospholine iodide (echothiophate iodide) or demecarium bromide, may have a 95% decrease in systemic pseudocholinesterase for up to 6 weeks after the drops are discontinued. If succinylcholine is used to facilitate anesthesia, this may result in prolonged apnea. Anesthesia personnel should be aware of the use of this medication, and ideally it should be discontinued 4 to 6 weeks before surgery.[10]

A number of medications used in the treatment of psychiatric patients are also contraindicated in the setting of general anesthesia. The combination of a monoamine oxidase inhibitor and a sympathomimetic used during anesthesia may lead to acute hypertensive attacks. Certain tricyclic antidepressants can cause arrhythmias when halothane and pancuronium are used, and lithium may prolong neurologic blockade.[10] If possible, these agents should also be discontinued before surgery or the plan for anesthesia altered to take them and any potential drug interactions into consideration.

Conversely, the treatment for other systemic conditions should not be discontinued before surgery, or serious consequences may arise. Insulin-dependent diabetics are advised to use one half of their usual morning dosage on arrival to the preoperative unit, and blood sugar levels are carefully monitored. Patients taking oral hypoglycemic drugs are best managed by holding the daily dose and providing insulin coverage for blood sugar levels on a sliding scale.[9] Hypertensive patients are advised to take their usual medications the morning of surgery with a small amount of water; attention is given to the hydration and electrolyte status of patients on diuretics. Bronchodilators are continued through the perioperative period, and theophylline levels are checked within 24 hours before surgery.[9] Similarly, patients on chronic systemic corticosteroids continue their medication and often receive a supplemental "stress" dose of up to 100 mg of hydrocortisone in the perioperative period.[9]

ANTICOAGULANTS

Few issues in the preoperative assessment of the patient attract more attention than the use of anticoagulants, including aspirin, dipyridamole, heparin, and warfarin. The risks of operating on an anticoagulated patient include retrobulbar hemorrhage, hyphema, and other intraocular hemorrhage, whereas the risks of discontinuing therapy include pulmonary embolism, stroke, and myocardial infarction.[11] A number of studies suggest that although bleeding, including hyphema, is more likely in an anticoagulated group,[12-14] serious vision-threatening hemorrhages are not seen more commonly than in controls.[12, 15] Further, discontinuation of therapy does not seem to alter the risk of patients on chronic anticoagulants and antiplatelet agents,[12] and the risk of systemic complications is not insignificant.[11] Coagulation profiles may be of value in identifying those patients with excessive levels of anticoagulation, although it is unclear whether even these patients are at more risk than those in a therapeutic range.[12] The use of peribulbar or retrobulbar injections with sharp needles is to be avoided, if possible. When extraocular muscle akinesia is required, the use of a blunt cannula[16] may decrease the risk of retrobulbar hemorrhage. When the anticipated surgery is extraocular or involves the use of a self-sealing incision, topical anesthesia with or without systemic sedation may be indicated. We advise a careful consideration of the risks and benefits associated with ocular surgery in an anticoagulated patient, with treatment tailored to each individual case. Communication and cooperation with the primary care physician and a discussion of the risks with the patient cannot be overemphasized.

DRUG ALLERGIES AND ADVERSE REACTIONS

A history of food or drug allergies must be obtained during the preoperative interview and any family or patient history of adverse reactions to anesthesia fully explored. A history of food sensitivity may alert the physician to allergies related to preservatives, such as benzoate, and metabisulphite, which are also present in some local anesthetic solutions. Sensitivity to the local anesthetic agent itself is extremely unusual in the amino amide class of drugs, which includes bupivacaine, lidocaine, and mepivacaine, but not uncommon in the amino ester class, represented by procaine, tetracaine, and cocaine.[17] An allergic reaction to an anesthetic agent is a contraindication to the use of other anesthetics of the same class. However, an allergic reaction in this group generally does not preclude the use of drugs in the other class of anesthetics. Skin testing for sensitivity to preservatives or the agents themselves may be helpful.

An investigation of previous anesthesia experiences in the patient or their family may reveal postoperative nausea and vomiting, agitation, urinary retention, or oversedation, which can be managed with alterations in the anesthetic approach. A history of agitation, palpitation, or tachycardia related to local anesthesia may be related to the direct effects of epinephrine used in conjunction with the anesthetic rather than an allergic reaction. More ominous, however, is a history of unexplained perioperative fever or family history of a death under anesthesia of unclear cause. This should alert the clinician to the possibility of malignant hyperthermia. Malignant hyperthermia, a rare defect in muscle metabolism resulting in more heat generation than the body can dissipate, is inherited in an autosomal dominant pattern with variable penetrance.[18] Succinylcholine and halothane have historically been the most common inciting agents,[10] but other volatile anesthetics—nitrous oxide, ketamine, epinephrine, calcium, potassium, and calcium channel blockers—should also be avoided in this setting.[18] Use of an amino amide local agent has been shown to be safe in patients with this disorder, but this does not rule out the possibility of its development during surgery.

Although anticipation and prevention are the optimal management techniques in malignant hyperthermia, prompt recognition and treatment of an episode is critical to patient survival. Early signs may include sweating, increased temperature, dramatic oxygen consumption with increased end-tidal carbon dioxide, muscle rigidity, cardiac arrhythmias, and unstable blood pressure.[10] Treatment consists of the prompt delivery of dantrolene, 2 mg/kg intravenously, with dosage repeated up to a level of 10 mg/kg, or until symptoms disappear, along with hyperventilation with 100% oxygen and management of the respiratory and metabolic acidosis.[19] The patient may require ice packing with stomach and colon irrigation, mannitol, and furosemide to maintain urine output and manage any hyperkalemia and procainamide to control cardiac arrhythmias. The optimal treatment remains clinical suspicion with special attention to children and strabismus patients. If suspicion exists, a muscle biopsy for contracture testing may be helpful but is rarely available. Pretreatment with dantrolene is advisable in these patients, with 2 mg/kg intravenously at the time of induction.[10]

ANESTHETIC SELECTION, SPECIAL CONSIDERATIONS

The tailoring of the anesthetic approach to the individual patient and surgical procedure to be performed is the ultimate goal of the preoperative evaluation. Although a complete listing of various circumstances is beyond the scope of this chapter, certain conditions may be of particular interest to the corneal surgeon.

THE PEDIATRIC PATIENT

The infant or young child is best managed under general anesthesia with surgery performed early in the day. Issues to be considered in children include any history of ocular abnormalities with possible systemic associations, such as seen in Riley-Day, or Sturge-Weber syndrome,[20] as well as a history of asthma, sleep apnea, or myotonic dystrophy.[9] Intraoperative bradycardia secondary to succinylcholine, halothane, or the oculocardiac reflex is common in children and safely managed with atropine in this group.[21] Temperature monitoring, hydration, and medication dosage within narrow therapeutic ranges must be carefully observed, particularly in infants.[10] Alternative induction techniques now exist, including sedation delivered rectally and fentanyl lollipops,[9] to ease some of the trauma of the anesthesia experience.

ANATOMIC CONSIDERATIONS

Diseases or syndromes altering the anatomy of the orbit, skull, or neck will impact on the ability to deliver effective and safe anesthesia. Patients with Apert's disease or other craniostenoses may have significantly altered orbital anatomy, complicating the delivery of retrobulbar or peribulbar anesthesia. Other patients with potential orbital abnormalities include those with fibrous dysplasia, previous orbital or sinus surgery, including the repair of an orbital blow-out fracture, or other orbital disease.

Patients with advanced arthritis or spinal conditions preventing neck extension may be poor candidates for general anesthesia as a result of intubation difficulties. The vertebral abnormalities and micrognathia seen in Goldenhar's syndrome patients may complicate intubation attempts, although these can be effectively overcome.[22] A variety of other conditions may affect the anatomy of the orbit, skull, spine, and oral pharynx and must be considered in the preoperative assessment of the patient. In most cases, these can be overcome with careful planning, anticipation, and cooperation.

THE OPEN GLOBE AND FULL STOMACH

Penetrating ocular trauma presents perhaps the most challenging clinical situation in anesthetic management. Two important issues are often in conflict: the stomach is full and aspiration of gastric contents is a real danger, and the eye is open and in need of repair with threatened extrusion of intraocular contents. Surgery often cannot be delayed the 6 to 8 hours needed for gastric emptying, but many maneuvers used to prevent aspiration can significantly elevate the intraocular pressure with an increased risk of further trauma to the already injured globe. Retrobulbar anesthesia carries the risk of increasing the intraocular pressure by direct pressure on the globe or by causing a retrobulbar hemorrhage, although one report noted success in a limited number of patients using a low-volume technique.[23] Regardless, the anesthesiologist should be informed of the existence of an open globe, and the vast majority of these patients will undergo repair under general anesthesia.

Although almost all anesthetic agents used in general anesthesia, with the exception of ketamine, will cause a decrease in intraocular pressure,[24] succinylcholine has been well documented to cause a significant rise in intraocular pressure.[25-28] Presumably this arises from initial contracture of the extraocular muscles followed by paralysis,[25] although one report suggests intraocular changes as well, causing elevation even with the extraocular muscles detached.[29] The classic teaching has followed for ocular surgery: succinylcholine should not be used in the setting of an open globe. This teaching has been seriously challenged on several fronts. First, pretreatment with a nondepolarizing muscle relaxant, such as d-tubocurarine or pancuronium, followed by succinylcholine appears to cause no elevation in intraocular pressure and allow a smooth induction and intubation.[30-32] Second, a number of reports now suggest that the elevation in intraocular pressure is not clinically significant and does not cause extrusion of intraocular contents or change the eventual visual outcome compared with groups not receiving succinylcholine.[30, 33, 34] Premedication with certain drugs, including intravenous lidocaine,[35] does not invariably blunt the increase in intraocular pressure with succinylcholine, whereas propofol and thiopentone are helpful.[36, 37] Although there is no doubt that succinylcholine causes a significant rise in intraocular pressure, one can be equally confident that if succinylcholine is otherwise the drug of choice for induction of general anesthesia, it can be used with little or no risk to the globe.

In a setting of an open globe and full stomach, the patient is often pretreated with mannitol and d-tubocurarine or gallamine, given intravenously to prevent muscle contracture. After preoxygenating, the patient is given thiopental sodium followed by succinylcholine. Cricoid pressure is applied until the endotracheal tube is placed to reduce the risk of reflux.[10] Although this technique may cause 90 to 100 seconds of apnea,[38] it appears safe in hands experienced with preoxygenation.

GENERAL VERSUS REGIONAL ANESTHESIA

The decision to use general or regional anesthesia requires a knowledge of the procedure to be performed and the clinical situation of the patient and consideration of the advantages and disadvantages inherent in general and retrobulbar or peribulbar anesthesia. Although significant progress has been made in regional anesthesia, particularly in sedation for both the block and the procedure, general anesthesia is also safer with fewer systemic side effects than just a few years ago.

BENEFITS OF GENERAL ANESTHESIA

The management of a patient under local anesthesia requires the ability to communicate effectively with the patient. A number of circumstances will interfere with the ability to elicit cooperation or provide reassurance to the patient, including mental retardation, deafness, language barriers, senility, confusion, extreme anxiety, and claustrophobia. Those patients who cannot be effectively managed and reassured are best considered as candidates for general anesthesia.

Certain involuntary responses, including cough and tremor, are best controlled in the setting of general anesthesia, in which tight control of respiratory status and muscular paralysis are possible. This control not only allows smooth performance of the surgical procedure but also may help to prevent complications, such as an expulsive choroidal hemorrhage,[39] but only if the patient is kept deeply anesthetized and paralyzed. Management of the hemodynamic and respiratory status of the patient also allows the performance of longer procedures than can be easily accomplished under local anesthesia, with freer communication between surgeon and operating room personnel. These advantages are further realized in a teaching hospital setting for resident training. Finally, the risks of regional anesthesia are avoided in general anesthesia. Globe perforation, retrobulbar hemorrhage, inadvertent anesthetic injection with local or systemic complications, and sedation risks are effectively eliminated. In highly myopic eyes in which there is an increased risk of globe perforation with retrobulbar anesthesia, general anesthesia is further indicated. Spontaneous orbital hemorrhage can rarely be seen after general anesthesia.[40]

RISKS OF GENERAL ANESTHESIA

Although general anesthesia is usually safe and effective, it is also true that the physiologic changes induced are far more profound than those seen in local anesthesia. Most authors agree that a recent myocardial infarction is a contraindication to general anesthesia; however, a number of studies have failed to document a higher mortality in the general anesthesia group compared with those undergoing ophthalmic surgery under local anesthesia.[41–44] These findings are somewhat confounded by potential bias from a lack of randomization, with "sicker" patients presumably having surgery under local anesthesia. Malignant hyperthermia is more common in general anesthesia but fortunately is quite rare.

Inhalational anesthetic agents, including halothane and enflurane, have significant effects on ocular blood flow in both the choroidal and retinal vascular beds. Whereas choroidal circulation is decreased in most studies, the retinal blood flow is more variably affected.[45–47] Similar decreases occur after local anesthesia, and it is unclear whether these blood flow changes are detrimental or protective against vascular events, such as expulsive choroidal hemorrhages.[47] Abnormal eye movements, inability to open the eyes, and total external ophthalmoplegia have also been described occurring transiently in the early postoperative period after general anesthesia with propofol, fentanyl, and atracurium. The authors speculate on a possible pons or midbrain effect of one or more of the agents.[48, 49] Patients undergoing general anesthesia are more likely to suffer from nausea and vomiting,[50] agitation, urinary retention, muscle pain, sore throat, dizziness, and airway trauma,[10] although current management techniques have made these less common.[51] The use of fine suture material and smaller, more secure wounds have also decreased the risks associated with postoperative coughing, vomiting, or other Valsalva maneuvers. Whereas patients undergoing surgery under local anesthesia often have prolonged postoperative pain relief, ocular pain can be significant after general anesthesia, unless supplemented at the end of the procedure with retrobulbar anesthetic injection.[52] The use of general anesthesia is also more time consuming in the operating room suite and requires a longer postoperative recovery period in the ambulatory setting.

BENEFITS OF REGIONAL ANESTHESIA

The benefits of a retrobulbar, peribulbar, or parabulbar block relate in large part to the ability to deliver the local anesthetic agent directly to the site of action with a minimal perturbation of the respiratory, cardiovascular, or endocrine status of the patient. A well-placed injection provides the rapid onset of anesthesia, akinesia, and amaurosis, with minimal systemic side effects. The current availability of longer acting anesthetic agents allows excellent postoperative pain relief, and the nausea and malaise seen after general anesthesia are avoided. Advances in sedation, both for the actual block and surgery, permit procedures on all but the most anxious patients with less danger of respiratory suppression. The technique is easy to perform, allows efficient use of operating room facilities, and is relatively safe.

The oculocardiac reflex can be seen in the setting of local or general anesthesia, but it is more common in the latter owing to an alteration in vagal tone associated with anesthesia.[10]

This reflex, resulting from ocular manipulation, traction on the extraocular muscles, or pressure on the globe or empty orbit, is characterized by cardiac arrhythmias, including a range from bradycardia to asystole, as well as nausea and faintness. A similar picture can be seen after stretching of the muscles of the eyelid[53] or cold irrigation of the eye.[54] The reflex is mediated through the trigeminal nerve through the brain stem to the visceral motor nuclei of the vagus nerve; the vagus nerve serves as the efferent limb of the reflex to the heart.[53] This reflex is particularly common in children and seen not infrequently in strabismus surgery. Effective control of the reflex has been reported with the use of intravenous atropine[55–58] or retrobulbar anesthesia[59–61]; incomplete success has been reported in some cases with either technique. It is estimated that retrobulbar block is successful in blocking the reflex approximately 50% of the time[10] and may cause the reflex in some patients by stretching and applying pressure to the orbital contents. Other reports document the failure of a peribulbar block or the combination of a retrobulbar block and intravenous atropine to prevent bradycardia.[62, 63] The use of atropine is contraindicated in adults with a history of significant heart disease or myocardial infarctions, because it may cause a mild dysrhythmia[64] or a lethal tachyrhythmia,[65, 66] but it appears well tolerated in children and healthy adults. Current recommendations include the judicious preoperative use of anticholinergic protection with atropine or glycopyrrolate,[57] ECG monitoring of the general or local anesthetic setting, cessation of surgical manipulation if an arrhythmia occurs, and treatment of arrhythmias as needed with intravenous atropine, retrobulbar block, or both.

RISKS OF REGIONAL ANESTHESIA

Despite the relative safety of retrobulbar and peribulbar anesthesia, the procedure is not without risks. The insertion of a needle into the orbital area threatens not only the globe but vascular structures, the optic nerve, and, by direct extension, the central nervous system. Anesthetic agents injected are potentially toxic locally and may have systemic effects manifested as toxic or allergic reactions.

Retrobulbar hemorrhage is perhaps the most commonly seen serious complication of retrobulbar injection, occurring in 0.1 to 1.7% of cases.[67–69] In one series the incidence was related to the experience of the physician delivering the block,[69] and in most series the surgery was canceled and later performed under general anesthesia. In one report of small-incision cataract cases, the surgery was performed after a period of observation without adverse sequelae.[68] If a hemorrhage is sufficiently severe to cause proptosis and elevated intraocular pressure or signs of retinal vascular compromise, a lateral canthotomy should be performed to decompress the orbital contents. No reports exist of the incidence of severe orbital hemorrhage in peribulbar anesthesia, but they are presumably rare and less threatening because they occur outside the confined space of the muscle cone.

Perforation of the globe can be seen after retrobulbar or peribulbar anesthesia.[70–74] Although Atkinson described the use of a blunt needle to prevent perforation, this complication has been reported after the use of sharp or blunt needles,[75] and if penetration does occur, the blunt needle may carry a poorer prognosis.[70] Studies have not been able to document consistently an increased risk in retrobulbar versus peribulbar injection or blunt versus sharp needles. Visual outcome is more closely related to the degree of initial trauma to the retina or optic nerve,[71, 74, 76–79] although intraocular lidocaine may be relatively well tolerated.[80, 81] The presence of axial myopia, previous scleral buckling surgery, and the use of multiple injection techniques may carry an increased risk of inadvertent ocular perforation.[74, 78, 82] Current technology in the area of virtual reality allows residents to practice their retrobulbar or peribulbar technique[83] and may assist in the training of anesthesia residents.[84] Early recognition of pain, visual symptoms, a firm globe, or change in the red reflex prompt examination with an indirect ophthalmoscope,[85] and appropriate referral to a vitreoretinal surgeon is recommended.[86]

Atkinson's original description of his retrobulbar technique[5] suggested the positioning of the eye in supranasal gaze during the injection. This was unchallenged until Unsöld, working with cadavers, pointed out the rotation of the optic nerve into a vulnerable position with this maneuver and suggested instead that the patient remain in primary gaze or look slightly downward.[87] These findings were confirmed by Liu and colleagues[88] using magnetic resonance imaging, and this group suggested a down-and-in gaze during retrobulbar injection. Numerous reports in the literature have documented the danger of direct injection of local anesthetic solution into the optic nerve sheath during retrobulbar block, with resultant optic nerve damage,[89] contralateral amaurosis, cranial nerve palsies,[90–95] drowsiness, shivering,[96] convulsions,[97] and respiratory or cardiac arrest.[98–105] Local anesthetic agents have been recovered from the spinal fluid in some of these patients,[98] and several experimental studies have supported direct subarachnoid spread from the optic nerve sheath.[106, 107] Other authors have reported convulsions, respiratory distress, or cardiac arrest after presumed injection into the ophthalmic artery with retrograde flow to the internal carotid and anterograde vascular flow to the central nervous system.[108–111]

A number of occlusive vascular events have also been described after retrobulbar injection, including central retinal artery occlusion,[112–114] combined vein and artery occlusion,[115–117] Purtscher-like retinopathy,[118] and direct embolization of retinal or choroidal vessels with local anesthetic or sub-Tenon corticosteroids.[115, 119] Whereas some events had an identifiable retrobulbar hemorrhage,[113] optic nerve sheath injection,[112, 116, 117] or direct vascular injection,[115, 119] others had no discernible cause, raising the possibility of some increased susceptibility in patients with advanced vascular disease.[114, 120] The volume injected during retrobulbar or peribulbar blocks may also directly impair blood flow[121] or venous return, with potential risks for vascular occlusion or intraocular hemorrhagic complications.[39] Whereas trauma to the optic nerve and direct vascular injection are rare in retrobulbar injection, they have not been described after peribulbar block.

Local anesthetic agents injected directly into a blood vessel or diffusing quickly into the systemic circulation from peripheral tissue can exhibit significant toxicity on both the cardiovascular and the central nervous systems. Local anesthetic agents tend to stabilize cell membranes in the myocardium with resultant bradycardia, decreased cardiac output, hypotension, and possible asystole. Disinhibition occurs in the pathways in the central nervous system with tingling, tinnitus, drowsiness, and disorientation, possibly progressing to myoclonic seizures, respiratory depression, and loss of consciousness.[10] Adequate monitoring, intravenous access, and availability of support personnel will permit prompt recognition and treatment of any adverse sequelae.

The muscles within the orbit are also susceptible to trauma from local anesthesia. Postoperative strabismus and ptosis have been reported,[122–129] with some documented cases of direct trauma to the involved muscle.[123] The incidence of postoperative ptosis has been variously ascribed to trauma, from the superior rectus bridle suture,[125] or the possible myotoxic effects of the local anesthetic agents themselves.[127, 130] Experiments in the rat and cynomolgus monkey suggest that the myotoxicity is most likely less important than direct trauma to the muscle, especially if combined with intramuscular injection of anesthetic.[131, 132] Postoperative ptosis seems to occur with equal frequency after peribulbar or retrobulbar techniques.[126]

GENERAL ANESTHESIA

A report of the technique of general anesthesia and specific agents used, beyond those already discussed, is beyond the scope of this chapter. The remainder of this chapter deals with the techniques involved in regional anesthesia for corneal surgery.

REGIONAL ANESTHESIA: ANATOMY OF THE EYE AND ORBIT

The safe and effective delivery of local anesthetic for ocular surgery requires some knowledge of orbital anatomy and the innervation of the globe and periocular structures. The bony orbit, shaped like a pear with the stem at the orbital apex, is approximately 40 to 50 mm deep with a volume of 30 mL. The medial walls of the two orbits are parallel, whereas the lateral walls are oriented approximately 45 degrees medially. The frontal sinus and anterior cranial fossa lie above the orbit, the maxillary sinus is below, and a thin medial wall separates the orbit from the ethmoid sinus and nasal cavity. The walls of the orbit are covered by the periorbita, the outer periosteal layer of the dura mater, and the anterior boundary of the orbit is formed by the orbital septum.

The eye is approximately 24 mm in diameter and has a volume of 6.5 mL. The optic nerve, with a diameter of 1.6 mm and intraorbital length of 25 mm, enters the orbit through the optic foramen and inserts on the globe slightly medially. The rectus muscles, four of the six extraocular muscles responsible for movement of the eye, arise from the annulus of Zinn, a tendon ring encircling the optic foramen (Fig. 2–1), and insert on the globe 5.5 to 7.5 mm posterior to the corneoscleral limbus. These muscles, together with a connecting intermuscular septum, create a "cone" between the orbital apex and the globe. Within the cone pass not only the optic nerve, ophthalmic artery and veins, and ciliary ganglion but also the oculomotor and abducens nerves and the ophthalmic branch of the trigeminal (see Fig. 2–1). All these structures are potentially vulnerable during retrobulbar injection.

The remaining extraocular muscles include (1) the superior oblique muscle, which originates superomedial to the optic foramen (see Fig. 2–1), runs along the medial wall to the trochlea and reverses, inserting on the globe below the superior rectus, and (2) the inferior oblique muscle, which originates from the lacrimal bone medially, passes below the inferior rectus and inserts posterolaterally on the globe. The levator palpebrae superioris muscle originates at the orbital apex and runs above the superior rectus muscle before inserting on the skin and tarsus of the upper lid.

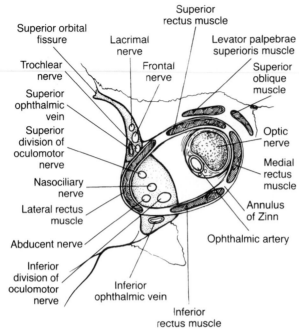

Figure 2–1. Posterior orbit and the annulus of Zinn. (From Albert DM, Jakobiec FA, eds. Principles and practice of ophthalmology, vol 3. Philadelphia: WB Saunders, 1994. Used with permission.)

NERVE SUPPLY OF EYE AND ORBIT

The oculomotor nerve provides innervation to the superior, medial, and inferior rectus, inferior oblique, and levator muscles, and the abducens nerve innervates the lateral rectus. The motor supply to the superior oblique is provided by the trochlear nerve, the only nerve controlling extraocular movement from outside the muscle cone and, thus, most frequently missed with low-volume retrobulbar injections. The upper zygomatic branch of the facial nerve supplies the frontalis and orbicularis oculi muscles of the upper lid, whereas the lower zygomatic branch supplies the lower lid orbicularis. The anatomy of the facial nerve is discussed in more detail during description of the facial nerve blocks.

The trigeminal nerve is a mixed nerve made up of a small motor and large sensory component and provides sensation to the eye and orbital contents. At the trigeminal ganglion, it separates into three divisions: mandibular, maxillary, and ophthalmic. The maxillary division provides sensation to the lower lid and medial and lateral canthal regions, the lateral wall of the orbit, and the temple region. All other innervation is provided by the ophthalmic division, which travels within the muscle cone and divides into a series of branches, including the frontal, nasociliary, and lacrimal. The conjunctiva is served by subbranches of all three, whereas the cornea derives most of its sensory input from the long and short ciliary branches of the nasociliary nerve (Fig. 2–2). The long ciliary nerves pass through the sclera near the optic nerve, whereas the short ciliary nerves penetrate a few millimeters posterior to the corneoscleral

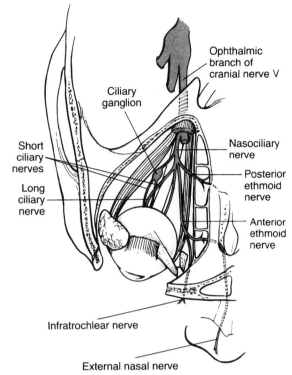

Figure 2-2. The ophthalmic division of cranial nerve V, which is the origin of the nasociliary nerve. (From Albert DM, Jakobiec FA, eds. Principles and practice of ophthalmology, vol 3. Philadelphia: WB Saunders, 1994. Used with permission.)

limbus. These form a plexus beneath Bowman's layer of the cornea and finally penetrate Bowman's layer to terminate in the corneal epithelium. Regeneration of corneal nerves is seen after damage at the limbus, but reinnervation may be limited after penetrating keratoplasty, with reduced central corneal sensation.[133]

Sympathetic innervation of the eye and orbit arises in the superior cervical ganglion through the long and short ciliary nerves, which then control the uveal vasculature, vasoconstriction, and motor stimulation to the iris dilator muscle (see Fig. 2-2). Parasympathetic innervation derives from fibers traveling with the oculomotor nerve to the ciliary ganglion through the short ciliary nerves to the ciliary body with motor impulses to the ciliary muscle and sphincter muscle of the iris.

SEDATION

Most techniques of ocular regional anesthesia involve some degree of patient discomfort, which adds to the anxiety of the patient in the perioperative period. A number of approaches varying in technique and medications allow patient comfort and sometimes amnesia of the peribulbar or retrobulbar block, a stable operative course, and prompt recovery and ambulation. Oral premedication with a benzodiazepine, such as diazepam or triazolam, provides excellent anxiolytic and sedative effects for a block, but triazolam may be overly sedating in the elderly.[134] Other oral agents, such as clonidine, have similar positive effects and also appear to lower the intraocular pressure when given preoperatively.[135] Intravenous sedation is also popular, and the most common agents, including propofol, midazolam, and methohexital, feature a relatively rapid onset of action, good sedation and amnesia for the block, depression of intraocular pressure, and rapid postoperative recovery.[136–138] Intravenous alfentanil or fentanyl, in combination with droperidol, also demonstrates similar benefits.[139] Droperidol may also have an antiemetic effect after local or general anesthesia.[51] Propofol, owing to a shorter half-life, is slightly better tolerated, allows more rapid postoperative recovery than other intravenous agents,[137, 138] and causes less respiratory depression than intravenous diazepam.[140] Some authors question whether continuous intravenous sedation during the surgery is more beneficial than simple oral premedication with a sedative agent,[141] whereas others suggest the use of a cold spray to numb the skin before regional block.[142] The value of simple patient reassurance and "hand-holding anesthesia" has also been emphasized.[143] We have had the opportunity to use most of these agents, and although we use bolus midazolam solely for the block most commonly, the ability of continuous intravenous propofol to keep an otherwise difficult patient smoothly sedated throughout surgery without respiratory depression and with a rapid postoperative recovery has been remarkable.

ANESTHETIC AGENTS: TOPICAL

A number of agents are available for eliminating the corneal and conjunctival reflex, but the most commonly used are proparacaine, tetracaine, and cocaine. Each agent has a relatively rapid onset of action of 30 to 60 seconds, with a duration of 10 to 20 minutes. The use of topical anesthesia allows one to take ocular measurements and apply lenses for examination of the eye as well as remove foreign bodies and perform minor surgical procedures on the surface of the eye. The chief limitation in the use of these medications is corneal epithelial toxicity, most marked with cocaine, and all three may cause delays in epithelial wound healing[144]; therefore, chronic use of these medications for symptomatic relief must be avoided. Cocaine is also useful in dacryocystorhinostomy surgery because it is the only local anesthetic providing pain relief, vasoconstriction, and shrinkage of mucous membranes.[145] On the ocular surface, it may be used as an adjunct to certain procedures by causing epithelial sloughing and constriction of scleral vessels.

Although allergic reactions are not rare with the topical agents, they are generally not severe. Systemic complications, seen only with the use of topical cocaine, can be serious and can occur with as little as 20 mg. Systemic absorption can occur rapidly with topical cocaine after drainage through the nasolacrimal duct onto the nasal mucosa. The blockage of catecholamine uptake and the sympathetic potentiating effects of cocaine may cause hypertensive crises in patients taking reserpine, guanethidine, methyldopa, or monoamine oxidase inhibitors.[145] The topical or intranasal use of this drug in ophthalmic surgery must be accompanied by careful attention to total dosage.

Bupivacaine has also been described for use as a topical anesthetic and appears to have slightly less epithelial toxicity and a similar duration of action to proparacaine.[146]

LOCAL ANESTHETIC AGENTS

The available agents for use in regional blocks in ophthalmology are listed in Table 2–1.[10, 147, 148] Cocaine and procaine are related to the molecule para-aminobenzoic acid and possess an ester linkage, are hydrolyzed by pseudocholinesterase in the plasma, and are referred to as the amino ester group of local anesthetics. The amino amide group, listed in Table 2–1, is structurally distinct, is degraded by the liver, and generally has a longer duration of action. The most popular agents for use in ophthalmic blocks are lidocaine and bupivacaine, usually in combination, to allow rapid onset and long duration of action.[149, 150] Some authors have questioned the use of this combination, believing that the dilution of both agents may decrease their effectiveness,[151] whereas others advocate the use of a small amount of 10% lidocaine in a bupivacaine solution to avoid dilution and provide the rapid onset that bupivacaine may lack.[152, 153] Etidocaine possesses the long-acting advantages of bupivacaine and appears to have a time of onset close to lidocaine.[154] Prilocaine and mepivacaine do not differ significantly from lidocaine in their performance.[155]

Certain agents have also been added to the anesthetic "cocktail" in an attempt to modify the duration of action or time of onset for various solutions. Epinephrine generally increases the duration of action of agents involved[156] presumably by causing local vasoconstriction with decreased systemic absorption and clearance. Epinephrine may cause systemic side effects, however, and at least one study suggests it may compromise ocular blood flow[121] when used in a block. Epinephrine does not appear to prolong the duration of action of bupivacaine or etidocaine in any clinically meaningful way and is most likely best avoided. Adjusting the pH of the anesthetic solution from approximately 5.0 to 6.5 with bicarbonate appears to speed the time to onset and decrease the pain on injection and may improve the success rate.[157–160]

Hyaluronidase is also frequently added to regional block solutions at

Table 2–1. Regional Anesthetic Agents[10, 147–148]

Agent		Concentration (%)	Chemical Class	Maximum Dose (mg)	Onset (Minutes)	Duration
Procaine	(Novocaine)	1–4	Ester	500	6–8	30–40 min
Lidocaine	(Xylocaine, Dalcaine)	1–2	Amide	500	4–6	30–60 min
Prilocaine	(Citanest)	1–2	Amide	600	3–5	60–90 min
Mepivacaine	(Carbocaine, Polarocaine)	1–2	Amide	500	3–5	1–2 hr
Etidocaine	(Duranest)	0.5–1	Amide	300	3–5	4–6 hr
Bupivacaine	(Marcaine, Sensorcaine)	0.25–0.75	Amide	175	3–5	4–12 hr

a concentration of 7.5 to 15 turbidity-reducing units per milliliter.[151] This enzyme dissolves the hyaluronic acid cement between cells and appears to provide rapid diffusion and a correspondingly faster time for onset of anesthetic effect and more complete block.[156, 159, 161, 162] This benefit is particularly essential in combination with bupivacaine or etidocaine and is additive to the effect of pH adjustment. Theoretically, this rapid diffusion may also result in a rapid systemic absorption with signs of anesthetic toxicity, as discussed previously, and careful monitoring of the patient during and after the regional block is valuable.

FACIAL NERVE AND EYELID BLOCKS

Paralysis of the orbicularis muscle is essential to the safe performance of intraocular surgery. Failure to block the eyelids makes surgery more technically difficult and increases the intraocular pressure with possible extrusion of the ocular contents. Local akinesia can be achieved by direct infiltration of the eyelids with anesthetic, as often occurs with peribulbar injection or more proximal blockade of the facial nerve and its appropriate branches. A number of these techniques have been described over the past 80 years.

In 1914, van Lint[4] described the blockade of the facial nerve with procaine at a point just temporal to the lateral canthal angle (Fig. 2–3). The needle is advanced below the orbital margin and 2 to 5 mL of anesthetic is deposited on withdrawal. A similar procedure is performed at the same site above the superior orbital rim. Digital pressure is applied to the area to promote the block, but lid edema and hemorrhage are common.[149] For this reason, the technique has been modified by moving the injection site back 1 to 2 cm from the lateral canthus.

The frequent development of lid edema after a van Lint lid block led O'Brien to describe a technique in 1927 for blocking the facial nerves at the mandibular condyle (Fig. 2–4).[163] The original description suggested depositing the anesthetic agent at this point, but anatomic variation in the course of the nerve frequently yielded incomplete akinesia. Later modifications included a second injection along the posterior border of the mandibular ramus (see Fig. 2–4), and Spaeth[164] later moved the injection more proximal, injecting anesthetic to block the nerve before it crosses the mandible (Fig. 2–5). Although the Spaeth modification in particular is quite effective, the O'Brien and Spaeth blocks can be quite

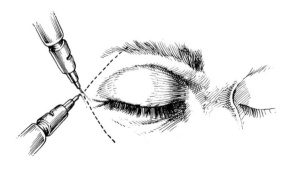

Figure 2–3. The van Lint block anesthetizes the facial nerve branches to the orbicularis muscle as they pass over the periosteum just lateral to the orbit. (From Spaeth GL, ed. Ophthalmic surgery: principles and practices. Philadelphia: WB Saunders, 1990. Used with permission.)

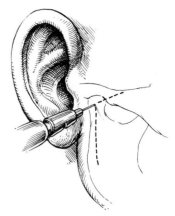

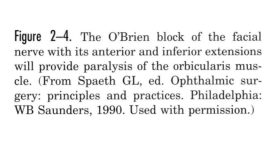

Figure 2–4. The O'Brien block of the facial nerve with its anterior and inferior extensions will provide paralysis of the orbicularis muscle. (From Spaeth GL, ed. Ophthalmic surgery: principles and practices. Philadelphia: WB Saunders, 1990. Used with permission.)

painful, and some patients are disturbed by the complete facial paralysis on the affected side. Rare cases of Bell's palsy lasting months have been described.[149, 165]

In 1953 Atkinson proposed blocking the facial nerve as it passed over the zygomatic arch (Fig. 2–6). The needle was inserted just below the lower margin of the zygomatic arch and directed toward the top of the ear, passing over the zygomatic arch. Anesthetic was again injected while withdrawing the needle.[166] Although excellent akinesia is generally obtained, this block can also be quite painful.

Although a great deal of anatomic variation is seen in the course of the facial nerve, there is consistency in the path from the nerve's emergence from the stylomastoid foramen to the parotid gland. Nadbath

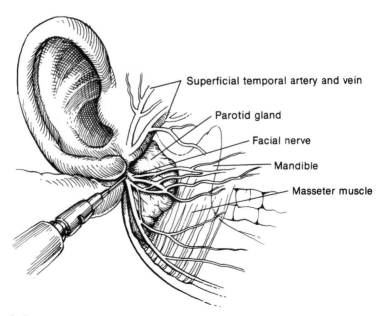

Superficial temporal artery and vein

Parotid gland

Facial nerve

Mandible

Masseter muscle

Figure 2–5. In the Spaeth modification of the O'Brien technique, the facial nerve is blocked where it crosses the posterior edge of the mandible, thus catching the nerve before it divides. (From Spaeth GL, ed. Ophthalmic surgery: principles and practices. Philadelphia: WB Saunders, 1990. Used with permission.)

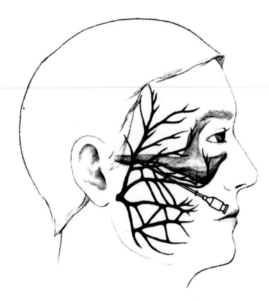

Figure 2–6. An alternative method of providing paralysis of the orbicularis muscle proposed by Atkinson intercepts the facial nerve fibers as they cross the zygomatic arch. (From Spaeth GL, ed. Ophthalmic surgery: principles and practices. Philadelphia: WB Saunders, 1990. Used with permission.)

and Rehman[167] advocated the use of a short (12-mm) needle inserted perpendicular to the skin and advanced to the hub, just below the external auditory meatus between the mandible and mastoid process (Fig. 2–7). Although this block yields excellent facial akinesia, it is painful and has caused respiratory obstruction in a number of cases[168–171] as a result of extension of the anesthetic to involve cranial nerves IX and X. Koenig and associates[172] advocated the use of short needles, small volumes of anesthetic, and avoidance of hyaluronidase to avert this complication and suggested patient positioning to manage the temporary unilateral airway obstruction.[173]

RETROBULBAR VERSUS PERIBULBAR

Once the patient's ophthalmologist and anesthesiologist have agreed that a given case may be safely performed under regional anesthesia, a number of technical options remain. Retrobulbar, peribulbar, parabulbar, or topical anesthesia may be optimal, depending on the patient and the procedure. Recommendations for specific corneal procedures are discussed later in this chapter. The use of a needle to introduce anesthetic solutions into the orbital space carries certain risks and benefits as previously described, and these are shared by retrobulbar and peribulbar techniques, although at somewhat different rates. The retrobulbar technique with direct injection of the anesthetic into the muscle cone generally requires a smaller volume and has rapid onset of anesthesia, excellent akinesia of the extraocular muscles, and amaurosis. This technique often requires a separate orbicularis block, however, and may carry a higher risk of perforation of the globe, serious retrobulbar hemorrhage, optic nerve injury, and inadvertent subarachnoid injection than peribulbar anesthesia. Needles longer than 3.125 cm (1¼ inch) may increase the risk of subarachnoid injection in both techniques.[174]

Although peribulbar injections theoretically avoid the many vital

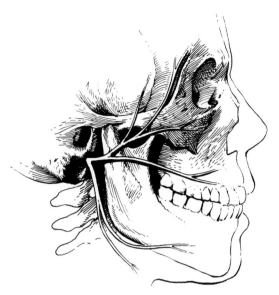

Figure 2–7. The Nadbath block catches the trunk of the facial nerve after its emergence from the stylomastoid foramen before it passes into the parotid gland. (From Spaeth GL, ed. Ophthalmic surgery: principles and practices. Philadelphia: WB Saunders, 1990. Used with permission.)

structures within the muscle cone, globe perforation may still occur, and incomplete akinesia of the extraocular muscles is common.[175, 176] A larger volume is generally injected, and patients often see during the operation. Excellent anesthesia and orbicularis blockade are the rule[177, 178] with this technique, and because it is less painful, sedation can often be avoided. A number of authors[67, 179–181] have reported large series of patients undergoing peribulbar versus retrobulbar anesthesia with no significant difference in effectiveness or complications with either technique when performed by experienced hands. Modifications in the original technique, as described by Davis and Mandel,[6] include transconjunctival injection,[182, 183] pH adjustment,[184] or warming of the solution to improve patient comfort.[185] A single injection technique to reduce the risks inherent in multiple injections into the peribulbar space has also been advocated.[186–188]

The injection of a small volume of anesthetic into the relatively small muscle cone, or a large volume into the peribulbar space, may have a significant effect on the intraocular pressure owing to direct pressure on the globe and possible compromise of venous outflow. The use of an external compression device, such as a "super pinkie,"[189] Honan balloon,[190, 191] mercury bag, or simple digital massage,[192] is critical to relieve the pressure on the globe. Ocular compression after the block may in itself compromise ocular blood flow,[193] and in cases of suspected ocular ischemia, external ocular compression before rather than after the block[189] or simple digital massage alone may be advisable. In all cases, ocular compression devices should be used no longer than 10 to 15 minutes to achieve orbital decompression[190] and augmentation of the regional block while minimizing potential side effects.

The risks inherent in the blind placement of a needle into the orbital or retrobulbar space have led to the development of a number of novel approaches to anesthesia for eye surgery. Straus[194, 195] described a curved needle that mimics the profile of the globe for delivery of retrobulbar anesthetic. Subconjunctival injections, particularly at the superior limbus, have been advocated for cataract surgery[196–199] with good anesthesia but poor ocular akinesia and the need for a supplemental orbicularis block. Sub-Tenon's injection, in which a dull[200–202] or flexible[16] cannula is inserted through a buttonhole in Tenon's capsule into the retrobulbar space, has been successfully used for retinal and cataract surgery and may not require a separate facial nerve block. Topical anesthesia delivered with drops,[203] a dissolving delivery medium,[204] or an ophthalmic rod[205] has been advocated as a safe delivery route but requires good patient cooperation and willingness to accept some sensation during the surgery. This technique also lacks control of the orbicularis or extraocular movements. Topical anesthetics also have significant corneal epithelial toxicity,[206] although new agents may be better tolerated. Although topical anesthesia is sufficient for removal of superficial corneal lesions and perhaps self-sealing intraocular procedures, the techniques of sub-Tenon's injections described by Greenbaum[16] and others appear to hold the most promise for good anesthesia and akinesia, with reduction of the risks of traditional peribulbar and retrobulbar injection.

TECHNIQUE: RETROBULBAR ANESTHESIA

Retrobulbar anesthesia can involve significant discomfort to the patient, and the use of sedation, as previously described, is recommended. ECG and pulse oximetry monitoring are also valuable to detect any complications of the block or sedation. The area to be injected is cleaned with a solution of iodine or alcohol, and the lower orbital rim is palpated. An anesthetic solution is prepared, most typically 0.75% bupivacaine, with 2 to 4% lidocaine and hyaluronidase. A skin wheal is raised at a point where the lateral one third of the infraorbital rim meets the medial two

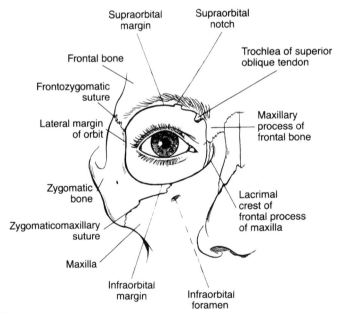

Figure 2–8. External landmarks of the bony orbit. (From Albert DM, Jakobiec FA, eds. Principles and practice of ophthalmology, vol 3. Philadelphia: WB Saunders, 1994. Used with permission.)

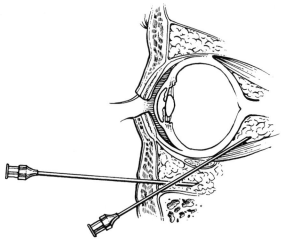

Figure 2–9. Retrobulbar block: the anesthetic agent is placed within the muscle cone. (From Spaeth GL, ed. Ophthalmic surgery: principles and practices. Philadelphia: WB Saunders, 1990. Used with permission.)

thirds (Fig. 2–8). The patient is instructed to maintain the eye in primary gaze, and a 23- to 25-gauge needle is inserted perpendicular to the skin and advanced between the eye and orbital floor to the equator of the globe. The needle is then redirected upward toward the orbital apex and advanced (Fig. 2–9). Mild resistance is sometimes felt as the needle penetrates the intramuscular septum. Gentle aspiration on the syringe helps rule out an intravascular or intraocular location, and 2 to 4 mL of solution is deposited. The needle is removed, and gentle ocular compression applied with digital massage or an external compression device. Supplemental retrobulbar or orbicularis blocks may be given as required, although the use of hyaluronidase in the solution seems to decrease the need for separate orbicularis blockade.[207]

TECHNIQUE: PERIBULBAR ANESTHESIA

After preparation of the anesthetic solution, monitoring and sedation of the patient, and sterile preparation of the injection site, a skin wheal is raised with a 25-gauge or finer needle at the supraorbital notch superiorly (see Fig. 2–8) and at the intersection of the lateral one third and medial two thirds of the inferior orbital rim (Fig. 2–10). The 3.125-cm (1¼ inch), 23- to 25-gauge dull needle is inserted perpendicular to the

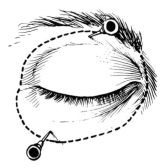

Figure 2–10. Posterior peribulbar block: anteroposterior view of needle position. (From Spaeth GL, ed. Ophthalmic surgery: principles and practices. Philadelphia: WB Saunders, 1990. Used with permission.)

skin, through the inferior site, and advanced along the orbital floor to the hub of the needle or until any resistance is felt if within 1.25 cm of the hub (Fig. 2–11). After gentle aspiration, 3 to 5 mL of solution is deposited and the needle is withdrawn. A similar approach is taken superiorly with another 3- to 5-mL deposit. Ocular compression is again applied. Supplemental peribulbar or retrobulbar blocks may be given for residual globe movement or subconjunctival–sub-Tenon's–topical supplements for anesthesia as needed. This block may take longer to be complete than a retrobulbar block, and adequate orbital decompression is essential. Administration of the injection is best performed in a monitored preoperative holding area before proceeding to the surgical suite.

SELECTION OF ANESTHESIA FOR SPECIFIC CORNEAL PROCEDURES

Anesthesia for corneal surgery can be divided into four distinct categories: topical, subconjunctival, peribulbar-retrobulbar, and general anesthesia. The first three categories may also be supplemented with systemic sedation when needed. Although surgical procedures may be performed with a variety of different anesthetic techniques, a general guide to anesthesia for corneal surgery follows.

TOPICAL ANESTHESIA

Topical anesthesia is generally reserved for extraocular, corneal, and conjunctival procedures. The topical agents available are proparacaine, tetracaine, and cocaine, although lidocaine and bupivacaine (Marcaine) may be used. Cocaine causes the most epithelial disruption and is generally the most difficult to obtain. In addition, cocaine is a potent vasoconstrictor. Topical cocaine is advantageous for corneal procedures in which epithelial debridement is important, such as epikeratophakia. However,

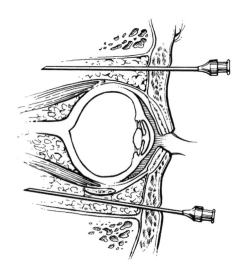

Figure 2–11. Posterior peribulbar block: lateral view of needle position. (From Spaeth GL, ed. Ophthalmic surgery: principles and practices. Philadelphia: WB Saunders, 1990. Used with permission.)

cocaine is generally not indicated for routine use. Proparacaine and tetracaine are more than adequate for removing corneal and conjunctival foreign bodies. In addition, with compliant patients, they can be used to suture small full-thickness corneal lacerations without the need for general anesthesia or the risk of retrobulbar injection causing pressure and extruding the intraocular contents. Topical anesthesia is usually more than adequate for incisional corneal surgeries, such as radial keratotomy, astigmatic keratotomies, and relaxing incisions. Ablative surgery, such as excimer laser phototherapeutic keratectomy and photo-refractive keratectomy, are generally performed with tetracaine or pro-paracaine as well. Extraocular corneal suturing may be performed with topical anesthetic in a compliant patient but is often reserved for peri-bulbar-retrobulbar or general anesthesia. These suturing procedures include partial-thickness corneal lacerations, replacing a suture in a penetrating keratoplasty, corneal wedge resections, and compression sutures for astigmatic procedures. Topical anesthesia is routinely used for corneal scrapings and anterior stromal puncture for recurrent ero-sions. Finally, topical anesthesia can be used to diagnose corneal infec-tions. Proparacaine is considered the least bacteriostatic of the topical anesthetics and is the anesthetic of choice for scraping corneal ulcers for culture or performing a corneal biopsy.

SUBCONJUNCTIVAL ANESTHESIA

Local subconjunctival injections of anesthetic agents are often used for conjunctival excisional surgery or episcleral suturing, in which topical anesthesia would not be sufficient. These procedures include pterygium excisions with or without suturing of the pterygium bed. Localized subconjunctival anesthesia is particularly useful when cautery or me-chanical scraping of the sclera is performed. Excision of conjunctival tumors is aided with the use of a subconjunctival injection of anesthetic to elevate the lesion. Excisional biopsies of small lesions and conjunctival biopsies for ocular cicatricial pemphigoid can often be performed with either topical or local anesthesia.

CORNEAL PROCEDURES: REGIONAL VERSUS GENERAL ANESTHESIA

The decision to use peribulbar-retrobulbar anesthesia, or general anes-thesia, is based on the need for anesthesia and akinesia. Conjunctival or corneal surgery that requires control of ocular motility is best per-formed with either of these two techniques. Procedures best performed with peribulbar-retrobulbar or general anesthesia include lysis of exten-sive symblepharon with conjunctival transplantation and conjunctival flaps, where large donor areas must be mobilized and excised with episcleral suturing. Bilateral corneal procedures such as free conjunc-tival grafts or keratoepithelioplasty from one eye to the other are best performed under general anesthesia, avoiding the risk and patient incon-venience of bilateral regional blocks.

Any time intraocular surgery with an open-sky or non-self-sealing full-thickness incision is contemplated, peribulbar-retrobulbar or general anesthesia is mandatory. Corneal indications for this type of anesthesia are predominantly penetrating keratoplasty, although general anesthesia as discussed previously is the anesthesia of choice for most corneal lacerations.

PENETRATING KERATOPLASTY

Adequate anesthesia and akinesia for penetrating keratoplasty in addition to patient comfort are often vital to the success of the procedure. Inadequate anesthesia can result in serious ocular morbidity. During a penetrating keratoplasty, from the point the recipient bed is trephined until the cardinal donor corneal sutures are placed, the eye is in a vulnerable position in which orbicularis pressure can extrude the intraocular contents.

Whereas a minor lid twitch might be insignificant in a small-incision cataract extraction, the same lid function can result in extrusion of the crystalline lens, vitreous loss, or even an expulsive choroidal hemorrhage during penetrating keratoplasty. Therefore, when peribulbar-retrobulbar anesthesia is used for penetrating keratoplasty anesthesia, akinesia of the globe and lids should be carefully examined before entering the anterior chamber. Supplementary anesthesia can always be given before this time. When general anesthesia is used, the anesthesiologist should be aware that, in addition to anesthesia, the patient should be paralyzed during penetrating keratoplasty while the eye is opened. A patient "bucking" on the intubation tube constitutes a Valsalva maneuver and increases the episcleral venous pressure, resulting in vitreous loss and a suprachoroidal hemorrhage. Once the corneal sutures are in place, the surgeon should inform the anesthesiologist that paralysis is no longer required. When general anesthesia is used for penetrating keratoplasty, increased vitreous pressure may push the lens-iris diaphragm forward. In addition to osmotic agents to shrink the vitreous volume, the surgeon can ask the anesthesiologist to hyperventilate the patient. By lowering the patient's carbon dioxide levels, the vitreous volume is osmotically reduced, and the vitreous pressure problem can be reversed.

During a penetrating keratoplasty, the patient's episcleral venous pressure should be lowered to reduce the risk of expulsive choroidal hemorrhage. This can be easily accomplished by positioning the patient on the operating table in a Fowler's position (reverse Trendelenburg). In this position, the patient's head is above the chest, and venous stasis will not result in increased episcleral venous pressure. When a peribulbar-retrobulbar injection of an anesthetic agent is used, at least 15 minutes should be allowed between the injection and trephination of the recipient bed. This time period allows the local anesthesia to diffuse into the adjacent tissues. Entering the eye without this delay may cause increased orbital volume and a significant increase in episcleral venous pressure, resulting in an increased risk of a suprachoroidal hemorrhage.[39]

Advances in local and general anesthesia have made corneal surgery safer and more comfortable for the patient and surgeon alike. Many corneal procedures can now be done in an office or outpatient setting with minimal risk or discomfort. Although the technology of corneal surgery has rapidly advanced, anesthesia for corneal surgery remains a science as well as an art. The ophthalmologist and patient, in conjunction with the anesthesiologist when needed, can individualize the anesthetic requirements of a procedure to the specific needs of the patient.

REFERENCES

1. Atkinson WS. The development of ophthalmic anesthesia. Am J Ophthalmol 1961;51:1.
2. Koller C. Über verwendung des kokains zur Anästhesierung am Auge. Wien Med Wochenschr 1884;43:461.
3. Knapp H. Cocaine and its use in ophthalmic and general surgery. Arch Ophthalmol 1884;13:402.
4. Van Lint A. Paralysie palpebrale temporaire provoquee dans l'operation de la cataracte. Ann Ocul (Paris) 1914;151:420.
5. Atkinson WS. Retrobulbar injection of anesthetic within the muscle cone. Arch Ophthalmol 1936;16:494.
6. Davis DB, Mandel MR. Posterior peribulbar anesthesia: an alternative to retrobulbar anesthesia. J Cataract Refract Surg 1986;12:182.
7. Rosen E. Anaesthesia for ophthalmic surgery. Br J Ophthalmol 1993;77:542.
8. Fisher SJ, Cunningham RD. The medical profile of cataract patients. Geriatr Clin North Am 1985;1:339.
9. Pasternak LR. Anesthetic considerations in otolaryngological and ophthalmological out-patient surgery. Intern Anesthesiol Clin 1990;28:89.
10. Wilson RP. Complications associated with local and general ophthalmic anesthesia. Int Ophthalmol Clin 1992;32:1.
11. Stone LS, Kline OR, Sklar C. Intraocular lenses and anticoagulation and antiplatelet therapy. Am Intraocular Implant Soc J 1985;11:165.
12. Gainey SP, Robertson DM, Fay W, et al. Ocular surgery on patients receiving long-term warfarin therapy. Am J Ophthalmol 1989;108:142.
13. Hall DL, Steen WH, Drummond JW, et al. Anticoagulants and cataract surgery. Ophthalmic Surg 1988;19:221.
14. Robinson GA, Nylander A. Warfarin and cataract extraction. Br J Ophthalmol 1989;73:702.
15. McMahan LB. Anticoagulants and cataract surgery. J Cataract Refract Surg 1988;14:569.
16. Greenbaum S. Parabulbar anesthesia. Am J Ophthalmol 1992;114:776.
17. Covino BG. Clinical pharmacology of local anesthetic agents. In: Cousins MJ, Bridenbaugh PO, eds. Neural blockade in clinical anesthesia and management of pain. Philadelphia: JB Lippincott, 1988, p 129.
18. Cousins MJ, Bromage PR. Epidural neural blockade. In: Cousins MJ, Bridenbaugh PO, eds. Neural blockade in clinical anesthesia and management of pain. Philadelphia: JB Lippincott, 1988, p 296.
19. Gromert GA. Malignant hyperthermia. Semin Anesth 1983;2:197.
20. McGoldrick KE. Considerations for pediatric eye surgery. Int Anesthesiol Clin 1990;28:78.
21. Steward DJ. Anticholinergic premedication for infants and children. Can Anaesth Soc J 1983;30:325.
22. Madan R, Trikha A, Venkataraman RK, et al. Goldenhar's syndrome: an analysis of anaesthetic management. Anaesthesia 1990;45:49.
23. Simonson D. Retrobulbar block for open-eye injuries: a report of 19 cases. Clin Reg Nurs Anesth 1992;3:35.
24. Murphy DF. Anesthesia and intraocular pressure. Anesth Analg 1985;64:520.
25. Lincoff HA, Breinin GM, DeVoe AG. The effect of succinylcholine on the extraocular muscles. Am J Ophthalmol 1957;43:440.
26. Varghese C, Chopra SK, Daniel R, et al. Intraocular pressure profile during general anesthesia. Ophthalmic Surg 1990;21:856.
27. Kovac AL, Bennets PS, Ohara S, et al. Effect of esmolol on hemodynamics and intraocular pressure response to succinylcholine and intubation following low dose alfentanil pre-medication. J Clin Anesth 1992;4:315.
28. Joshi C, Bruce DL. Thiopental and succinylcholine: action on intraocular pressure. Anesth Analg 1975;54:471.
29. Kelly RE, Dinner M, Turner LS, et al. Succinylcholine increases intraocular pressure in the human eye with the extraocular muscles detached. Anesthesiology 1993;79:948.
30. Wang ML, Seiff SR, Drasner K. A comparison of visual outcome in open-globe repair:

succinylcholine with d-tubocurarine versus nondepolarizing agents. Ophthalmic Surg 1992;23:746.

31. Abdulla WY. The synergistic effect of two different nondepolarizing muscle relaxants on intraocular pressure. J Clin Anesth 1993;5:5.

32. Konchigeri HN, Lee YE, Venugopal K. Effect of pancuronium on intraocular pressure changes induced by succinylcholine. Can Anesth Soc J 1979;26:479.

33. Moreno RJ, Kloess P, Carlson DW. Effect of succinylcholine on the intraocular contents of open globes. Ophthalmology 1991;98:636.

34. Libonati MM, Leahy JJ, Ellison N. The use of succinylcholine in open eye surgery. Anesthesiology 1985;62:637.

35. Smith RB, Babinski M, Leano N. The effect of lidocaine on succinylcholine-induced rise in intraocular pressure. Can Anesth J 1979;26:482.

36. Mirakhur RK, Shepherd WFI, Darrah WC. Propofol or thiopentone: effects on intraocular pressure associated with induction of anaesthesia and tracheal intubation (facilitated with suxamethonium). Br J Anaesth 1987;59:431.

37. Abdulla WY, Flaifil HA. Intraocular pressure changes in response to endotracheal intubation facilitated by atracurium or succinylcholine with or without lidocaine. Acta Anaesthesiol Belg 1992;43:91.

38. Calobrisi BL, Lebowitz P. Muscle relaxants and the open globe. Int Anesth Clin 1990;28:83.

39. Ingraham HJ, Donnenfeld ED, Perry HD. Massive suprachoroidal hemorrhage in penetrating keratoplasty. Am J Ophthalmol 1989;108:670.

40. Anderson KK, Larson NH, Saga-Rumley SA, et al. Spontaneous orbital hemorrhage during general anesthesia and arthroplasty. J Clin Anesth 1994;6:145.

41. Quigley HA. Mortality associated with ophthalmic surgery: a 20-year experience at the Wilmer Institute. Am J Ophthalmol 1974;77:517.

42. Duncalf D, Gartner S, Carol B. Mortality in association with ophthalmic surgery. Am J Ophthalmol 1970;69:610.

43. Petruscak J, Smith RB, Breslin P. Mortality related to ophthalmological surgery. Arch Ophthalmol 1973;89:106.

44. Heinze J, Rohrbach M. Cataract surgery: general anesthesia versus retrobulbar block. A randomized trial of high risk patients. Anaesthetist 1992;41:481.

45. Roth S. The effects of halothane on retinal and choroidal blood flow in cats. Anesthesiology 1992;76:455.

46. Roth S, Pietrzyk Z, Crittenden AP. The effects of enflurane on ocular blood flow. J Ocular Pharmacol 1993;9:251.

47. Hessemer V. Anesthesia effects on ocular circulation: synopsis of a study. Fortschritte der Ophthalmologie 1991;88:577.

48. Marsch SCU, Schaefer HG. Problems with eye opening after propofol anesthesia. Anesth Analg 1990;70:127.

49. Marsch SCU, Schaefer HG. External ophthalmoplegia after total intravenous anaesthesia. Anaesthesia 1994;49:525.

50. Lynch S, Wolf GL, Berlin I. General anesthesia for cataract surgery: a comparative review of 2,217 consecutive cases. Anesth Analg 1974;53:909.

51. Iwamoto K, Schwartz H. Antiemetic effect of droperidol after ophthalmic surgery. Arch Ophthalmol 1978;96:1378.

52. Duker JS, Nielsen J, Vander JF, et al. Retrobulbar bupivacaine irrigation for postoperative pain after scleral buckling surgery. Ophthalmology 1991;98:514.

53. Anderson RL. The blepharocardiac reflex. Arch Ophthalmol 1978;96:1418.

54. Arndt GA, Stock MC. Bradycardia during cold ocular irrigation under general anaesthesia: an example of the diving reflex. Can J Anaesth 1993;40:511.

55. Moonie GT, Rees DL, Elton D. The oculocardiac reflex during strabismus surgery. Can Anaesth Soc J 1964;11:621.

56. Alexander JP. Reflex disturbances of cardiac rhythm during ophthalmic surgery. Br J Ophthalmol 1975;59:518.

57. Meyers EF, Tomeldan FA. Glycopyrrolate compared with atropine in prevention of the oculocardiac reflex during eye muscle surgery. Anesthesiology 1979;51:350.

58. Bosomworth PP, Ziegler C, Jacoby J. The oculo-cardiac reflex in eye muscle surgery. Anesthesiology 1958;19:7.

59. Taylor C, Wilson FM, Roesch R, et al. Prevention of the oculocardiac reflex in children: comparison of retrobulbar block and intravenous atropine. Anesthesiology 1963;24:646.

60. Kirsch RE, Samet P, Kugel V, et al. The electrocardiographic changes during ocular surgery and their prevention by retrobulbar injection. Arch Ophthalmol 1957;58:348.

61. Berler DK. Oculocardiac reflex. Am J Ophthalmol 1963;56:954.

62. Batterbury M, Wong D, Williams R, et al. Peribulbar anaesthesia: failure to abolish the oculocardiac reflex. Eye 1992;6:293.

63. Smith RB, Douglas H, Petruscak J. The oculocardiac reflex and sino-atrial arrest. Can Anaesth Soc J 1972;19:138.

64. McGoldrick KE. Transient left bundle branch block during local anesthesia. Anesthesiol Rev 1981;8:36.
65. Massumi RA, Mason DT, Amsterdam EA, et al. Ventricular fibrillation and tachycardia after intravenous atropine for treatment of bradycardias. N Engl J Med 1972;287:336.
66. Horgan J. Atropine and ventricular tachyarrhythmia. JAMA 1973;223:693.
67. Hamilton RC, Gimbel HV, Strunin L. Regional anesthesia for 12,000 cataract extraction and intraocular lens implantation procedures. Can J Anaesth 1988;35:615.
68. Cionni RJ, Osher RH. Retrobulbar hemorrhage. Ophthalmology 1991;98:1153.
69. Ruben S. The incidence of complications associated with retrobulbar injection of anaesthetic for ophthalmic surgery. Acta Ophthalmol 1992;70:836.
70. Grizzard WS, Kirk NM, Pavan PR, et al. Perforating ocular injuries caused by anesthesia personnel. Ophthalmology 1991;98:1011.
71. Hay A, Flynn HW, Hoffman JI, et al. Needle penetration of the globe during retrobulbar and peribulbar injections. Ophthalmology 1991;98:1017.
72. Zaturansky B, Hyams S. Perforation of the globe during the injection of local anesthesia. Ophthalmic Surg 1987;18:585.
73. Kimble JA, Morris RE, Witherspoon CD, et al. Globe perforation from peribulbar injection. Arch Ophthalmol 1987;105:749.
74. Duker JS, Belmont JB, Jenson WE, et al. Inadvertent globe perforation during retrobulbar and peribulbar anesthesia. Ophthalmology 1991;98:519.
75. Waller SG, Taboada J, O'Connor P. Retrobulbar anesthesia risk: do sharp needles really perforate the eye more easily than blunt needles? Ophthalmology 1993;100:506.
76. Vestal KP, Meyers SM, Zegarra H. Retinal detachment as a complication of retrobulbar anesthesia. Can J Ophthalmol 1991;26:32.
77. Seelenfreund MH, Freilich DB. Retinal injuries associated with cataract surgery. Am J Ophthalmol 1980;89:654.
78. Schneider ME, Milstein DE, Oyakawa RT, et al. Ocular perforation from a retrobulbar injection. Am J Ophthalmol 1988;106:35.
79. Rinkoff JS, Doft BH, Lobes LA. Management of ocular penetration from injection of local anesthesia preceding cataract surgery. Arch Ophthalmol 1991;109:1421.
80. Schechter RJ. Management of inadvertent intraocular injections. Ann Ophthalmol 1985;17:771.
81. Lincoff H, Zweifach P, Brodie S, et al. Intraocular injection of lidocaine. Ophthalmol 1985;92:1587.
82. Ramsay RC, Knobloch WH. Ocular perforation following retrobulbar anesthesia for retinal detachment surgery. Am J Ophthalmol 1978;86:61.
83. Merril JR, Notaroberto NF, Laby DM, et al. The ophthalmic retrobulbar injection simulator: an application of virtual reality to medical education. Proc Comput Appl 1993;4:702.
84. Miller-Meeks MJ, Bergstrom T, Karp KO. Prevalent attitudes regarding residency training in ocular anesthesia. Ophthalmology 1994;101:1353.
85. Feibel RM. Ocular penetration by anesthetic injection. Ophthalmology 1992;99:301.
86. Boniuk V, Nockowitz R. Perforation of the globe during retrobulbar injection: medico-legal aspects of four cases. Surv Ophthalmol 1994;39:141.
87. Unsöld R, Stanley JA, DeGroot J. The CT-topography of retrobulbar anesthesia: anatomic/clinical correlation of complications and suggestions of a modified technique. Arch Klin Ophthalmol 1981;217:125.
88. Liu C, Youl B, Moseley I. Magnetic resonance imaging of the optic nerve in extremes of gaze: implications for the positioning of the globe for retrobulbar anaesthesia. Br J Ophthalmol 1992;76:728.
89. Pautler SE, Grizzard WS, Thompson LN, et al. Blindness from retrobulbar injection into the optic nerve. Ophthalmic Surg 1986;17:334.
90. Rodgers R, Orellana J. Cranial nerve palsy following retrobulbar anaesthesia. Br J Ophthalmol 1988;72:78.
91. Javitt JC, Addiego R, Friedberg HL, et al. Brain stem anesthesia after retrobulbar block. Ophthalmology 1987;94:718.
92. Ahn JC, Stanley JA. Subarachnoid injection as a complication of retrobulbar anesthesia. Am J Ophthalmol 1987;103:225.
93. Antoszyk AN, Buckley EG. Contralateral decreased visual acuity and extraocular muscle palsies following retrobulbar anesthesia. Ophthalmology 1986;93:462.
94. Friedberg HL, Kline OR. Contralateral amaurosis after retrobulbar injection. Am J Ophthalmol 1986;101:688.
95. Follette JW, LoCascio JA. Bilateral amaurosis following unilateral retrobulbar block. Anesthesiology 1985;63:237.
96. Nicoll JMV, Acharya PA, Edge KR, et al. Shivering following retrobulbar block. Can J Anaesth 1988;35:671.

97. Meyers EF, Ramirez RC, Boniuk I. Grand mal seizures after retrobulbar block. Arch Ophthalmol 1978;96:847.
98. Kobet KA. Cerebral spinal fluid recovery of lidocaine and bupivacaine following respiratory arrest subsequent to retrobulbar block. Ophthalmic Surg 1987;18:11.
99. Ruusuvaara P, Setala K, Tarkkanen A. Respiratory arrest after retrobulbar block. Acta Ophthalmol 1988;66:223.
100. McGalliard JN. Respiratory arrest after two retrobulbar injections. Am J Ophthalmol 1988;105:90.
101. Smith JL. Retrobulbar bupivacaine can cause respiratory arrest. Ann Ophthalmol 1982;14:1005.
102. Nicoll JMV, Acharya PA, Ahlen K, et al. Central nervous system complications after 6,000 retrobulbar blocks. Anesth Analg 1987;66:1298.
103. Brookshire GL, Gleitsmann KY, Schenk EC. Life-threatening complications of retrobulbar block: a hypothesis. Ophthalmology 1986;93:1476.
104. Meyers EF. Brain-stem anesthesia after retrobulbar block. Arch Ophthalmol 1985;103:1278.
105. Hamilton RC. Brain stem anesthesia following retrobulbar blockade. Anesthesiology 1985;63:688.
106. Drysdale DB. Experimental subdural retrobulbar injection of anesthetic. Ann Ophthalmol 1984;16:716.
107. Shantha TR. The relationship of retrobulbar local anesthetic spread to the neural membranes of the eyeball, optic nerve, and arachnoid villi in the optic nerve. Anesthesiology 1990;73:A850.
108. Rosenblatt RM, May DR, Barsoumian K. Cardiopulmonary arrest after retrobulbar block. Am J Ophthalmol 1980;90:425.
109. Rodman DJ, Notaro S, Peer GL. Respiratory depression following retrobulbar bupivacaine: three cases and literature review. Ophthalmic Surg 1987;18:768.
110. Fletcher SJ, O'Sullivan G. Grand mal seizure after retrobulbar block. Anaesthesia 1990;45:696.
111. Aldrete JA, Romo-Salas F, Arora S, et al. Reverse arterial blood flow as a pathway for central nervous system toxic responses following injection of local anesthetics. Anesth Analg 1978;57:428.
112. Brod RD. Transient central retinal artery occlusion and contralateral amaurosis after retrobulbar anesthetic injection. Ophthalmic Surg 1989;20:643.
113. Kraushar MF, Seelenfreund MH, Freilich DB. Central retinal artery closure during orbital hemorrhage from retrobulbar injection. Trans Am Acad Ophthalmol Otolaryngol 1974;78:65.
114. Klein ML, Jampol LM, Condon PI, et al. Central retinal artery occlusion without retrobulbar hemorrhage after retrobulbar anesthesia. Am J Ophthalmol 1982;93:573.
115. Morgan CM, Schatz H, Vine AK, et al. Ocular complications associated with retrobulbar injections. Ophthalmology 1988;95:660.
116. Sullivan KL, Brown GC, Forman AR, et al. Retrobulbar anesthesia and retinal vascular obstruction. Ophthalmology 1983;90:373.
117. Mieler WF, Bennett SR, Platt LW, et al. Localized retinal detachment with combined central retinal artery and vein occlusion after retrobulbar anesthesia. Retina 1990;10:278.
118. Lemagne J, Michiels X, Van Causenbroeck S, et al. Purtscher-like retinopathy after retrobulbar anesthesia. Ophthalmology 1990;97:859.
119. McLean EB. Inadvertent injection of corticosteroid into the choroidal vasculature. Am J Ophthalmol 1975;80:835.
120. Cowley M, Campochiaro PA, Newman SA, et al. Retinal vascular occlusion without retrobulbar or optic nerve sheath hemorrhage after retrobulbar injection of lidocaine. Ophthalmic Surg 1988;19:859.
121. Horven I. Ophthalmic artery pressure during retrobulbar anaesthesia. Acta Ophthalmol 1978;56:574.
122. Schipper I, Luthi M. Diplopia after retrobulbar anesthesia and cataract surgery: a case report. Klin Monatsbl Augenheilkd 1994;204:176.
123. Hamed LM. Strabismus presenting after cataract surgery. Ophthalmology 1991;98:247.
124. Hamilton SM, Elsas FJ, Dawson TL. A cluster of patients with inferior rectus restriction following local anesthesia for cataract surgery. J Pediatr Ophthalmol Strabismus 1993;30:288.
125. Kaplan LJ, Jaffe NS, Clayman HM. Ptosis in cataract surgery: a multivariant computer analysis of a prospective study. Ophthalmology 1985;92:237.
126. Feibel RM, Custer PL, Gordon MO. Postcataract ptosis: a randomized double-masked comparison of peribulbar and retrobulbar anesthesia. Ophthalmology 1993;100:660.
127. Rainin EA, Carlson BM. Postoperative diplopia and ptosis: a clinical hypothesis based on the myotoxicity of local anesthetics. Arch Ophthalmol 1985;103:1337.

128. Erie JC. Acquired Brown's syndrome after peribulbar anesthesia. Am J Ophthalmol 1990;109:349.
129. Esswein MB, Von Noorden GK. Paresis of a vertical rectus muscle after cataract extraction. Am J Ophthalmol 1993;116:424.
130. Rao VA, Kawatra VK. Ocular myotoxic effects of local anesthetics. Can J Ophthalmol 1988;23:171.
131. Foster AH, Carlson BM. Myotoxicity of local anesthetics and regeneration of the damaged muscle fibers. Anesth Analg 1980;58:727.
132. Carlson BM, Emerick S, Komorowski TE, et al. Extraocular muscle regeneration in primates: local anesthetic-induced lesions. Ophthalmology 1992;99:582.
133. Rao GN. Recovery of corneal sensation in grafts following penetrating keratoplasty. Ophthalmology 1985;92:1408.
134. Kontinen VK, Maunuksela E, Sarvela J. Premedication with sublingual triazolam compared with oral diazepam. Can J Anaesth 1993;40:829.
135. Filos KS, Patroni O, Goudas LC, et al. A dose-response study of orally administered clonidine as pre-medication in the elderly: evaluating hemodynamic safety. Anesth Analg 1993;77:1185.
136. Senn P, Johr M, Kaufmann S, et al. Brief narcosis with propofol/ketamine for administering retrobulbar anesthesia. Klin Monatsbl Augenheilkd 1993;202:528.
137. Ferrari LR, Donlon JV. A comparison of propofol, midazolam, and methohexital for sedation during retrobulbar and peribulbar block. J Clin Anesth 1992;4:93.
138. Pratila MG, Fischer ME, Alagesan R, et al. Propofol versus midazolam for monitored sedation: a comparison of intraoperative and recovery parameters. J Clin Anesth 1993;5:268.
139. Coley S, Jones GW, Lassey D, et al. A comparison of the effects of alfentanil/droperidol or fentanyl/droperidol on intraocular pressure. Anaesthesiology 1990; 45:477.
140. Holas A, Faulborn J. Propofol versus diazepam for sedation of patients undergoing ophthalmic surgery under local anaesthesia. Anaesthetist 1993;42:766.
141. Salmon JF, Mets B, James MFM, et al. Intravenous sedation for ocular surgery under local anaesthesia. Br J Ophthalmol 1992;76:598.
142. Shibata K, Inage K, Takayama T, et al. Use of cold spray for relieving pain from local anesthetic injections in ocular surgery. J Ophthalmic Nurs Tech 1993;12:23.
143. Havener WH. Hand-holding anesthesia. Ophthalmic Surg 1990;21:375.
144. Man WG, Wood R, Senterfit L, et al. Effect of topical anesthetics on regeneration of the corneal epithelium. Am J Ophthalmol 1957;43:606.
145. Meyers EF. Cocaine toxicity during dacryocystorhinostomy. Arch Ophthalmol 1980;98:842.
146. Liu JC, Steinemann TL, McDonald MB, et al. Topical bupivacaine and proparacaine: a comparison of toxicity, onset of action, and duration of action. Cornea 1993;12:228.
147. Feitl ME, Krupin T. Neural blockade for ophthalmologic surgery. In: Cousins MJ, Bridenbaugh PO, (eds). Neural blockade in clinical anesthesia and management of pain. Philadelphia: JB Lippincott, 1988, p 577.
148. Seifert HA, Nejman AM, Barron M. Regional anesthesia of the eye and orbit. Dermatol Clin 1992;10:701.
149. Wong DH. Regional anaesthesia for intraocular surgery. Can J Anaesth 1993;40:635.
150. House PH, Hollands RH, Schulzer M. Choice of anesthetic agents for peribulbar anesthesia. J Cataract Refract Surg 1991;17:80.
151. Feibel RM. Current concepts in retrobulbar anesthesia. Surv Ophthalmol 1985;30:102.
152. Laaka V, Nikki P, Tarkkanen A. Comparison of bupivacaine with and without adrenalin and mepivacaine with adrenalin in intraocular surgery. Acta Ophthalmol 1972;50:229.
153. Graham SL, Lawrence J. Peribulbar blockade—an alternative anaesthetic "cocktail." Aust N Z J Ophthalmol 1992;20:273.
154. Smith PH, Smith ER. A comparison of etidocaine and lidocaine for retrobulbar anesthesia. Ophthalmic Surg 1983;14:569.
155. Schimek F, Steuhl KP, Fahle M. Retrobulbar blockade of somatic, motor and visual nerves by local anesthetics. Ophthalmic Surg 1993;24:171.
156. Sarvela J, Nikki P, Paloheimo M. Orbicular muscle akinesia in regional ophthalmic anesthesia with pH-adjusted bupivacaine: effects of hyaluronidase and epinephrine. Can J Anaesth 1993;40:1028.
157. Lewis P, Hamilton RC, Liken R, et al. Comparison of plain with pH-adjusted bupivacaine with hyaluronidase for peribulbar block. Can J Anaesth 1992;39:555.
158. Zahl K, Jordan A, McGroarty J, et al. pH-adjusted bupivacaine and hyaluronidase for peribulbar block. Anesthesiology 1990;72:230.
159. Zahl K, Jordan A, McGroarty J, et al. Peribulbar anesthesia: effect of bicarbonate on mixtures of lidocaine, bupivacaine, and hyaluronidase with or without epinephrine. Ophthalmology 1991;98:239.

160. Eccarius SG, Gordon ME, Parelman JJ. Bicarbonate-buffered lidocaine-epinephrine-hyaluronidase for eyelid anesthesia. Ophthalmology 1990;97:1499.
161. Abelson MB, Mandel E, Paradis A, et al. The effect of hyaluronidase on akinesia during cataract surgery. Ophthalmic Surg 1989;20:325.
162. Nicoll JMV, Treuren B, Acharya PA, et al. Retrobulbar anesthesia: the role of hyaluronidase. Anesth Analg 1986;65:1324.
163. O'Brien CS. Akinesia during cataract extraction. Arch Ophthalmol 1929;1:447.
164. Spaeth GL. A new method to achieve complete akinesia of the facial muscles of the eyelids. Ophthalmic Surg 1976;7:105.
165. Spaeth GL. Total facial nerve palsy following modified O'Brien facial nerve block. Ophthalmic Surg 1987;18:518.
166. Atkinson WS. Akinesia of the orbicularis. Am J Ophthalmol 1953;36:1255.
167. Nadbath RP, Rehman I. Facial nerve block. Am J Ophthalmol 1963;55:143.
168. Wilson CA, Ruiz RS. Respiratory obstruction following the Nadbath facial nerve block. Arch Ophthalmol 1985;103:1454.
169. Rabinowitz L, Livingston M, Schneider H, et al. Respiratory obstruction following the Nadbath facial nerve block. Arch Ophthalmol 1986;104:1115.
170. Shoch D. Complications of the Nadbath facial nerve block. Arch Ophthalmol 1986;104:114.
171. Cofer HF. Cord paralysis after Nadbath facial nerve block. Arch Ophthalmol 1986;104:337.
172. Koenig SB, Snyder RW, Kay J. Respiratory distress after a Nadbath block. Ophthalmology 1988;95:1285.
173. Lawson NW. The lateral decubitus position: anesthesiologic considerations. In: Martin JT, ed. Positioning in anesthesia and surgery, 2nd ed. Philadelphia: WB Saunders, 1987, p 171.
174. Katsev DA, Drews RC, Rose BT. An anatomic study of retrobulbar needle path length. Ophthalmology 1989;96:1221.
175. Ali-Melkkila TM, Virkkila M, Jyrkkio H. Regional anesthesia for cataract surgery: comparison of retrobulbar and peribulbar techniques. Reg Anesth 1992;17:219.
176. Murdoch IE. Peribulbar versus retrobulbar anaesthesia. Eye 1990;4:445.
177. Agrawal K, Saxena RC, Nath R, et al. Local anesthesia by peribulbar block for cataract extraction in an eye relief camp: a double-masked randomized control trial. Online J Curr Clin Trials 1993; doc no 40.
178. Davis DB, Mandel MR. Efficacy and complication rates of 16,224 consecutive peribulbar blocks: a prospective multi-center study. J Cataract Refract Surg 1994;20:327.
179. Shriver PA, Sinha S, Galusha JH. Prospective study of the effectiveness of retrobulbar and peribulbar anesthesia for anterior segment surgery. J Cataract Refract Surg 1992;18:162.
180. Weiss JL, Deichman CB. A comparison of retrobulbar and periocular anesthesia for cataract surgery. Arch Ophthalmol 1989;107:96.
181. Saunders DC, Sturgess DA, Pemberton CJ, et al. Peribulbar and retrobulbar anesthesia with prilocaine: a comparison of two methods of local ocular anesthesia. Ophthalmic Surg 1993;24:842.
182. Sweeney EJ, Barber K, Prosser JA. A comparison of percutaneous and perconjunctival routes of administration of periocular anaesthesia for day case cataract surgery. Anaesthesia 1993;48:336.
183. Ismail F, Brighouse D, Wainwright AC. Peribulbar anaesthesia and aspirin. Anaesthesia 1993;48:1109.
184. Pollock AN, Mercer JD, McKenzie AJ. Peribulbar anaesthesia for intraocular surgery. Anaesth Intensive Care 1992;20:543.
185. Bloom LH, Scheie HG, Yanoff M. The warming of local anesthetic agents to decrease discomfort. Ophthalmic Surg 1984;15:603.
186. Arnold PN. Prospective study of a single-injection peribulbar technique. J Cataract Refract Surg 1992;18:157.
187. Saini JS, Roysarkar TK, Grewal SP, et al. Efficacy and timed sequence analyses of modified single injection peribulbar anesthesia. J Cataract Refract Surg 1993;19:646.
188. Teichmann KD. Single-injection peribulbar local anaesthesia. Aust N Z J Ophthalmol 1992;20:144.
189. Zabel RW, Clarke WN, Shirley SY, et al. Intraocular pressure reduction prior to retrobulbar injection of anesthetic. Ophthalmic Surg 1988;19:868.
190. Quist LH, Stapleton SS, McPherson SD. Preoperative use of the Honan intraocular pressure reducer. Am J Ophthalmol 1983;95:536.
191. Jay WM, Carter H, Williams B, et al. Effect of applying the Honan intraocular pressure reducer before cataract surgery. Am J Ophthalmol 1985;100:523.
192. Palay DA, Stulting RD. The effect of external ocular compression on intraocular pressure following retrobulbar anesthesia. Ophthalmic Surg 1990;21:503.
193. Morin Y, Renard-Charalabidis C, Haut J. Definitive transient monocular blindness

caused by ocular compression during general anesthesia. J Fr Ophtalmol 1993;16:680.

194. Straus JG. A new retrobulbar needle and injection technique. Ophthalmic Surg 1988;19:134.

195. Straus JG. Retrobulbar anesthesia and safety. Ophthalmic Surg 1990;21:149.

196. Smith R. Cataract extraction without retrobulbar anaesthetic injection. Br J Ophthalmol 1990;74:205.

197. Petersen WC, Yanoff M. Subconjunctival anesthesia: an alternative to retrobulbar and peribulbar techniques. Ophthalmic Surg 1991;22:199.

198. Redmond RM, Dallas NL. Extracapsular cataract extraction under local anaesthesia without retrobulbar injection. Br J Ophthalmol 1990;74:203.

199. Furuta M, Toriumi T, Kashiwagi K, et al. Limbal anesthesia for cataract surgery. Ophthalmic Surg 1990;21:22.

200. Buys YM, Trope GE. Prospective study of subtenons versus retrobulbar anesthesia for inpatient and day-surgery trabeculectomy. Ophthalmology 1993;100:1585.

201. Friedberg MA, Spellman FA, Pilkerton AR, et al. An alternative technique of local anesthesia for vitreoretinal surgery. Arch Ophthalmol 1991;109:1615.

202. Hansen EA, Mein CE, Mazzoli R. Ocular anesthesia for cataract surgery: a direct subtenon's approach. Ophthalmic Surg 1990;21:696.

203. Kershner RM. Topical anesthesia for small incision self-sealing cataract surgery: a prospective evaluation of the first 100 patients. J Cataract Refract Surg 1993;19:290.

204. Lawrenson JG, Edgar DF, Gudgeon AC, et al. A comparison of the efficacy and duration of action of topically applied proxymetacaine using a novel ophthalmic delivery system versus eye drops in healthy young volunteers. Br J Ophthalmol 1993;77:713.

205. Alani SD. The ophthalmic rod: a new ophthalmic drug delivery system. G Arch Ophthalmol 1990;4:297.

206. Marr WG, Wood R, Senterfit L, et al. Effect of topical anesthetics on regeneration of the corneal epithelium. Am J Ophthalmol 1957;43:606.

207. Gills JP, Loyd TL. A technique of retrobulbar block with paralysis of orbicularis oculi. Am Intraocular Implant Soc J 1983;9:339.

CHAPTER 3

ANESTHESIA FOR REFRACTIVE SURGERY

CRAIG H. KLIGER, MD
ROBERT K. MALONEY, MD, MA (Oxon)

Recent surgical advances have made permanent correction of refractive errors of the eye more practical and, therefore, more common.

Because these procedures have primarily been regarded as elective, patients must usually bear the full cost on their own. This, combined with advances such as the development of clear corneal cataract surgery and the fact that refractive surgery is usually performed on otherwise normal eyes, has served to raise patient expectations regarding anesthesia for such procedures and made those physicians who emphasize convenience and comfort somewhat more appealing to patients.

Yet those involved in modern refractive surgery must carefully balance factors patients may regard as "inconveniences" with potential risk. Although certain individuals will test the resolve and composure of even the most patient surgeon or anesthesiologist, maintaining patient safety as the primary concern is of the utmost importance. Toward this end, a thorough knowledge of the impact of each surgical step on the involved tissues and careful patient assessment regarding threshold of pain and cooperation by both the surgeon and anesthesiologist are especially important in this population of patients, who, experience has shown, appear from a psychological standpoint to have higher expectations regarding comfort and less tolerance of complications.

SURGICAL TREATMENT OF REFRACTIVE ERRORS: AN OVERVIEW

Because this text is intended for a wide range of professionals, a brief discussion of basic ophthalmic optics and an overview of the various refractive surgical procedures currently being performed are appropriate.

BASIC OPHTHALMIC OPTICS

Three factors are primarily responsible for the ability of the eye to focus an image on the retina: the refractive power of the corneal surface (related to its degree of curvature), the refractive power of the crystalline lens, and the axial length of the eye, which determines the physical location of the retina with respect to the refractive elements.

When the sum of these factors does not focus an image sharply on the retina, a relative refractive error exists. Myopia (nearsightedness) occurs when the image formed by the refractive components of the eye falls in front of the retina and is, therefore, perceived as blurred. Hyperopia (farsightedness) is the analogous condition when the image forms behind the retina. Astigmatism exists when the refractive elements are asymmetric and allow the image to come into focus over a range of distances in front of, behind, or straddling the retina, resulting in a characteristic distortion.

Some degree of hyperopia can be tolerated because the crystalline lens is capable of becoming more spherical through accommodation (i.e., increasing its refractive power through contraction of intrinsic eye musculature) and bringing an image located behind the retina to the retinal surface. No similar change can correct myopia because bringing an image located in front of the retina into focus requires decreasing the refractive power of the lens, a task for which no intrinsic eye musculature exists. Net astigmatism is unaffected by accommodation because the resulting uniform change in lens shape cannot correct the asymmetry of the refractive elements (or rarely the retina) and, therefore, cannot collapse into a single plane, the range over which the image is formed.

With age, changes to the responsible musculature or the lens itself limit this accommodative ability, resulting in presbyopia (loss of near vision associated with aging).

REFRACTIVE SURGERY TECHNIQUES

Of the three factors that determine whether an image comes into sharp focus on the retina, only the refractive power of the corneal surface and the refractive power of the lens lend themselves to modification from a practical standpoint, and this forms the basis for refractive surgery.

Corneal Surgery. Various surgical methods of flattening or steepening the cornea, thereby reducing or increasing its refractive power, respectively, have been described.[1–3]

Radial keratotomy (RK) is a means of surgically correcting mild to moderate myopia. In this procedure, a series of evenly spaced, almost full-depth, radial incisions are placed in the cornea, permitting peripheral protrusion and resultant flattening of the central cornea to achieve the requisite loss of dioptric power[4] (Fig. 3–1A). Astigmatic keratotomy (AK) uses arc-shaped or straight incisions perpendicular to the steepest optical meridian to achieve net "rounding" of the central cornea, flattening it in the steepest meridian and steepening it in the flattest meridian[4] (Fig. 3–1B).

Photorefractive keratectomy (PRK) flattens the central cornea by controlled ablation of the superficial layers of a disk-shaped area of stroma with an excimer laser after removal of the epithelium (Fig. 3–1C).[5–13] Elliptical treatment areas have been used to improve astigmatism,[14, 15] and treatments for hyperopia have been proposed.[16]

Lamellar corneal surgery has benefited from major improvements in instrumentation, increasing the popularity of various forms of keratomileusis for the correction of myopia. In myopic keratomileusis in situ, a lamellar lenticule of approximately 15% depth is created with a microkeratome. A second pass of the same device excises additional tissue of a smaller diameter (the refractive cut), and when the initial lenticule is draped over the reshaped surface, the lenticule assumes the required flattened shape[17] (Fig. 3–1D). Alternatively, the refractive "cut" can be performed by tissue ablation with the excimer laser of either the lenticule or the corneal bed.[5, 18–22]

In hyperopic lamellar keratoplasty, the lamellar lenticule created is approximately 70% of the corneal thickness. The remaining 30% or so of the corneal tissue is structurally weaker than the original full-thickness tissue, and the presence of a positive intraocular pressure permits an ectasia in the form of an anterior protrusion. The lenticule is then draped over this ectatic base and acquires its shape, making the anterior surface steeper with a higher dioptric power (Fig. 3–1E). Varying the diameter of the lenticule permits control of the amount of refractive change.

Treatment for hyperopia has the potential to treat presbyopia by intentionally creating a limited amount of myopia, permitting the eye to see clearly (only) at near. This is usually performed in one eye with the other eye corrected for distance ("monovision").

Radial thermokeratoplasty has been proposed as a means of treating hyperopia.[23–26] A circular pattern of photocoagulation "spots" is performed with a hot needle or a holmium laser centered on the visual axis of the cornea at a fixed diameter. Because photocoagulation causes contraction of corneal collagen, this shortens the diametric arc passing through a given spot, similar to that caused by placement of a tight suture in a given axis in cataract surgery. Evenly spaced contractures in a circular pattern yield uniform central steepening (Fig. 3–1F). Spots placed along a specific axis may prove useful in treating astigmatism.

Intracorneal rings add volume to corneal tissue where they are inserted. The circular pattern of this thickening (essentially a "tissue addition") combined with subsequent epithelial hyperplasia within the depression inside the ring creates a gradual flattening of the central cornea that corrects myopia[27] (Fig. 3–1G).

Lenticular Surgery. The other optical element of the eye that can be surgically manipulated to address refractive errors is the crystalline lens.

Clear lens extraction has been described as a means of treating severe myopia because removal of the crystalline lens, by eliminating a significant refractive element of the eye, results in movement of an image focused anterior to the retina to a position closer to (or possibly behind) its surface. Placement of an appropriate intraocular lens permits refinement of this procedure, limiting the need for ultimate spectacle correction and allowing treatment of hyperopia as well[28–30] (Fig. 3–1H).

The disadvantage of clear lens extraction in a young person is the loss of accommodative ability that results, requiring the use of bifocals or progressive lenses to perform near work. This has prompted investigators to develop innovative intraocular methods of altering the refractive power of the eye without disturbing the crystalline lens.

Phakic intraocular lenses are currently being investigated for this purpose.[31, 32] The prototype of these is an anterior chamber device: the Worst-Fechner Iris "Claw" Lens.[33, 34] It is a biconcave intraocular lens designed to straddle the pupil and is secured by fixation haptics that attach to the anterior surface of the iris (Fig 3–1I). Complications have included cataract formation, hyphema, and endothelial cell loss.[35, 36] Alternatively, a lens can be fixated in the anterior chamber angle (Baikoff),[37] which may increase the risk of glaucoma.

Posterior chamber intraocular lenses are also being studied. Fyodorov described what is essentially an "intraocular contact lens," which is draped directly over the anterior surface of the crystalline lens and held in place by iris constriction (Fig. 3–1J). Experience with this has been mixed, with some recipients developing cataracts, likely through microtrauma to the crystalline lens capsule from movement of the device.

Other techniques are likely on the horizon. Nonetheless, they will

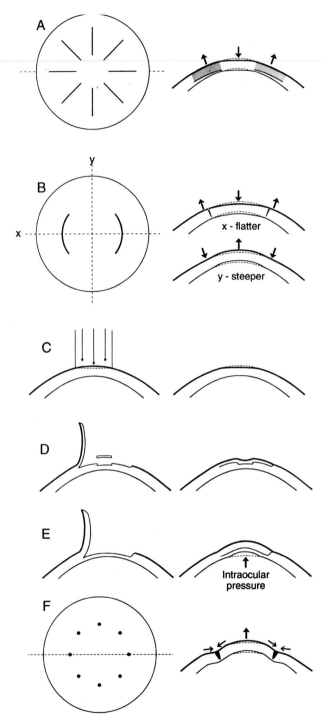

Figure 3–1. Schematic representations of various refractive surgery techniques. *A*, Radial keratotomy. *B*, Astigmatic keratotomy. *C*, Photorefractive keratectomy. *D*, Myopic keratomileusis in situ. *E*, Hyperopic lamellar keratoplasty. *F*, Radial thermokeratoplasty.

Illustration continued on opposite page

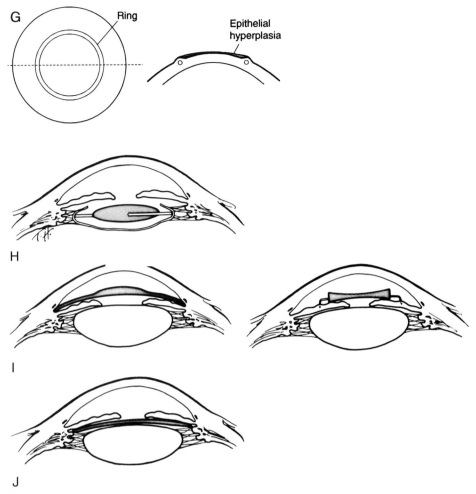

Figure 3–1 *Continued. G,* Intracorneal ring. *H,* Clear lens extraction. *I,* Anterior chamber phakic intraocular lens. *J,* Posterior chamber phakic intraocular lens.

almost certainly fall in one of the two prior general categories, which, as discussed later, will tend to determine the appropriate level of required anesthesia.

ANESTHESIA FOR REFRACTIVE SURGERY

Three ocular tissues are sources of pain while performing refractive surgery: the cornea, the conjunctiva, and the uvea. In general, corneal refractive surgeries tend to require anesthesia of the cornea and frequently the conjunctiva, and lenticular refractive surgeries, being intraocular, in addition require anesthesia of the uvea through blockade of the long ciliary nerves (branches of the first division of the trigeminal nerve). Table 3–1 summarizes the tissues primarily involved for each of the just-described procedures.

Although primarily a corneal refractive surgery, keratomileusis is unique in its potential requirements. Because the suction ring used to

Table 3–1. Tissues Primarily Involved in Refractive Surgery

Refractive Surgery	Tissues Impacted	Typical Anesthesia Requirements
Corneal surgeries		
Photorefractive keratectomy	Cornea	Topical (mild)
Radial-astigmatic keratotomy	Cornea, conjunctiva	Topical (mild)
Keratomileusis	Cornea, conjunctiva, uvea*	Topical (mild); also local (mild) in extreme circumstances
Holmium laser photocoagulation	Cornea, conjunctiva	Topical (mild)
Intracorneal ring	Cornea, conjunctiva	Topical (mild); also local (mild) in extreme circumstances
Lenticular surgeries		
Clear lens extraction	Cornea, conjunctiva, uvea	Local (mild), MAC (moderate); also general in extreme circumstances
Phakic intraocular lens	Cornea, conjunctiva, uvea	Local (mild), MAC (moderate); also general in extreme circumstances

*Indirect effect.
MAC = monitored anesthesia care.

stabilize and center the microkeratome as it passes over the cornea raises the intraocular pressure above 65 mm Hg, uveal pain receptors are indirectly stimulated (i.e., without direct contact with uveal tissues), creating a sensation described by various patients as "someone sticking their thumb" in their eye. Although this is usually well tolerated with appropriate pre- and intraoperative counseling, anesthesia of the uvea may be required in a select few patients even though the surgery is not intraocular.

Procedures that may directly stimulate the uvea require retro- or peribulbar local anesthetic blocks (or in rare cases general anesthesia), essentially the same anesthetic requirements as for other anterior segment intraocular surgeries (e.g., cataract extraction). However, the limited length of some refractive procedures (e.g., placement of phakic intraocular lenses) may permit the use of a shorter acting anesthetic agent such as lidocaine alone as opposed to a combination of lidocaine and bupivacaine (Marcaine). Because the anesthetic techniques for intraocular surgery are well described in other areas of this text (Chapter 1), the remainder of this chapter is restricted to anesthesia for corneal refractive surgery.

ANESTHESIA FOR CORNEAL REFRACTIVE SURGERY

GOALS OF ANESTHESIA

As with all surgical procedures, successful anesthesia for refractive surgery should produce adequate analgesia, sedation, and in some cases akinesia. Achieving such anesthesia in an efficient manner requires excellent communication between the surgeon and anesthesiologist because the degree of anesthesia required is often a subjective judgment of their combined assessments.

One should recognize that it may be necessary to rethink and continually reassess both the surgical and anesthesia aspects of a given method as well as the order in which steps are performed. In this way, one can achieve an optimal technique meeting specific, often individual, requirements.

ASSESSMENT OF ANESTHESIA REQUIREMENTS

The ability of a patient to cooperate, the perception of his or her threshold of pain, and the level of patient (and possibly surgeon) anxiety all play important roles in decision making regarding anesthesia requirements. Such decision making is facilitated by an intimate familiarity with the applicable procedure or technique, its impact on the involved tissues, and the consequences of small patient movements.

Two steps common to all corneal refractive surgeries deserve special attention. It is, therefore, illustrative to address them individually to understand the potential advantages and disadvantages of the different degrees of anesthesia for each method.

Locating the Entrance Pupil. Because most refractive procedures achieve optimal results if the surgical treatment is centered on the patient's entrance pupil, a means of ensuring such centration is useful. This always involves enlisting the patient's cooperation to fixate on a target while various markings are made.

Anesthetics that hinder the patient's voluntary eye movements or sedatives that alter the level of concentration or consciousness can adversely affect the surgeon's ability to mark the entrance pupil accurately. Should such akinesia or sedation be desirable in a given set of circumstances, it may necessary to locate the entrance pupil before the onset of action of the involved medications.

Fixating the Eye. Stabilization of the corneal tissue during surgery permits precise placement of surgical treatment. In addition, it is necessary to minimize inadvertent patient movements that may result in suboptimal surgical results, including catastrophic injury to the visual axis.

With the exception of PRK, in which the patient uses his or her eye musculature to align the eye with the beam of the excimer laser, this requires manipulation of the conjunctiva through the use of a limbal fixation ring or special forceps. Painful stimuli to this ocular tissue, which is often difficult to anesthetize completely, may induce unintentional eye movements in the patient as well. Thus, it is vital that adequate analgesia of all impacted tissues be maintained throughout the procedure and that consideration be given to local anesthetic blocks when these would minimize risk to the patient.

As described, keratomileusis offers a special challenge with regard to globe fixation. Although also requiring anesthesia of the conjunctiva, because the suction ring used raises the intraocular pressure to at least 65 mm Hg, the resulting stimulation of uveal pain receptors typically produces an uncomfortable sensation. This is usually well tolerated; however, retro- or peribulbar anesthesia may be required in certain patients.

MODES OF ANESTHESIA

Although not all modes of anesthesia are equally suited for refractive surgery, any of the various means of ocular anesthesia that are routinely relied on in general ophthalmic practice can prove useful in a given situation. Taking into account the initial comments of this chapter, however, some of these may be more acceptable than others. Table 3–1 outlines the typical anesthesia requirements for each type of refractive surgery discussed previously, although individual circumstances may necessitate deviation from these suggestions.

The specifics of local ocular and general anesthesia are described in excellent detail elsewhere in this text (Chapter 1) and are not duplicated here. Salient points regarding each of these in relation to refractive surgery are discussed next.

Topical Anesthesia. This is by far the most widely used anesthesia technique in refractive surgery. Not only is it simple to perform and usually adequate for the typical patient, but it also requires no special equipment and only minimal monitoring. Nonetheless, adequate precautions for handling emergencies inherent in the administration of any medication (e.g., anaphylaxis) or for addressing cardiopulmonary arrest must be taken should refractive surgery under topical anesthesia be performed in an office setting. Anesthetic agents commonly used for this method have largely been selected on the basis of functionality and availability.[38]

Cocaine has been used in the past and provides excellent analgesia. Given its current medicolegal implications (e.g., it may be detected on a routine toxicology screen now required by many employers and governmental agencies in various circumstances) and significant documentation requirements, as well as the availability of other agents that produce equally acceptable anesthesia, it is rarely used today.

Proparacaine is commonly available in an office setting and provides corneal and superficial conjunctival analgesia for periods of 10 to 15 minutes.[39] The difficulty with this agent for use in refractive surgery arises from the current nonavailability of a sterile dispensing system; the multiuse bottles it comes in are subject to contamination of the contents, and its use requires a second person to introduce a single drop in a sterile manner onto the surgical field. Thus, it is commonly used as an initial agent before preparing the skin around the eyes to minimize irritation from the antimicrobials used in this process as well as from the subsequent instillation of one of the other anesthetic agents, which tend to cause more initial discomfort.

Tetracaine is likely the most commonly used agent for corneal refractive surgeries. Although its duration and depth of analgesia are clinically somewhat poorer than those of proparacaine, especially on conjunctiva, it is commercially available in single-use sterile containers that may remain on the surgical field and permit the surgeon to apply additional anesthetic at will.

Of the topical agents, lidocaine (2% or 4%) likely produces the most complete analgesia and clinically appears to anesthetize the conjunctiva better than tetracaine. Combinations with epinephrine provide vasoconstriction, which minimizes bleeding from conjunctival manipulation and increases the duration of action. Because lidocaine must be drawn up from a stock bottle into a syringe—no single-use container is currently available—it is less convenient to use than tetracaine and is commonly reserved for a procedure demanding maximal anesthesia of the ocular coverings, such as keratomileusis, in which the conjunctiva and episclera are transiently incarcerated between the suction ring and the sclera.

All of these agents tend to soften the epithelium and thus promote the formation of epithelial defects during corneal refractive surgery.[38] This issue turns out to be less important in the case of PRK because most surgeons remove the epithelium before the ablation step and can use the softening produced by repeated application of anesthetic to their advantage. That specific case notwithstanding, because patients complain almost exclusively of conjunctival manipulation rather than corneal pain during a procedure after a single administration of topical anesthetic, one should avoid repeated indiscriminate application of such medication over the entire surface of the eye but rather should concentrate the agent where it is specifically required. This can be accomplished by saturating a cellulose sponge and placing it directly on a specific point of conjunctival contact (Fig. 3–2).

Local Anesthetic Blocks. Because of their relatively short lengths compared to intraocular surgery, corneal refractive surgeries rarely require blocks. When the added control they offer would benefit the patient from the standpoint of potential surgical outcome, however, consideration should be given to their use.

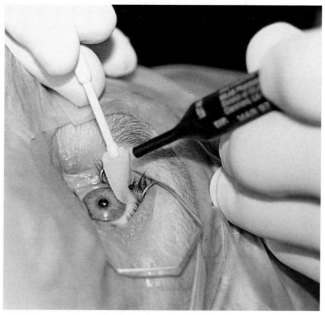

Figure 3–2. Cellulose sponges concentrate topical anesthetic at points of direct conjunctival manipulation. This maximizes analgesia where it is needed and minimizes contact of extraneous anesthetic with the corneal surface, which can soften the epithelium and lead to defects during surgery.

Blocks for intraocular surgery tend to be performed with mixtures of lidocaine and bupivacaine, the latter to prolong the length of anesthesia. Again, because the time course of a typical corneal refractive surgery is comparatively shorter, lidocaine as a single agent is usually adequate under these circumstances. Work performed in 1991 indicates that pH adjustment by the addition of bicarbonate to the anesthetic may speed the onset of action of such local anesthetic blocks.[40]

Retrobulbar anesthesia, in which a relatively blunt needle is used to introduce anesthetic into the extraocular muscle cone, offers maximal control of the eye, usually without the loss of higher motor functions and consciousness. Unfortunately, the akinesia achieved eliminates the possibility of patient cooperation after anesthetic administration. In addition, the effects on the optic nerve, even if a short-acting agent is used, may result in transient blindness that will likely be troubling to the patient postoperatively.

This method carries rare but serious risks. Retrobulbar hemorrhage can lead to globe compression and, in the extreme case, occlusion of the central retinal artery. Inadvertent injection of local anesthesia into the optic nerve sheath can cause seizures and respiratory arrest. Optic nerve trauma can lead to permanent vision loss, which has been reported in a patient who underwent RK.[41] Furthermore, penetration or perforation of the globe can have devastating retinal consequences and is especially common in axial myopes, whose higher-than-average eye lengths coincidentally make them excellent candidates for refractive surgery.

Peribulbar anesthesia relies on injection of a larger amount of anesthetic outside the muscle cone, requiring diffusion to reach its site of action, usually adding to the procedure length. Although its risks and benefits are similar to those of retrobulbar anesthesia, its primary advantage is a lower risk of optic nerve or globe trauma and retrobulbar hemorrhage, although this risk cannot be completely eliminated. Although this can be performed with a relatively short 1.56-cm (5/8 inch) needle and injections can be made both superiorly and inferiorly to the globe to limit the proximity of the needle to vital structures behind the eye, the resultant lid swelling that commonly occurs may interfere with smooth performance of various refractive surgeries. We therefore prefer a single "deep" peribulbar block inferiorly using an Atkinson needle that is passed along the orbital floor but not angled into the muscle cone before injection (Fig. 3–3).

In 1992 Greenbaum introduced a flexible cannula for performing parabulbar anesthesia.[42] The device is inserted through an anterior incision in Tenon's capsule and passed posteriorly a short distance, hugging the sclera, allowing anesthetic to then track along the globe to gain access to the retrobulbar space. This technique has the advantages of a retrobulbar injection while posing minimal risk to the globe or optic nerve because no needle is involved.

If the bulk of the fluid volume used to create a local anesthetic block is placed posterior to the globe, such as with the retrobulbar and deep peribulbar techniques, this may move it forward, serendipitously improving corneal exposure during a refractive procedure. Note, however, that if this fluid tracks forward subconjunctivally, increasing lid swelling and causing conjunctival chemosis, this may actually decrease exposure

Figure 3–3. Deep peribulbar anesthesia. The Atkinson needle maintains close apposition with the orbital floor rather than entering the muscle cone. This technique minimizes the potential for injury to the globe, especially in the case of axial myopes (in which eyes are of longer than average length), and the optic nerve.

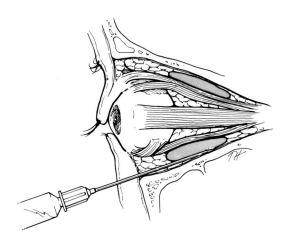

or result in blockage of the vacuum port on the suction ring when performing keratomileusis, preventing firm adherence of the microkeratome base. Furthermore, increased extraocular pressure created by the volume of fluid anesthetic placed behind or around the eye is transmitted to the corneal tissue, modifying the tensile forces acting on it. Thus, it can alter the effect of a given surgeon's technique because increased pressure frequently makes the keratotomy incisions deeper, thereby increasing the risk of corneal perforation.

Monitored Anesthesia Care. For patients with established histories of cardiopulmonary disease or other medical conditions that may raise the question of instability during surgery, topical anesthesia or local anesthetic blocks administered under appropriate monitoring in an outpatient surgery center or hospital setting may be indicated. Such monitored care may also permit administration of more powerful sedatives than might be safely given in an office practice and may be appropriate for patients with extreme anxiety.

General Anesthesia. This has the advantage of providing the highest level of control for the surgeon from the perspective of the surgery itself as well as greatest protection of the patient's airway and ventilation. In addition, because the anesthetic interventions involved do not directly impact the eye, the surgeon is offered essentially pristine ocular tissues with which to work.

Yet, attractive as these features may sound, postoperative complications such as nausea, vomiting, and throat irritation from the placement of an endotracheal tube and decreased overall comfort, combined with the small, yet real, inherent risk of death, make this mode of anesthesia difficult to justify in a purely elective procedure, except in the most extreme of circumstances (e.g., an extremely anxious patient or one who becomes easily disoriented and might attempt to sit up during surgery).

As with the local anesthetic blocks, the absence of patient consciousness makes patient assistance in locating the entrance pupil during the procedure impossible, and this must be done either before entering the surgical suite or immediately before administering the general anesthetic.

ADJUVANT SEDATION

As with any surgical procedure, patient anxiety may interfere with the ability to execute smoothly a given refractive surgical technique, especially because in most circumstances the patient retains voluntary control of the eye. Obviously, a calm, reassuring voice can work wonders in a patient who has significant trust in his or her surgical team. Nonetheless, pharmacologic assistance in this area tends to create a baseline level of relaxation, making the overall experience more pleasant for all concerned.

Anxiolytics[38] such as diazepam (Valium) have a relatively short onset of action and long duration and are, therefore, ideal for refractive surgery. It should be kept in mind, however, that although the administration of such substances usually serves to relax an anxious patient, certain individuals may fall asleep or, in the opposite extreme, become combative, especially if overmedicated.

For patients who display a high level of anxiety, or in the rare circumstance in which patient safety is at risk, more extreme measures may be required. As stated, monitored anesthesia care offers the possibility of intravenous sedation with more potent agents than might safely be used in a less structured environment such as an office or minor surgery suite.

General anesthesia eliminates patient awareness and voluntary patient movements. It should be kept in mind, however, that during periods of anesthesia "lightness" or when paralysis is incomplete, unpredictable patient movements or contractures of eye musculature are a real possibility, defeating the purpose of such anesthesia from the standpoint of refractive surgery. Thus, a surgeon should not be lulled into a false sense of security simply because the patient is under general anesthesia but should communicate his or her surgical needs to the anesthesiologist to ensure they are met during crucial parts of the procedure.

ADJUVANT FACIAL BLOCKS

Although likely not as significant clinically as injection of local anesthetic around the eye, squeezing of the lids has the potential to increase intraocular pressure and, therefore, can modify the surgical outcome in radial and astigmatic keratotomy. Furthermore, significant orbicularis activity on the part of the patient may limit exposure at crucial times during each of the described procedures. Thus, any of the various types of facial blocks (e.g., van Lint, Nadbath, O'Brien) that yield lid akinesia, although rarely indicated, may be useful in selected patients and are described in detail elsewhere in this text.

The benefits of such lid blocks must be balanced with the potential complications, which include ecchymoses and nerve damage (leading to partial or complete palsy). If administered, the temporary facial paralysis produced will eliminate the protective functions of the lids long after the procedure is over and will necessitate postoperative patching to protect the cornea and globe from exposure damage.

ANESTHESIA PROTOCOLS FOR CORNEAL REFRACTIVE SURGERY

Although each surgeon and anesthesiologist team will develop its own refinements to any approach presented, the following methods have worked well in our experience and provide a reasonable starting point for those performing corneal refractive surgery.

PRK

1. Diazepam, 5 mg, can be given to achieve mild sedation, taking care not to overmedicate because patient cooperation is required for centration of the ablation zone on the patient's cornea.
2. If pachymetry is performed as a separate step, an additional drop of proparacaine is given immediately before this measurement.
3. Before any surgical preparation, another drop of proparacaine is instilled to minimize irritation from the antiseptic (e.g., povidone iodine) as well as stinging from any subsequent tetracaine, which is usually more pronounced than with proparacaine.
4. During the procedure itself, tetracaine is administered as necessary to maintain anesthesia.

RK, AK, HOLMIUM LASER PHOTOCOAGULATION, AND INTRACORNEAL RING PLACEMENT

1. Diazepam, 10 mg, can be given to achieve sedation, keeping in mind that patient cooperation is usually required for locating the center of the visual axis.
2. If pachymetry is performed as a separate step, an additional drop of proparacaine is given immediately before this measurement. If desired, location of the visual axis can be performed at this point as well before the onset of effect of any sedation.
3. Before any surgical preparation, another drop of proparacaine is instilled to minimize irritation from the antiseptic (e.g., povidone-iodine) as well as stinging from any subsequent tetracaine, which is usually more pronounced than with proparacaine.
4. During the procedure itself, tetracaine is administered as necessary to maintain anesthesia. Points of direct conjunctival manipulation receive a concentrated application using anesthetic-soaked cellulose sponges.

KERATOMILEUSIS

1. If desired, diazepam, 10 to 20 mg, based on the patient's weight and level of anxiety, can be given to achieve sedation, keeping in mind that patient cooperation is usually required for locating the center of the visual axis.
2. If pachymetry is performed as a separate step, an additional drop

of proparacaine is given immediately before this measurement. If necessary, the visual axis can be located at this point as well before the onset of effect of any sedation.

3. Before any surgical preparation, another drop of proparacaine is instilled to minimize irritation from the antiseptic (e.g., povidone-iodine) as well as stinging from any subsequent tetracaine, which is usually more pronounced than with proparacaine.

4. Once the preparation has been completed, approximately 2 mL of 2% lidocaine without epinephrine is carefully applied to the conjunctival surfaces of the surgical eye.

5. During the procedure itself, additional lidocaine is administered as necessary to maintain analgesia.

CONCLUSIONS

Anesthesia for refractive surgery offers special challenges because unexpected patient movements precipitated by inadequate analgesia can have devastating consequences. This chapter has attempted to offer insight into the impact of various surgical manipulations involved in refractive surgical procedures, facilitating both pre- and intraoperative counseling. Well-informed patients who expect potential discomfort are much better able to repress sudden movements than those who are caught off guard, and it is hoped that these comments will assist participating surgeons and anesthesiologists to anticipate the anesthetic needs of refractive surgery patients, minimizing both their discomfort and surgical risk.

REFERENCES

1. Aquavella JV. Major refractive surgical techniques. Ophthalmic Surg 1994;25:573.
2. Choyce DP. The correction of high myopia. Refract Corneal Surg 1992;8:242.
3. Thompson V. The surgical correction of myopic and hyperopic astigmatism. Int Ophthalmol Clin 1994;34:87.
4. Waring GO III, ed. Refractive keratotomy for myopia and astigmatism. St. Louis, MO: Mosby-Year Book, 1992.
5. Salz JJ, ed. Corneal laser surgery. St. Louis, MO: CV Mosby, 1995.
6. Epstein D, Fagerholm P, Hamberg-Nystrom H, Tengroth B. Twenty-four-month follow-up of excimer laser photorefractive keratectomy for myopia: refractive and visual acuity results. Ophthalmology 1994;101:1558.
7. Heitzmann J, Binder PS, Kassar BS, Nordan LT. The correction of high myopia using the excimer laser. Arch Ophthalmol 1993;111:1627.
8. Kim JH, Hahn TW, Lee YC, Sah WJ. Excimer laser photorefractive keratectomy for myopia: two-year follow-up. J Cataract Refract Surg 1994;20(suppl):229.
9. Maguen E, Salz JJ, Nesburn AB, et al. Results of excimer laser photorefractive keratectomy for the correction of myopia. Ophthalmology 1994;101:1548.
10. McDonald MB, Beuerman R, Falzoni W, et al. Refractive surgery with the excimer laser. Am J Ophthalmol 1987;103:469.
11. Seiler T, Specht H, Matallana M, Bende T. Principles of refractive corneal surgery with the 193 nm excimer laser. Biomedizinische Technik 1990;35(suppl 3):12.
12. Sher NA, Hardten DR, Fundingsland B, et al. 193-nm excimer photorefractive keratectomy in high myopia. Ophthalmology 1994;101:1575.
13. Talley AR, Hardten DR, Sher NA, et al. Results one year after using the 193-nm excimer laser for photorefractive keratectomy in mild to moderate myopia. Am J Ophthalmol 1994;118:304.
14. Colliac JP, Shammas HJ, Bart DJ. Photorefractive keratectomy for the correction of myopia and astigmatism. Am J Ophthalmol 1994;117:369.
15. Taylor HR, Kelly P, Alpins N. Excimer laser correction of myopic astigmatism. Cataract Refract Surg 1994;20(suppl):243.

16. Dausch D, Klein R, Schroder E. Excimer laser photorefractive keratectomy for hyperopia. Refract Corneal Surg 1993;9:20.
17. Pallikaris IG, Papatzanaki ME, Siganos DS, Tsilimbaris MK. A corneal flap technique for laser in situ keratomileusis: human studies. Arch Ophthalmol 1991;109:1699.
18. Buratto L, Ferrari M, Genisi C. Keratomileusis for myopia with the excimer laser (Buratto technique): short-term results. Refract Corneal Surg 1993;9(suppl 2):S130.
19. Buratto L, Ferrari M, Genisi C. Myopic keratomileusis with the excimer laser: one-year follow up. Refract Corneal Surg 1993;9:12.
20. Buratto L, Ferrari M, Rama P. Excimer laser intrastromal keratomileusis. Am J Ophthalmol 1992;113:291.
21. Kliger CH, Maloney RK. Excimer laser myopic keratomileusis. In: Salz JJ, ed. Corneal laser surgery. St. Louis, MO: CV Mosby, 1995.
22. Pallikaris IG, Siganos DS. Excimer laser in situ keratomileusis and photorefractive keratectomy for correction of high myopia. J Refract Corneal Surg 1994;10:498.
23. Durrie DS, Schumer DJ, Cavanaugh TB. Holmium:YAG laser thermokeratoplasty for hyperopia. J Refract Corneal Surg 1994;10(suppl 2):S277.
24. Neumann AC, Sanders D, Raanan M, DeLuca M. Hyperopic thermokeratoplasty: clinical evaluation. J Cataract Refract Surg 1991;17:830.
25. Neumann AC, Fyodorov S, Sanders DR. Radial thermokeratoplasty for the correction of hyperopia. Refract Corneal Surg 1990;6:404.
26. Seiler T, Matallana M, Bende T. Laser thermokeratoplasty by means of a pulsed holmium:YAG laser for hyperopic correction. Refract Corneal Surg 1990;6:335.
27. Assil KK, Barrett AM, Fouraker BD, Schanzlin DJ. One-year results of the intrastromal corneal ring in nonfunctional human eyes: Intrastromal Corneal Ring Study Group. Arch Ophthalmol 1995;113:159.
28. Colin J, Robinet A. Clear lensectomy and implantation of low-power posterior chamber intraocular lens for the correction of high myopia. Ophthalmology 1994;101:107.
29. Lyle WA, Jin GJ. Clear lens extraction for the correction of high refractive error. Cataract Refract Surg 1994;20:273.
30. Siganos DS, Siganos CS, Pallikaris IG. Clear lens extraction and intraocular lens implantation in normally sighted hyperopic eyes. J Refract Corneal Surg 1994;10:117.
31. Praeger DL, Momose A, Muroff LL. Thirty-six month follow-up of a contemporary phakic intraocular lens for the surgical correction of myopia. Ann Ophthalmol 1991;23:6.
32. Praeger DL. Innovations and creativity in contemporary ophthalmology: preliminary experience with the phakic myopic intraocular lens. Ann Ophthalmol 1988;20:456.
33. Fechner PU, Strobel J, Wicchmann W. Correction of myopia by implantation of a concave Worst-iris claw lens into phakic eyes. Refract Corneal Surg 1991;7:286.
34. Fechner PU, van der Heijde GL, Worst JG. The correction of myopia by lens implantation into phakic eyes. Am J Ophthalmol 1989;107:659.
35. Mimouni F, Colin J, Koffi V, Bonnet P. Damage to the corneal endothelium from anterior chamber intraocular lenses in phakic myopic eyes. Refract Corneal Surg 1991;7:277.
36. Saragoussi JJ, Cotinat J, Renard G, et al. Damage to the corneal endothelium by minus power anterior chamber intraocular lenses. Refract Corneal Surg 1991;7:282.
37. Baikoff G, Joly P. [Surgical correction of severe myopia using an anterior chamber implant in the phakic eye: concept—results]. Bull Soc Belg Ophtalmol 1989;233:109.
38. American Medical Association. Drug evaluations, annual 1994. Chicago: American Medical Association, 1994.
39. Jordan A, Baum J. Basic tear flow: does it exist? Ophthalmology 1980;87:920.
40. Zahl K, Jordan A, McGroarty J, et al. Peribulbar anesthesia: effect of bicarbonate on mixtures of lidocaine, bupivacaine, and hyaluronidase with or without epinephrine. Ophthalmology 1991;98:239.
41. O'Day DM, Feman SS, Elliott JH. Visual impairment following radial keratotomy. Ophthalmology 1986;93:319.
42. Greenbaum S. Parabulbar anesthesia (letter). Am J Ophthalmol 1992;114:776.

CHAPTER 4

ANESTHESIA FOR GLAUCOMA SURGERY

DAVID J. PINHAS, MD
JEFFREY M. LIEBMANN, MD
ROBERT RITCH, MD

Anesthesia for glaucoma surgery should follow the same basic principles as for all ophthalmic surgery: adequate anesthesia to allow for smooth performance of the procedure while maintaining the well-being of the patient. In particular, anesthesia in the glaucoma patient should minimize the risk of further compromise of optic nerve function. Several reports have described alternative techniques to traditional methods of anesthesia.[1–9] We strongly believe that minimal amounts of localized anesthetic are much safer than retrobulbar or peribulbar anesthesia in glaucoma patients with moderate or advanced damage. In this chapter, we review the traditional methods with their benefits and untoward effects and present the more recent techniques with their advantages and limitations.

GENERAL ANESTHESIA

At present, general anesthesia for anterior segment procedures is reserved primarily for infants and children and those patients who are unable to cooperate during regional anesthesia. In children, diagnostic evaluation can be performed under ketamine anesthesia, whereas therapeutic procedures generally require inhalation anesthetics and intubation. Confused or extremely nervous patients who cannot cooperate under local anesthesia can be more safely managed under general anesthesia. The same applies to patients with whom communication is not possible (e.g., deafness, foreign language speaking only).

There are certain advantages to general anesthesia. The risk of orbital or ocular complications from the local anesthetic are avoided. The anesthesiologist's total control of the patient allows for better operating conditions for the surgeon and a more relaxed atmosphere for the operating room staff. Because of their longer duration or complexity, certain procedures (i.e., seton implantation, combined procedures) may be better performed under general anesthesia in restless patients. In specific regard to surgery for glaucoma patients, the avoidance of sudden, often extreme intraocular pressure (IOP) elevation that can occur after administration of anesthetic agents into the orbit is especially important in preventing further damage to compromised optic nerves.[2]

PREOPERATIVE EVALUATION

Patients who are to undergo general anesthesia should have a history and physical examination no more than 1 to 2 weeks before the scheduled surgery.[10, 11] In addition, a full list of current ocular and systemic medications and allergies must also be included. Echothiophate iodide and demecarium bromide, occasionally used for IOP control, may deplete plasma pseudocholinesterase levels.[12] This enzyme hydrolyzes succinylcholine and ester-type local anesthetics, and a lack of pseudocholinesterase may lead to prolonged muscle relaxation and respiratory depression if these anesthetics are used. It can take as long as 6 weeks for pseudocholinesterase levels to return to normal after discontinuing these drugs. One should, therefore, avoid the use of succinylcholine or ester-type anesthetics during this period.[10] Anesthesiologists may neglect to ask or parents may forget to reveal the use of these medications before pediatric surgery.

Laboratory work should include a complete blood count, serum electrolytes, and, in patients older than 40 years, electrocardiogram (ECG). An ECG is required in all patients with known cardiovascular disease regardless of age. Depending on the patient's age and physical condition, a chest x-ray film may also be indicated. Patients who are using anticoagulants or aspirin preparations may require bleeding-clotting profiles in their preoperative evaluation.[11] Because ocular bleeding may have adverse effects on the success of glaucoma surgery, it has been taught that medications that interfere with clotting should be stopped (with the internist's consent) long enough before surgery to allow clotting mechanisms to normalize. This is probably more important in patients with neovascular glaucoma, elevated episcleral venous pressure, nanophthalmos, pre-existing ciliochoroidal effusions, and conditions in which increased risk of intraoperative, intraocular, and orbital bleeding exists. All chronic medical conditions should be under the best possible control before undergoing general anesthesia.

IOP AND GENERAL ANESTHETICS

The effect of medications used in general anesthesia on IOP is especially important in infants or children undergoing diagnostic or follow-up examination under anesthesia, in which accurate determination of IOP is essential. Intramuscular or intravenous ketamine is the anesthetic of choice for general anesthesia without intubation because of its lack of respiratory depression.[13] It has been taught that following administration, ketamine tends to elevate IOP.[14, 15] This IOP rise is thought to be secondary to an increase in extraocular muscle tone and may be as high as 10 mm Hg, lasting up to 30 minutes after injection, with a peak at 15 minutes.[14] Other reports found that ketamine does not increase IOP,[16, 17] suggesting that the results of the previous studies may have been affected by differences in premedication as well as the use of indentation tonometry, which is generally considered less accurate than the applanation tonometers. We have found that to maximize the likelihood that IOP after administration resembles the unmedicated state as much as possible, it is reasonable to wait approximately 5 minutes after initiation of ketamine anesthesia and to measure the IOP with an applanation tonometer.

The depolarizing muscle relaxant succinylcholine raises IOP.[18] This agent causes extraocular muscle contraction in the depolarization phase of anesthesia and should be avoided in childhood eye diseases and in cases of suspected ocular trauma. This rise is similar in magnitude and duration as that previously described with ketamine.[19] This IOP effect may be blunted by deeper anesthesia at the time of delivery or the preoperative use of acetazolamide,[13, 20] nifedipine,[21] or β-blockers.[13]

Other than succinylcholine and possibly ketamine, nearly all other general anesthetic agents either lower IOP or have a minimal effect on it.[22, 23] All inhalation anesthetics reduce IOP[24–27] and most central nervous system depressants have a similar effect.[10, 28, 29] This is theorized to be secondary to depression of brain centers, which maintain extraocular muscle tone. The intravenous anesthetics propofol,[30, 31] thiopental,[32] and etimodate[32] reduce IOP. Narcotics,[33–35] benzodiazepines,[29, 36] as well as droperidol[37] also lower IOP approximately 10 to 15%.[38] In contrast to succinylcholine, the nondepolarizing muscle relaxants such as pancuronium and vecuronium reduce IOP.[39–45] It is questionable as to whether nitrous oxide has any effect at all on IOP. One study has found that it may raise IOP slightly.[23] The combined use of ketamine with another general anesthetic, most frequently a benzodiazepine or a narcotic agent, may mimic the natural-state IOP, an important issue in evaluations under anesthesia, although the administration of medications that both lower and raise the IOP make pressure measurements less reliable.

Besides direct drug effects, a number of other factors may influence IOP. Physiologic factors, including a marked elevation of heart rate or systemic arterial pressure, can cause an increased IOP.[29, 46] Hypercarbia and hypoxia resulting from hypoventilation during anesthesia may cause IOP elevation,[47] whereas the opposite situation leads to a lowering of IOP by diminishing choroidal blood flow through vasoconstriction of the precapillary arterioles.

Maneuvers that increase central venous pressure, such as coughing, straining, or vomiting, may raise episcleral venous pressure by as much as 35 mm Hg.[48] (This holds true for patients who are placed in the Trendelenburg position or in whom a tourniquet effect exists when a surgical gown is tied tightly around the patient's neck, limiting venous return.)

Endotracheal intubation causes a marked rise in IOP as well as arterial blood pressure and heart rate.[21, 22, 38, 49–51] This elevation may reach 50 mm Hg. In an attempt to attenuate this effect, a number of agents have been used. Lidocaine has met with limited success.[52] Nifedipine has been found to be more effective[21] in ameliorating IOP rise and tachycardia. Propofol has been found to blunt IOP elevation in 62% of patients with glaucoma when administered before tracheal intubation.[30] This study also found that patients who underwent laryngeal mask insertion had an IOP that was significantly lower than baseline values when induction was performed with propofol. This may be a preferred anesthetic technique in patients with advanced glaucoma, markedly elevated preoperative IOP, or ruptured globes.

General anesthesia is not without its potential ocular complications because it has been implicated in delayed suprachoroidal hemorrhage (SCH).[53–56] A major potential problem of general anesthesia is a postextubation increase in episcleral venous pressure. Elevated venous pressure resulting from nausea and vomiting or a Valsalva maneuver is a particular threat.[55, 57] Ariano and Ball[58] reported delayed nonexpulsive SCH after trabeculectomy in five patients; four had general anesthesia and three had strained and bucked at extubation. Van Meurs and van den Bosch[59] described a man who had undergone a scleral buckling procedure 3 years previously in whom postoperative SCH developed after vomiting. Girard and colleagues[60] described a similar episode after coughing and straining.

The complications of general anesthesia such as cardiac arrest, myocardial infarction, apnea, malignant hyperthermia, and arterial hypertension are not specific to glaucoma surgery and are not discussed here.

LOCAL ANESTHETICS

The most commonly used local anesthetics for glaucoma surgery include the amide anesthetics lidocaine, bupivacaine, mepivacaine, and, less commonly, the ester-linked anesthetic procaine. Surgeons frequently use a combination of these anesthetics to take advantage of the rapid onset of action of one (i.e., lidocaine or mepivacaine) and the long duration of action of another (i.e., bupivacaine).[61] Many surgeons also include the enzyme hyaluronidase in an attempt to promote rapid diffusion of the anesthetic agents as well as to increase the area of tissue anesthetized.[62]

Some surgeons also include dilute concentrations of epinephrine (1:100,000–1:200,000) for its vasoconstrictive effect in an attempt at decreasing systemic absorption of anesthetic, thereby prolonging its duration of action and decreasing its systemic effects.[63, 64] This is unnecessary and may even be detrimental to the patient with glaucomatous optic nerve damage. First, the duration of action of bupivacaine has been shown not to be extended by the use of epinephrine.[65, 66] Second, the vasodilatory effect of local anesthetics, which may be beneficial to optic nerve blood flow in patients with pre-existing nerve damage, is negated by epinephrine's vasoconstrictive effect. Finally, epinephrine has been shown to decrease ophthalmic artery pulse pressure significantly,[67] further decreasing optic nerve blood flow.

In addition to avoiding epinephrine in anesthesia for the glaucoma patient, one should use a higher concentration of anesthetic to minimize the total volume of fluid placed in the retrobulbar or peribulbar space, thereby limiting the secondary rise in IOP after injection.

One may also tailor the type of anesthetic used to the procedure performed. For instance, mepivacaine 2% or lidocaine 2% usually has a sufficient duration of action for trabeculectomy. The addition of bupivacaine 0.50 to 0.75% is often beneficial in longer procedures such as combined cataract extraction–trabeculectomy or seton implant surgery.

REGIONAL ANESTHESIA

As in all intraocular surgery, adequate akinesia of the eyelids is a necessity in all intraocular glaucoma procedures because it allows for a smoother intraoperative course, reducing the risk of complications, which may affect the overall outcome of the surgery. For instance, a limbus-based conjunctival peritomy requires maximal exposure. If this exposure is not obtained, one risks buttonholing the conjunctiva or placing the peritomy too far anteriorly.[68]

Large volumes of anesthetic in the periorbital tissues should be avoided to minimize inadvertent dissection of anesthetics into the lids. Excellent exposure is also required in fornix-based conjunctival flaps when adjuvant topical mitomycin C or 5-fluorouracil is used. These procedures require more extensive sub-Tenon's dissection for application of the antimetabolite-soaked sponge.

Maximal lid exposure is most necessary for seton implant surgery,[69, 70] especially if a double-plate device is used. These devices typically require sub-Tenon's dissection of 15 mm or more because the leading edge is placed 10 to 12 mm posterior to the limbus.

In addition to exposure of the operative site, lid akinesia reduces the risk of repetitive intraoperative shallowing of the anterior chamber from squeezing. This shallowing increases the risk of corneal endothelial damage[71, 72] and lens capsule manipulation, which increases the possibility of postoperative cataract formation and prolongs the operative procedure. Furthermore, lid squeezing has a pronounced effect on IOP and has been shown to cause a pressure rise to greater than 90 mm Hg.[73]

EYELID ANESTHESIA

The facial nerve has five branches, only the superior two of which—the temporal and zygomatic nerves—subserve motor function to the orbicularis oculi muscle and other muscles of eyelid closure.[74] The various techniques commonly used for lid block differ in respect to where along its course the facial nerve is blocked and which portions are blocked. For instance, the O'Brien,[75] Spaeth,[76] and Nadbath[77] blocks are meant to block the facial nerve immediately after its exit from the cranial vault through the stylomastoid foramen. These often achieve excellent eyelid paralysis, avoid periorbital edema, and allow for maximal surgical exposure. This occurs at the expense of a hemifacial paralysis and the risks of postoperative pain on jaw movement at the injection site[77] (which may last for weeks) possible respiratory distress,[78–81] as well as dysphonia and dysphagia associated with the Nadbath block.

In contrast, the classic van Lint block[82] affects the facial nerve at its fibers entering the orbicularis oculi. This avoids the hemifacial paralysis and the complications of the other methods of lid block but may lead to periorbital edema and, rarely, tracking of anesthetic into the subconjunctival space, both of which limit exposure of the operative field. A modification of this technique (Fig. 4–1), however, places the anesthetic more temporal to the lateral canthus and further away from the supra- and infraorbital rims, thereby avoiding lid edema. It is important to involve the corrugator supercilii muscle in the modified van Lint block because this muscle is often not affected by the classic block.

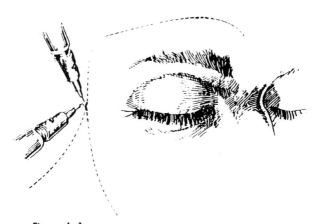

Figure 4–1. Modified van Lint facial nerve block.

RETROBULBAR ANESTHESIA

The use of a retrobulbar block to achieve anesthesia of the conjunctiva, cornea, and uvea as well as akinesia of the extraocular muscles was standard in ocular surgery for the past 50 years and is still very widely used. In the past decade, it has been supplanted to a large extent, at least for cataract surgery, by peribulbar anesthesia, which we do not recommend for routine use in filtration surgery. More recently, topical anesthesia and localized anesthesia have been shown to be both safe and effective.

Retrobulbar anesthesia may be considered in certain situations for the patient with glaucoma (Fig. 4–2). If the glaucoma is of recent onset or if the patient has not yet experienced severe optic nerve or visual field damage but still requires surgical intervention for control of IOP, this form of regional block should not add to the risk of further glaucomatous damage. A retrobulbar injection is also useful in cyclodestructive procedures because it affords more reliable anesthesia and analgesia from these often painful procedures. The volume of retrobulbar injection should be limited to 2 mL to avoid overexpansion of the muscle cone and rise in retrobulbar pressure.

However, for patients with advanced optic nerve damage and visual field loss, especially those that approach or even include fixation, retrobulbar injection may increase the risk of worsening existing damage, including loss of central fixation ("snuff out"). A number of factors may play a role in this phenomenon. An immediate increase in IOP after retrobulbar injection has been reported.[83] Patients with glaucoma experienced higher and more persistent increases than those without glaucoma.[83] Orbital pressure elevation after injection of anesthetic can com-

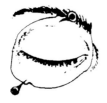

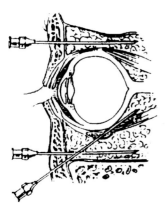

Figure 4–2. Positioning of needles for retrobulbar and peribulbar injection.

promise optic nerve blood flow, potentially exacerbating existing glaucomatous damage. This is more so likely should a retrobulbar hemorrhage occur, because such pressure elevation would be sustained.

Preoperative elevation of IOP has been identified as a risk factor for intraoperative suprachoroidal expulsive hemorrhage.[84, 85] Any procedure, including retrobulbar injection, that increases orbital pressure and thus IOP, however transient, may increase the risk of expulsive suprachoroidal hemorrhage. Retrobulbar block has also been associated with such complications as globe perforation, brain stem anesthesia, and blindness (Table 4–1).[86–103] Systemic complications, such as respiratory arrest,[104–106] cardiopulmonary arrest,[87, 106, 107] as well as generalized seizure activity[108] can also occur. To reduce these risks of retrobulbar anesthesia to the glaucoma patient, one should use a higher concentration of anesthetic to limit the volume injected, avoid the use of epinephrine in the anesthetic mixture, inject the anesthetic slowly to prevent the sudden rise in pressure, and, if possible, use a different technique of regional anesthesia.

PERIBULBAR ANESTHESIA

Posterior peribulbar blocks were first popularized by Kelman[109] as a safer alternative to retrobulbar anesthesia. As originally described, peribulbar anesthesia and akinesia of the globe and eyelids are achieved without a separate lid block while avoiding the retrobulbar space. This negates the risk of intraoptic nerve injection, which could lead to blindness[96, 101] and brain stem paralysis,[89, 93, 95] and significantly reduces the risk of ocular perforation,[88, 90, 94, 102, 103] although perforation has been described with peribulbar anesthesia.[90, 94, 110] It also reduces the risk of ipsilateral and contralateral amaurosis associated with retrobulbar injection,[86, 91, 92] especially in late glaucoma patients.[99]

Peribulbar anesthesia affords specific advantages to retrobulbar block in glaucoma patients. As previously described, it avoids the placement of a relatively high volume of fluid in the muscle cone, which increases the IOP as well as retrobulbar pressure, limiting optic nerve blood flow and possibly causing more damage to pre-existing glaucomatous optic neuropathy. Additionally, the risk of the extreme rise of IOP associated with retrobulbar hemorrhage is avoided.

The technique usually uses two injections (see Fig. 4–2)—one in the inferior peribulbar space and the other in the superior peribulbar

Table 4–1. Complications of Retrobulbar Injection

Retrobulbar hemorrhage
Globe perforation[92–97]
Optic nerve sheath laceration[87, 88]
Central retinal artery occlusion[87, 88]
Central retinal vein occlusion[87]
Vitreous hemorrhage[87]
Extraocular muscle dysfunction[98]
Respiratory arrest[82, 83]
Cardiopulmonary arrest[82, 83]
Brain stem anesthesia[89, 91]
Grand mal seizures[85]

space—placing 6 to 8 mL of anesthetic into the orbit, which may, although less likely than intraconal injection, lead to further damage of a severely affected optic nerve. Another potential disadvantage to peribulbar injection is the frequent eyelid edema and subconjunctival chemosis, both of which limit exposure of the surgical field, making trabeculectomy or seton implantation technically more difficult.

To improve the usefulness of peribulbar anesthesia in glaucoma surgery, a proposed modification of the two-injection technique, consisting of a single injection of 3 to 4 mL of anesthetic into the inferior peribulbar space, achieved complete akinesia in 90% of patients.[9] This may be especially well suited for glaucoma patients with advanced visual field loss, although it does not prevent conjunctival chemosis, which occurred in 80% of patients. Although injection of this small an amount of anesthetic may achieve akinesia of the globe, it often is not sufficient to obtain adequate eyelid akinesia, necessitating a separate facial nerve block. Alternatively, separate 2-mL injections into the superior and inferior peribulbar spaces may be adequate for ocular akinesia and anesthesia without causing conjunctival chemosis.

SUBCONJUNCTIVAL ANESTHESIA

In an attempt to reduce the risks of retrobulbar and peribulbar anesthesia, a number of investigators have proposed the use of subconjunctival anesthesia in ocular surgery.[1–7] Advocates of this technique for glaucoma surgery suggest that subconjunctival injection avoids the sudden increases in orbital pressure caused by retrobulbar or peribulbar anesthesia, which can compromise optic nerve head blood flow, exacerbating damage in patients with pre-existing advanced glaucomatous optic nerve atrophy. Second, the risks of retrobulbar injection, including retrobulbar hemorrhage, with its marked elevation of IOP, is eliminated. Third, the decreased exposure of the surgical field associated with peribulbar anesthesia is avoided.

A number of different techniques for subconjunctival block have been described. Peterson and Yanoff[1] injected 0.5 mL of lidocaine with hyaluronidase and epinephrine using a 27-gauge needle beneath the superior conjunctiva, 5 mm posterior to the limbus, supplementing it with topical anesthetics as required. Redmond Smith[8] suggested a similar technique for cataract extraction and intraocular lens implantation in which the anesthetic is injected under the limbal conjunctiva. No superior rectus stay suture was used in that technique.

Ritch and Liebmann[111] reported a technique for trabeculectomy that has now been used successfully in a series of more than 800 patients. After a modified van Lint–type eyelid block and placement of the speculum, topical tetracaine 0.5% solution is applied topically to the eye. An 8-0 polyglactin (Vicryl) traction suture (Fig. 4–3) is placed midthickness through clear cornea, approximately 1 mm anterior to the limbus. This traction suture has several advantages. It eliminates the need for large needle openings at the level of the superior rectus muscle and prevents trauma to the muscle itself. It also decreases the risk of subconjunctival hemorrhage. The eye can then be moved in any direction or fixated in any position by taping it to the operative drape. This flexibility limits

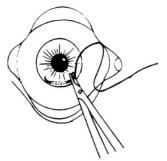

Figure 4–3. Placement of corneal traction suture using an 8-0 polyglactin suture.

the tension on the stretched conjunctiva and reduces the chance of inadvertently buttonholing it. At this point, approximately 1 mL of mepivacaine (Carbocaine) 2% or lidocaine (Xylocaine) 2% without epinephrine via a 30-gauge needle is injected beneath Tenon's capsule over the anterior portion of the superior rectus muscle (Fig. 4–4). One-half milliliter is then injected over the medial and lateral rectus muscles. Leaving the inferior rectus muscle unanesthetized allows for spontaneous infraduction, further improving exposure of the superior conjunctiva.

Concerns regarding sensation during iridectomy have proven to be unfounded, and only rarely do patients complain of discomfort at the time of iridectomy. Sensation at other points of the procedure, such as cauterization of scleral vessels or conjunctival closure, also seem not to be problematic because topical tetracaine has sufficed to relieve the discomfort, as is often done when retrobulbar or peribulbar anesthesia is used.

Although subconjunctival anesthesia has proven to be quite safe, complications can occur. Yanoff and Redovan[112] described a case of ocular perforation during subconjunctival injection. Rupture of the lens capsule as a result of unexpected motion of the eye has also been reported.[5] To prevent the risk of postoperative leak of the filtering bleb, one should use as small a needle as possible and enter the subconjunctival space at some distance from the proposed filtering site.

ANESTHESIA FOR OTHER PROCEDURES

For patients undergoing argon laser trabeculoplasty, laser iridotomy, peripheral iridoplasty, or laser goniosynechiolysis, nearly all authors

Figure 4–4. Sub-Tenon injection over the superior rectus muscle with the globe infraducted by the corneal traction suture. Injection over the medial and lateral rectus muscles can be performed in a similar manner.

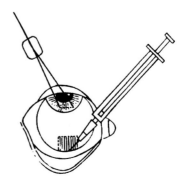

agree that topical anesthesia with proparacaine or tetracaine is sufficient. Cyclocryotherapy and cyclophotocoagulation, however, are painful procedures and, therefore, require more effective and longer acting anesthesia of sensory fibers of the ciliary body and conjunctiva. This may be achieved most readily by retrobulbar injection of a long-acting anesthetic such as bupivacaine 0.5% in an even mixture with a fast-acting agent such as lidocaine 2%. No eyelid block is necessary.

In an attempt to re-establish flow to a failed filtering procedure because of subconjunctival scarring, scleral flap scarring, or Tenon's cyst formation, the glaucoma surgeon may wish to perform transconjunctival needling of the surgical site. This can be performed by first applying topical tetracaine 0.5% and phenylephrine 2.5% to constrict the conjunctival vessels and reduce the risk of subconjunctival hemorrhage, which can limit visualization. With a 30-gauge needle on a tuberculin syringe filled with lidocaine 2%, the subconjunctival space is entered with the needle approximately 5 mm from the surgical site. The subconjunctival space is then expanded with the anesthetic as the needle is advanced to prevent inadvertent formation of a buttonhole. The needle tip is then used to separate any adhesions or to rupture a Tenon's cyst wall. To prevent any sudden movements that may lead to a conjunctival buttonhole, the patient should be informed that he or she may experience a mild burning sensation on injection of the anesthetic.

REFERENCES

1. Peterson WC, Yanoff M. Subconjunctival anesthesia: an alternative to retrobulbar and peribulbar techniques. Ophthalmic Surg 1991;22:199.
2. Ritch R, Liebmann JM. Sub-Tenon's anesthesia for trabeculectomy. Ophthalmic Surg 1992;23:502.
3. Furuta M, Toriumi T, Kashiwagi K, et al. Limbal anesthesia for cataract surgery. Ophthalmic Surg 1990;21:22.
4. Redmond RM, Dallas NL. Extracapsular cataract extraction under local anesthesia without retrobulbar injection. Br J Ophthalmol 1991;74:203.
5. Lichter PR. Avoiding complications from local anesthesia. Ophthalmology 1988; 95:565.
6. Diamond GR. Topical anesthesia for strabismus surgery. J Pediatr Ophthalmol Strabismus 1989;26:86.
7. Steele MA, Lavrich JB, Nelson LB, Koller HP. SubTenon's infusion of local anesthetic for stabismus surgery. Ophthalmic Surg 1992;23:40.
8. Redmond Smith JH. Why retrobulbar anesthesia? Br J Ophthalmol 1988;72:1.
9. Kishore K, Agarwal HC, Sood NN, Mandal AK. A modified technique of anterior peribulbar anesthesia. Indian J Ophthalmol 1991;39:166.
10. Bruce AB, McGoldrick KE, Oppenheimer P. Anesthesia for ophthalmology. Birmingham, AL: Aesculapius, 1982.
11. Barash PG, Cullen BF, Stoelting RK. Handbook of clinical anesthesia. Philadelphia: JB Lippincott, 1991.
12. Ellis EP, Esterdahl M. Echothiophate iodide therapy in children: effect upon blood cholinesterase levels. Arch Ophthalmol 1967;77:598.
13. Litwiller RW, DiFazio C, Rushia EL. Pancuronium and intraocular pressure. Anesthesiology 1975;42:750.
14. Yoshikawa K, Murai Y. The effect of ketamine on intraocular pressure in children. Anesth Analg 1971;50:199.
15. Purschke RI, Hassouna I. Der Einfluss von Ketamin auf den intraokularen Druck. Z Prakt Anaesth 1973;8:227.
16. Ausinsch B, Rayburn RL, Munson ES, et al. Ketamine and intraocular pressure in children. Anesth Analg 1976;55:773.
17. Peuler M, Glass DD, Arens JF. Ketamine and intraocular pressure. Anesthesiology 1975;43:575.
18. Miller RD, Way WL, Hickey RF. Inhibition of succinylcholine-induced intraocular pressure by non-depolarizing muscle relaxants. Anesthesiology 1968;29:123.

19. Eakins KE, Katz RL. The action of succinylcholine on the tension of extraocular muscle. Br J Pharmacol 1966;26:205.
20. Carballo AS. Succinylcholine and acetazolamide in anesthesia for ocular surgery. Can Anaesth Soc J 1986;12:486.
21. Indu B, Batra YK, Puri GD, et al. Nifedipine attenuates the intraocular pressure response to intubation following succinylcholine. Can J Anaesth 1989;36:269.
22. Magora F, Collins VJ. The influence of general anesthetic agents on intraocular pressure in man. Arch Ophthalmol 1962;66:806.
23. Holloway KB. Control of the eye during general anesthesia for intraocular surgery. Br J Anaesth 1980;52:671.
24. Ausinsch B, Graves GA, Munson ES, et al. Intraocular pressure in children during isoflurane and halothane anesthesia. Anesthesiology 1975;42:167.
25. Duncalf D, Foldes FF. Effect of anesthetic drugs and muscle relaxants on intraocular pressure. Int Ophthalmol Clin 1973;13:21.
26. Radtke N, Waldman J. The influence of enflurane anesthesia on intraocular pressure in youths. Anesth Analg 1975;54:212.
27. Tammisto T, Halalainen L, Tarkkanen L. Halothane and methoxyflurane in ophthalmic anesthesia. Acta Anaesthesiol Scand 1965;9:173.
28. Von Sallmann L, Lowenstein O. Responses of intraocular pressure, blood pressure and cutaneous vessels to electrical stimulation in the diencephalon. Am J Ophthalmol 1955;39:11.
29. Murphy DF. Anesthesia and intraocular pressure. Anesth Analg 1985;64:520.
30. Barclay K, Wall T. Intra-ocular pressure changes in patients with glaucoma: comparison between the laryngeal mask airway and tracheal tube. Anaesthesia 1994;49:159.
31. Mirakhur RK, Shepherd WFI. Intraocular pressure changes with propofol (Diprivan): comparison with thiopentone. Postgrad Med J 1985;61(suppl 3):41.
32. Badrinath SK, Vazurz A, McCarthy RJ, et al. The effect of different methods of inducing anesthesia on intraocular pressure. Anesthesiology 1986;65:431.
33. de Roetth A Jr, Schwartz H. Aqueous humor dynamics in glaucoma. Arch Ophthalmol 1956;55:755.
34. Leopold IH, Comroe JH. Effect of intramuscular administration of morphine, atropine, scopolamine and neostigmine on the human eye. Arch Ophthalmol 1948;40:285.
35. Mostafa SM, Lockhart A, Kumar D. Comparison of effects of fentanyl and alfentanyl on intraocular pressure. Anaesthesia 1986;41:493.
36. Al-Abrak MH. Diazepam and intraocular pressure. Br J Anaesth 1978;50:866.
37. Ivankovich AD, Lowe HJ. The influence of methoxyflurane and neurolepanalgesia on intraocular pressure. Br J Anaesth 1978;50:866.
38. Stoelting RK. Endotracheal intubation. In: Miller RD, ed. Anesthesia, vol 1. New York: Churchill Livingstone, 1986.
39. Blamoutos NG, Tsakona H, Tsakona H. Alcuronium and intraocular pressure. Anesth Analg 1983;62:521.
40. Cunningham AJ, Kelly PC, Kelly PC. Effect of metocurine pancuronium combination on IOP. Can Anaesth Soc J 1982;29:617.
41. Agarwal LP, Mathur SP. Curare in ocular surgery. Br J Ophthalmol 1952;36:603.
42. Van Aken H. Prevention of hypertension at intubation with intravenous lidocaine. Anesthesia 1982;37:82.
43. Sellick BA. Cricoid pressure to control regurgitation of stomach contents during induction of anesthesia, preliminary communication. Lancet 1961;2:404.
44. Calobrisi BL, Lebowitz P. Muscle relaxants and the open globe. Int Anesthesiol Clin 1990;28:83.
45. Schneider MJ, Stirt JA, Finholt DA. Atacurium, vecuronium, and intraocular pressure in humans. Anesth Analg 1986;65:877.
46. PrysRoberts C, Meloche R, Foex P. Studies of anesthesia in relation to hypertension: 1. Cardiovascular responses of treated and untreated patients. Br J Anaesth 1971;43:122.
47. Libonati MM, Leahy JJ, Ellison N. The use of succinylcholine in open eye surgery. Anesthesiology 1985;62:637.
48. Cunningham AJ, Barry P. Intraocular pressure physiology and implications for anesthesia management. Can Anaesth Soc J 1986;33:195.
49. Libonati MM. Complications of general anesthesia. In: Spaeth GL, Katz LJ, ed. Current therapy in ophthalmic surgery. Philadelphia: BC Decker, 1989.
50. Adams A, Fordham RMM. General anesthesia in adults. Int Ophthalmol Clin 1973;13:83.
51. Rosen DA. Anesthesia in ophthalmology. Can Anesth J 1962;9:545.
52. Drenger B, Pe'er J, Ben Ezra D. The effect of intravenous lidocaine on the increase in intraocular pressure induced by tracheal intubation. Anesth Analg 1985;64:1211.
53. Wheeler TM, Zimmerman TJ. Expulsive choroidal hemorrhage in the glaucoma patient. Ann Ophthalmol 1987;19:165.

54. Taylor DM. Expulsive hemorrhage: some observations and comments. Trans Am Ophthalmol Soc 1974;82:157.
55. Campbell JK. Expulsive choroidal hemorrhage and effusion—a reappraisal. Ann Ophthalmol 1980;12:332.
56. Frenkel REP, Shin DH. Prevention and management of delayed suprachoroidal hemorrhage after filtration surgery. Arch Ophthalmol 1986;104:1459.
57. Cantor LB, Katz LJ, Spaeth L. Complications of surgery in glaucoma: suprachoroidal expulsive hemorrhage in glaucoma patients undergoing intraocular surgery. Ophthalmology 1985;92:1265.
58. Ariano ML, Ball SF. Delayed nonexpulsive suprachoroidal hemorrhage after trabeculectomy. Ophthalmic Surg 1987;18:661.
59. Van Meurs JC, van den Bosch WA. Suprachoroidal hemorrhage following a Valsalva maneuver. Arch Ophthalmol 1993;111:1025.
60. Girard LJ, Spak KE, Hawkins RS, et al. Expulsive hemorrhage during intraocular surgery. Trans Am Acad Ophthalmol Otol 1973;77:119.
61. Gills JP, Rudisill JEL. Bupivacaine in cataract surgery. Ophthalmic Surg 1974;5:67.
62. Mindel JS. Value of hyaluronidase in ocular surgical akinesia. Am J Ophthalmol 1978;85:643.
63. Adraiani J. Newer anesthetics, sedatives, preoperative regimens. In: Symposium on Ocular Pharmacology and Therapeutics. St. Louis: CV Mosby, 1970.
64. Bryant JA. Local and topical anesthetics in ophthalmology. Surv Ophthalmol 1969;13:263.
65. Lufstrom B. Aspects of pharmacology of local anesthetic agents. Anaesthesiology 1970;42:194.
66. Lufstrom B, Green K, Jansson O, et al. An evaluation of bupivacaine (Marcaine) without adrenaline. Acta Anaesth Scand 1970;37(suppl):282.
67. Hørven I. Ophthalmic artery pressure, retrobulbar anesthesia. Acta Ophthalmol 1978;56:574.
68. Liebmann JL. Complications of glaucoma filtering surgery. In: Ritch R, Shields MB, Krupin T, eds. The glaucomas. St. Louis: CV Mosby, 1995, p 1704.
69. Krupin T, Ritch R, Camras CB, et al. A long Krupin-Denver valve implant attached to a 180° scleral explant for glaucoma surgery. Ophthalmology 1988;95:1174.
70. Schocket SS, Nivankari VS, Lakhanpal V, et al. Anterior chamber tube shunt to an encircling band in the treatment of neovascular glaucoma and other refractory glaucomas: a long-term study. Ophthalmology 1985;92:553.
71. Fiore PM, Richter CV, Arzeno G, et al. The effect of anterior chamber depth on endothelial cell count after filtration surgery. Arch Ophthalmol 1989;107:1609.
72. Smith DL, Skuta GL, Lindenmuth KA, et al. The effect of glaucoma filtering surgery on corneal endothelial cell density. Ophthalmic Surg 1991;22:251.
73. Coleman DJ, Trokel SL. Direct-recorded intraocular pressure variations in a human subject. Arch Ophthalmol 1969;82:637.
74. Katz LJ, Spaeth GL. Filtration surgery. In: Ritch R, Shields MB, Krupin T, eds. The glaucomas. St. Louis: CV Mosby, 1989, 653–657.
75. O'Brien CS. Akinesia during cataract extraction. Arch Ophthalmol 1929;1:447.
76. Spaeth GL. A new method to achieve complete akinesia of the facial nerve muscles of the eyelids. Ophthalmic Surg 1976;7:105.
77. Nadbath RP, Rehman I. Facial nerve block. Am J Ophthalmol 1963;55:143.
78. Wilson CA, Ruiz RS. Respiratory obstruction following the Nadbath facial nerve block. Arch Ophthalmol 1985;103:1454.
79. Schoch D. Complications of the Nadbath facial nerve block. Arch Ophthalmol 1986;104:1115.
80. Rabinowitz L, Livingston M, Schneider H, et al. Respiratory obstruction following the Nadbath facial nerve block. Arch Ophthalmol 1986;104:1115.
81. Lindquist TL, Kopietz LA, Spigelman AV, et al. Complications of Nadbath facial nerve block and a review of the literature. Ophthalmic Surg 1988;19:271.
82. Van Lint A. Paralysie palpébrale temporaire provoquée dans l'opération de la cataracte. Ann Ocul (Paris) 1914;151:420.
83. O'Donoghue E, Batterbury M, Lavy T. Effect on intraocular pressure of local anaesthesia in eyes undergoing intraocular surgery. Br J Ophthalmol 1994;78:605.
84. Fluorouracil Filtering Surgery Study Group T. Risk factors for suprachoroidal hemorrhage after filtering surgery. Am J Ophthalmol 1992;113:501.
85. Speaker MG, Guerriero PN, Met JA, et al. A case-control study of risk factors for intraoperative suprachoroidal expulsive hemorrhage. Ophthalmology 1991;98:202.
86. Antoszyk AN, Buckley EG. Contralateral decreased visual acuity and extraocular muscle palsies following retrobulbar anesthesia. Ophthalmology 1986;93:462.
87. Beltranena HP, Vega MJ, Garcia JJ, Blankenship G. Complications of retrobulbar marcaine injection. J Clin Neuroophthalmol 1982;2:159.
88. Berg P, Kroll P, Küchle HJ. Iatrogenic perforation of the globe during parabulbar and retrobulbar injections. Klin Monatsbl Augenheilkd 1986;93:1476.

89. Chang JL, Gonzalez-Abola E, Larson CE, Lobes L. Brainstem anesthesia following retrobulbar block. Anesthesiology 1984;16:716.
90. Duker JS, Belmont JB, Benson WE, et al. Inadvertant globe perforation during retrobulbar and peribulbar anesthesia: patient characteristics, surgical management and visual outcome. Ophthalmology 1991;98:519.
91. Follette JW, LoCasio JA. Bilateral amaurosis following unilateral retrobulbar block. Anesthesiology 1985;63:238.
92. Friedberg HL, Kline OR. Contralateral amaurosis after retrobulbar injection. Am J Ophthalmol 1986;101:688.
93. Hamilton RC. Brainstem anesthesia following retrobulbar blockade. Anesthesiology 1985;63:688.
94. Hay A, Flynn HWJ, Hoffman JI, Rivera AH. Needle penetration of the globe during retrobulbar and peribulbar injections. Ophthalmology 1991;98:1017.
95. Javitt JC, Addiego R, Friedberg HL, et al. Brain stem anesthesia after retrobulbar block. Ophthalmology 1987;94:718.
96. Jindra LF. Blindness following retrobulbar anesthesia for astigmatic keratotomy. Ophthalmic Surg 1989;20:433.
97. Labelle PF. Ocular complications associated with retrobulbar anesthesia. Ophthalmology 1988;95:1595.
98. Meyers EF. Brain-stem anesthesia after retrobulbar block. Arch Ophthalmol 1985;103:1278.
99. Mo XJ. Temporary amaurosis from retrobulbar lidocaine injection in late glaucoma patients. Chung Hua Yen Ko Tsa Chih 1991;27:265.
100. Morgan CM, Schatz H, Vine AK, et al. Ocular complications associated with retrobulbar injections. Ophthalmology 1988;95:660.
101. Pautler SE, Grizzard WS, Thompson LN, Wing GL. Blindness from retrobulbar injection into the optic nerve. Ophthalmic Surg 1986;17:334.
102. Ramsay RC, Knobloch WH. Ocular perforations following retrobulbar anesthesia for retinal detachment surgery. Am J Ophthalmol 1978;86:61.
103. Schneider ME, Milstein DE, Oyakawa RT, et al. Ocular perforation from a retrobulbar injection. Am J Ophthalmol 1988;106:35.
104. Rodman DJ, Notaro S, Peer GL. Respiratory depression following retrobulbar bupivacaine: three case reports and literature review. Ophthalmic Surg 1987;18:768.
105. McGalliard JN. Respiratory arrest after two retrobulbar injections. Am J Ophthalmol 1988;105:90.
106. Smith JL. Retrobulbar Marcaine can cause respiratory arrest. J Clin Neuroophthalmol 1981;1:171.
107. Rosenblatt RM, May DR, Barsoumian K. Cardiopulmonary arrest after retrobulbar block. Am J Ophthalmol 1980;90:425.
108. Meyers EF, Ramirez RC, Boniuk I. Grand mal seizures after retrobulbar block. Arch Ophthalmol 1978;96:847.
109. Wilson RP. Anesthesia. In: Spaeth GL, ed. Ophthalmic surgery: principles and practice. Philadelphia: WB Saunders, 1990, p 87.
110. Kimble JA, Morris RE, Witherspoon CD, et al. Globe perforation from peribulbar injection. Arch Ophthalmol 1987;105:749.
111. Ritch R, Liebmann JM. SubTenon's anesthesia for trabeculectomy. Ophthalmic Surg 1992;23:502.
112. Yanoff M, Redovan EG. Anterior eyewall perforation during subconjunctival cataract block. Ophthalmic Surg 1990;21:262.

CHAPTER 5

ANESTHESIA FOR EYE MUSCLE SURGERY

RENÉE RICHARDS, MD, FACS
STEPHEN N. LIPSKY, MD

The understanding and treatment of ocular misalignment, or strabismus, have evolved tremendously since the early studies of Fallopius in the 16th century. As techniques for correcting strabismus have progressed, so too have the methods of providing anesthesia to such patients.

Modern anesthesia can trace its roots to Dr. Karl Koller, an Austrian ophthalmologist, who in 1884 observed that cocaine could be used as a topical anesthetic for eye surgery. Strabismus surgery can be documented before this critical date. John Taylor is credited with the earliest surgical procedure to correct strabismus in 1739. Taylor proved simply to be a showperson and his procedure a ruse. Taylor would merely snip the conjunctiva of the deviating eye, patch the sound eye, and leave town before the chicanery was discovered.[1] Modern strabismus surgery began in 1838 with Stromeyer, who performed an extraocular muscle tenotomy on a cadaver eye, and Dieffenbach, who performed a myotomy of the medial rectus muscle of a 7-year-old child for esotropia. Anesthesia for these procedures consisted of little more than a good meal and good wine, combined with a firm restraint and a swift surgeon.[1]

Anesthesia has evolved from topical agents to ether to the modern methods of anesthesia used today. Many modern texts that serve the strabismologist and general ophthalmologist provide little detail on anesthesia techniques for strabismus patients. They often assume a skilled anesthesiologist will take charge of this aspect of surgery. Although the complexity of modern anesthesia demands the skill and training of anesthesiologists, ophthalmologists should understand the anesthesia techniques required by their specialty. The goal of this chapter is to acquaint ophthalmologists further with the complex nature of anesthesia for this condition so they can better choose the proper anesthesia for their patients.

Controversy exists surrounding the age at which local anesthesia can be substituted for general anesthesia and for what procedures each method should be used. Atkinson suggested that all patients younger than 10 years undergo general anesthesia and patients older than 65 years receive local anesthesia because of their increased medical risk.[2] Von Noorden indicated that apprehensive or nervous patients and those undergoing reoperation, surgery on the inferior rectus muscle as a result of thyroid disease, and surgery on the muscles of both eyes should have general anesthesia.[3]

It is paramount to consider that the proper anesthesia choice for each case is dictated by what will best suit the patient. This decision is further tempered by the experience and training of the particular surgeon, the complexity and duration of the case, and the suggestions and rules of the anesthesiologist.

GENERAL ANESTHESIA FOR PEDIATRIC STRABISMUS PATIENTS

The majority of strabismus surgery is performed on very young patients. Thus, general anesthesia is often used. Local anesthesia may be considered for an extremely cooperative older child. However, one must be cognizant of the fact that the alien environment of the operating suite combined with separation from parents may provoke uncontrolled anxiety and agitation in the most cooperative child, thus compromising the surgical situation.

General anesthesia in the pediatric population requires the ophthalmologist to have a mindful understanding of the procedures used. Furthermore, the ophthalmologist must be sensitive to the anxieties and conceptions of patient and parents. A dynamic and educational relationship between physician and family is advantageous. The care of the pediatric patient requires a team approach involving the pediatrician, ophthalmologist, and anesthesiologist. Communication among the three must be clear and concise to avoid confusion.

Anesthesia in the pediatric age group begins the moment the family enters the ophthalmologist's office. The setting should be pleasant to both parents and child and provide an atmosphere of comfort and confidence.[4] The child should be allowed as much autonomy as possible during the examination and given choices whenever possible. The child must be treated as an active member of the care team, regardless of age, and reference to the child in the third person should be avoided. Parents should be encouraged to ask questions and be given the opportunity to speak with the anesthesiologist. They can be reassured that the morbidity rate associated with elective ophthalmic procedures is extremely low.

MEDICAL EVALUATION OF THE PEDIATRIC STRABISMUS PATIENT

Children must be evaluated by a pediatrician once a decision to perform surgery using general anesthesia has been made. The examination should take place within 2 weeks of surgery because a child's health status may change suddenly. The evaluation is designed to identify risk factors that may compromise the outcome, determine the presence of acute or chronic medical problems, and determine whether the child is healthy enough to undergo the planned procedure.

Attention to recent exposure to infectious diseases is an essential component of the history. A child with a runny nose and no other systemic symptoms may suffer from allergic rhinitis. Although excessive secretions secondary to this condition may complicate general anesthesia, it is not a contraindication to surgery.[4] If antihistamines are being used before surgery, they should be continued until the day of surgery. Surgery on a patient with a history of exposure to infectious agents such as chickenpox within the prior 3 weeks and strep throat within 3 to 5 days probably should be postponed.[4]

Other systemic symptoms such as high temperature, lethargy, anorexia, purulent rhinorrhea, or productive cough may suggest the presence of a more serious infection, and surgery should be postponed until symptoms have resolved. A review of pediatric cases with upper respiratory tract infections (URIs) demonstrated that the risk of respiratory complications was increased two to seven times in children with a URI compared with those without.[5] These children should be re-evaluated before elective surgical intervention.

Otitis media often affects the pediatric patient and should be carefully checked. Acute otitis media should be resolved before any elective surgical intervention and should be assessed by a pediatrician. A child taking prophylactic medication for chronic otitis media usually can undergo general anesthesia safely.[4]

MEDICATIONS

A drug history is vital in the pediatric population. Phospholine Iodide (echothiophate iodide) is often used in the management of strabismus. This medication interferes with systemic pseudocholinesterase activity and makes patients sensitive to prolonged effects from depolarizing agents such as succinylcholine and ester-based local anesthetics. This medication should be discontinued 4 to 6 weeks before surgery.[1] Residual effects from this medication can persist for months after discontinuation. If any question remains, these agents should not be used. Nondepolarizing agents should be used for neuromuscular blockade. Most other medications should be continued up until surgery. This is vital in patients with conditions such as asthma, seizures, delayed gastric emptying, and so on. A history of second-hand smoke is also pertinent.

Postoperative nausea and emesis are responsible for the majority of admissions after ambulatory strabismus surgery.[6–8] Often these children are found to have a history of motion sickness preoperatively. A history of motion sickness should be noted and can alert the surgeon to the need for perioperative emesis control.

A history of easy bruising, bleeding gums, bleeding into deep tissues or joints, and excessive bleeding with previous surgery should alert the physician to a possible bleeding disorder. One should also inquire about aspirin use. A positive history of anesthesia complications should also be noted and communicated to the anesthesiologist.

FAMILY HISTORY

Family history is important for investigating bleeding disorders, allergies, asthma, congenital anomalies, and possible adverse reactions to anesthesia. Malignant hyperthermia has been found to be a familial trait. Helveston[1] recommended that patients with a family history of malignant hyperthermia be pretreated with dantrolene and the anesthesia equipment be purged with oxygen for 24 hours before surgery to remove any traces of halothane. Phenylketopyruvate serum levels, muscle biopsy, and the in vitro caffeine halothane contracture test may be indicated.[9] Halothane should be avoided, and fentanyl, nitrous oxide, and nondepolarizing muscle relaxants should be substituted. A link among blepharoptosis, strabismus, and malignant hyperthermia has been proposed,[4] and the presence of ptosis and strabismus should raise a suspicion for malignant hyperthermia.

SYSTEMIC DISEASE

Certain systemic conditions are common to the pediatric population and require special attention. Both pediatricians and anesthesiologists may communicate the systemic status of a patient using the American Society of Anesthesiologists (ASA) Physical Status Ranking (Table 5–1).

Table 5–1. American Society of Anesthesiologists Physical Status Ranking

Class	Description
I	Healthy patient
II	Mild systemic disease* (no functional limitation)
III	Severe systemic disease* (definite functional limitation)
IV	Severe systemic disease that is a constant threat to life
V	Moribund patient not expected to survive 24 hours with or without operation

*Regardless of whether the systemic disease is cause of surgery.

Subacute Bacterial Endocarditis

A history of congenital or acquired cardiac abnormalities may necessitate prophylaxis for subacute bacterial endocarditis. These include valvular heart disease (rheumatic and acquired), prosthetic heart devices, previous bacterial endocarditis, mitral valve prolapse (with regurgitation), idiopathic hypertrophic subaortic stenosis, congenital heart disease (except for isolated secundum atrial septal defect), patent ductus arteriosus (less than 6 months after repair), atrial septal defect without patch (less than 6 months after repair), and possibly cardiac transplantation.[10] Current recommendations for prophylaxis include ampicillin, 50 mg/kg intravenously (maximum 2 g), 30 minutes before surgery and half the initial dose in 6 hours. In penicillin-allergic patients, clindamycin, 10 mg/kg (maximum 300 mg), can be substituted. Oral prophylaxis includes amoxicillin, 50 mg/kg (maximum 3 g), and erythromycin, 20 mg/kg (maximum 800 mg), or clindamycin, 10 mg/kg (maximum 300 mg), in the penicillin-allergic patient. See Table 5–2.

Asthma

The incidence of asthma in children is increasing, necessitating an increased awareness of this condition by surgeons and anesthesiologists.[11] The goal of the anesthesiologist in these patients is to avoid triggering bronchospasm, which may induce an asthmatic attack. It is recommended that relatively deep halothane anesthesia be used in these patients to avoid inciting an attack. The degree of concern is dependent on the preoperative asthmatic control in each patient. Patients under good control often tolerate routine anesthesia well. Those patients with a recent history of a steroid-dependent episode or those on chronic steroids may have a blunted steroid stress response and may require supplemental steroids at the time of surgery. The effect of inhaled corticosteroids is not completely understood at this time, and their use should be considered in the preoperative assessment. It is advisable to consider postponing elective surgery in asthmatics if wheezing is discovered preoperatively.[4] The presence of an early URI must be ruled out, especially if it is associated with other symptoms. A chest x-ray film is recommended in the preoperative evaluation of the asthmatic.[4]

Diabetes Mellitus

Pediatric diabetic patients often are difficult to control in the operative setting. Care must be taken to prevent hypoglycemia during surgery

Table 5–2. Subacute Bacterial Endocarditis Guidelines

Dosing Regimen		Dose	Max	Timing
Patient NPO				
Standard	Ampicillin IM, IV	50 mg/kg	2 g	30 min prior
PCN allergic	Clindamycin	10 mg/kg	300 mg	Follow-up dose should be one-half the initial dose in 6 hr
Patient NPO and High Risk				
Standard	Ampicillin IM, IV and	50 mg/kg	2 g	30 min prior
	Gentamicin IM, IV	2 mg/kg	80 mg	Follow-up dose should be one-half the initial dose in 8 hr
PCN allergic	Vancomycin IV over 1 hr	20 mg/kg	1 g	No follow-up dose
Patient NPO for GU or GI Procedures				
Standard	Ampicillin IM, IV and	50 mg/kg	2 g	30 min prior and in 8 hr IV (alternate follow-up)
	Gentamicin IM, IV	2 mg/kg	80 mg	and 25 mg/kg amoxicillin PO every 6 hr
PCN allergic	Vancomycin IV over 1 hr and	20 mg/kg	1 g	1 hr prior and repeat in 8 hr
	Gentamicin IV	2 mg/kg	80 mg	
Patient Can Take Oral Medication				
Standard	Amoxicillin PO	50 mg/kg	3 g	Follow-up dose should be one-half the initial dose in 6 hr
PCN allergic	Erythromycin PO or	20 mg/kg	800 mg	
	Clindamycin PO	10 mg/kg	300 mg	

Indicated for	*Not Recommended for*
Prosthetic cardiac valves	Isolated secundum ASD
Previous bacterial endocarditis	Postrepair ASD, VSD, or PDA (>6 mo postrepair)
Surgically constructed systemic-pulmonary shunts	Mitral valve prolapse without regurgitation
Most congenital cardiac malformations	Innocent heart murmurs
Rheumatic and acquired valvular dysfunction	Previous Kawasaki syndrome without valvular dysfunction
Hypertrophic cardiomyopathy	Previous rheumatic fever without valvular dysfunction
Mitral valve prolapse with regurgitation	Endotracheal intubation

GI = gastrointestinal; GU = genitourinary; PCN = penicillin; NPO = nothing by mouth; IM = intramuscular; IV = intravenous; PO = oral; ASD = atrial septal defect; VSD = ventricular septal defect; PDA = patent ductus arteriosus.
Adapted from Dajani AS, Bisno AL, Chung KJ, et al. Prevention of bacterial endocarditis: a statement for health professionals from the Committee on Rheumatic Fever, Endocarditis, and Kawasaki Disease of the Council on Cardiovascular Disease in the Young, the American Heart Association. JAMA 1990;264:2919. Copyright 1990, American Medical Association.

while avoiding ketosis and diabetic ketoacidosis. Juvenile diabetics with good metabolic control may be admitted the morning of surgery. A normal meal and midnight snack should be consumed the day before surgery along with normal insulin doses. The ambulatory juvenile diabetic should receive two thirds of the long-acting insulin and no short-acting insulin the morning of surgery. These patients should be placed on the surgical schedule as early as possible. Careful intraoperative monitoring of blood glucose levels should be performed and maintenance fluids provided. The blood glucose levels should be checked postoperatively and adjusted as needed. If glucose control is achieved and the patients are able to take oral liquids well, they may be discharged into the care of a competent adult.

Brittle juvenile diabetics should be admitted the night before surgery for proper management of carbohydrates, insulin, and fluids. These patients should also be placed first on the operative schedule with careful intraoperative fluid, insulin, and glucose control. Less stable diabetics should be monitored postoperatively until they are stable. A preoperative urinalysis for ketones is advisable in these patients.[4]

Down Syndrome

Down syndrome may be associated with ophthalmic disorders such as strabismus. Several systemic malformations and ailments should be kept in mind when performing surgery on a child with Down syndrome. Most notable is an increased incidence of C1-2 instability. If present, these patients are at risk for spinal cord trauma during the extension of the neck during intubation. Radiologic evaluation of the cervical spine should be conducted to detect asymptomatic atlantoaxial instability if unknown before surgery.[4] If present, excessive extension of the neck should be avoided. Jaw thrust methods or fiberoptic laryngoscopes should be used for intubation.

Down syndrome patients have an increased incidence of congenital cardiac abnormalities, and these should be addressed as discussed later. Facial and airway abnormalities are also common. Down syndrome patients are at increased risk of airway obstruction as a result of macroglossia, subglottic stenosis, frequent URIs, and hypertrophied tonsillar and adenoid tissues. Therefore, it is recommended that these patients be fully awake before extubation so that the airway musculature is functioning.[4] Furthermore, these patients have an increased incidence of thyroid disease, malabsorption, and leukemia. Although it is controversial, patients with Down syndrome may demonstrate an increased sensitivity to atropine, which should be taken into account when choosing premedication and in the face of the oculocardiac reflex. Preoperative assessment for all the associated conditions just listed is mandatory to ensure safe anesthesia in Down syndrome patients.

Sickle-Cell Disease

Sickle-cell disease should be sought in all patients with an ethnic predisposition: blacks and Mediterranean populations. Preoperative evaluation should include hemoglobin electrophoresis and hematocrit. If the hemoglobin S is greater than 40%, transfusions are recommended to keep it below this level. Perioperative dehydration and hypoxia, which may promote sickling and operative stress, should be prevented.

Cerebral Palsy

Cerebral palsy patients are at an increased anesthesia risk because of recurrent seizures, gastroesophageal reflux, and joint contractures. Optimization of the antiseizure regimen is mandatory before any elective surgical procedure. Because of increased incidence of gastroesophageal reflux, a longer period of preoperative fasting is recommended.[4]

Congenital Syndromes

Many congenital syndromes produce craniofacial or airway abnormalities, which may complicate anesthesia in these patients. The anesthesiologist should be made aware of the presence of these conditions so that special equipment, such as fiberoptic bronchoscopes, can be made available and the possible need for tracheostomy or intensive care unit admission can be discussed with the parents.

The majority of pediatric patients undergoing strabismus surgery can be admitted the same day as surgery. The rare patient with systemic disease as discussed previously should be admitted the night before for stabilization of the disease process (e.g., diabetic control, subacute bacterial endocarditis prophylaxis). Discharge the same day as surgery is possible in the majority of strabismus patients. Again, patients manifesting any complications from systemic illnesses should be observed. Children younger than 1 year should be operated on in a facility that can easily support admission for observation if necessary.

PREOPERATIVE LABORATORY EVALUATION

Preoperative laboratory assessment in the pediatric strabismus patient is controversial. Many authorities believe that if the child is healthy and is monitored by a pediatrician, no preoperative laboratory tests are needed. Laboratory tests rarely alter the decision to perform surgery; rather, the systemic evaluation described previously is primarily used to determine whether a patient is suitable for surgery. The authors believe that a complete blood count (CBC) should be performed on all patients. This will provide a baseline hemoglobin and hematocrit and help rule out occult anemia. This also allows the white blood count (WBC) to be evaluated after a recent URI. As discussed, asthmatics should have a preoperative chest x-ray film. Patients with congenital heart disease should have a cardiology evaluation and testing. Juvenile diabetics require preoperative glucose levels and possibly hemoglobin A_{1c} testing to check control. Preoperative urinalysis in diabetic patients can detect ketone spilling. Trisomy 21 syndrome patients should have cervical spine films, thyroid function tests, vitamin A level tests, and a WBC to rule out leukemia. Blacks and Mediterranean patients should have hemoglobin electrophoresis in addition to a CBC. Cerebral palsy patients should have serum levels of anticonvulsant drugs measured to ensure therapeutic levels.

PREOPERATIVE FAST

The current recommendations for pediatric preoperative fasting at our institution is restriction of solid food for 8 hours before surgery and clear liquids (water, flat soda, Kool-Aid, dilute apple juice) up to 3 hours before surgery. Patients with delayed gastric emptying should be restricted from all oral intake for at least 8 hours before surgery.

On the day of surgery, it is essential that the child not get lost in the activity. The child's questions and fears should be given special care and attention, with answers he or she can comprehend. It is the surgeon's responsibility to make sure the child is at ease and feels in control. This can often be accomplished by taking time to educate the parents fully about the procedure. Parental anxiety is easily picked up by the child. The child should be allowed to bring his or her favorite toy to the operating room so that the experience is not completely foreign. At our institution, children are given a strawberry- or bubble gum–scented mask to play with preoperatively, which they bring to the operating room with them. When induction is begun via mask anesthesia, the child is familiar with his or her mask.

Parents should be given the opportunity to be present for induction and recovery because this will serve to calm an anxious child. We have observed that postoperative pain control and sedation are required less often when a parent is present. Parents should be made aware of what to expect during these procedures and at what point their exit will be requested. This will prevent confusion and distress in the operating room.

These techniques are not without failure, and often a child is inconsolable and must be restrained to induce anesthesia. Again, parents should be aware of this possibility, and all efforts should be made to comfort the child. Conversation in the operating room should be professional and aimed at reassuring the child. Humor is inappropriate while anesthesia is being administered. A child may interpret comments as being directed toward him or her, which can intensify the insecurity and psychological trauma associated with the event. It is important to be aware that an unpleasant experience may affect the child's future responses to health care providers.

General anesthesia and the complex monitoring required are primarily the responsibility of the anesthesiologist. Anesthesia often begins with premedication. With the shift toward outpatient surgery, premedication of pediatric patients is often omitted.[1] Excessive premedication can produce extended sedation of the young patient, and preoperative narcotics have been associated with an increased incidence of postoperative nausea and vomiting. Atropine, .01 mg/kg, has been recommended for preoperative anesthesia in infants, with a maximum dose of .4 mg and a minimum of .1 mg. If premedication is necessary, oral midazolam (Versed) administered in a grape-flavored liquid has replaced diazepam for outpatient surgery.[1] The dose of midazolam ranges from .5 to .75 mg/kg and should be adjusted for the patient. Patients with potential airway obstruction as a result of congenital malformation, Down syndrome, tonsillar hypertrophy, and so on should not receive premedication. A patient with a depressed respiratory drive should probably not receive any premedication.

Controversy exists as to whether antiemetic medication should be part of premedication.[7, 8, 12] A study by Lin and Furst[12] showed that patients medicated with droperidol, .075 mg/kg, or metoclopramide, .25 mg/kg, had a significantly decreased incidence of postoperative nausea without excessive sedation. Studies have shown these medications to be superior to lidocaine for control of nausea.

In preparation for induction, it is important to be aware of the equipment that should be available to provide safe anesthesia to children. Auscultation of the patient's heart and lungs and monitoring of an electrocardiogram and the patient's blood pressure and temperature should be performed. Pulse oximetry with an audible pulse tone will allow the surgeon to recognize bradycardia associated with the oculocardiac reflex rapidly. End-tidal carbon dioxide is essential for monitoring for malignant hyperthermia.

Mask anesthesia of an inhalational agent such as halothane, fluroxene, or desflurane is often used for induction. As mentioned, this is often facilitated by allowing the child to play with the mask in the preoperative area. As soon as the child is asleep, intravenous access should be achieved. If bradycardia or hypotension is encountered during induction, the anesthetic agent should be discontinued, and atropine, .01 to .02 mg/kg, along with intravenous fluids, calcium, and epinephrine should be used. Intramuscular ketamine, 1 to 3 mg/kg, is reserved for the uncooperative child. Ketamine is associated with nystagmus, increased secretions, and loss of airway reflexes. Atropine may aid in decreasing excessive secretions.

Intubation should proceed with a proper sized (RAE) endotracheal tube (see Chapter 11, Figs. 11–2, 11–3) to protect the airway. This J-shaped tube allows maintenance of the airway while keeping the endotracheal tube and anesthesia lines away from the surgical field. The uncuffed construction of the RAE tube helps to decrease tracheal trauma in children younger than 10 years and allows for a slight leak around the tube. Gauze may be placed between the lips to decrease the escape of the volatile agents into the operating room. Depolarizing neuromuscular blocking agents such as succinylcholine have fallen out of favor. Among other problems, succinylcholine interferes with forced duction testing by increasing the force necessary to move the globe.[9] Neuromuscular blockade is frequently not used. A nondepolarizing agent such as pancuronium may be used to ease intubation.

A major development for pediatric anesthesia is the laryngeal mask. This mask-like device covers the entrance to the trachea without cannulating the trachea. It has been found to be less irritating to the airway and is not associated with an increase in intraocular pressure, which is observed with standard endotracheal intubation.[4] The risk of aspiration of gastric contents may be increased slightly with this device. The laryngeal mask is not recommended for long procedures.

Propofol (Diprivan) represents a new method of providing general anesthesia through an intravenous route. Diprivan has been associated with less postoperative emesis and a shorter time from extubation to discharge.[13–15] Induction can be achieved through mask anesthesia described previously or with propofol alone. The induction dose is 2 to 3 mg/kg, and maintenance anesthesia is achieved with an intravenous drip of 160 to 200 μg/kg/min.[16] This may be supplemented with an inhalational agent.

Alternatively, inhalational agents can be used for maintenance of anesthesia. Intraoperative administration of analgesics, muscle relaxants, and antiemetic medications is based on duration of surgery, the practices of the institution or anesthesiologist, and the particular patient. Desflurane is becoming a more popular inhalational agent for outpatient general anesthesia in adults because of its rapid recovery profile.[13]

Emergence from anesthesia can be aided by the surgeon's informing the anesthesiologist of the expected duration of the procedure. Removal of the endotracheal tube will be associated with less coughing if the child is under deep anesthesia, because laryngeal reflexes are reduced. This may be associated with an increased risk of airway complications such as laryngospasm if secretions irritate the larynx.[17] Some anesthesiologists suggest that infants younger than 6 months and patients with

Down syndrome or cerebral palsy be awake before extubation because all active reflexes will be present.[4]

Each patient should be observed in the recovery area until the baseline level of alertness has returned. Pain, nausea, bleeding, and airway problems should be controlled before discharge, and the patient should be afebrile. If these variables cannot be controlled, the child may need to be admitted for observation and control. Controversy exists about oral intake of fluids in the pediatric patient. Oral intake earlier than 8 hours after general anesthesia has been associated with an increased incidence of nausea and vomiting.[6-8] Some anesthesiologists, however, insist on oral intake by children before discharge. This practice may produce nausea and vomiting in some children. Transportation home from ambulatory surgery may induce nausea and vomiting in children, and parents should be aware of this. Antiemetics may be suggested before long automobile trips home from the hospital.

Although present, morbidity associated with anesthesia for strabismus surgery is extremely low. A study by Romano and Robinson[18] showed no incidences of mortality or permanent morbidity. Reversible morbidity was found in 11.6% of cases.

POSTOPERATIVE CROUP

A barking cough postoperatively is suggestive of constriction of the airway and is referred to as postoperative croup. This condition is manifested by cough, stridor, chest retractions, wheezing, and cyanosis. The small radius of a child's airway is responsible for this condition.[4] The resistance to flow in a cylinder is inversely proportional to the radius of the lumen raised to the fourth power. Thus, as little as 1 mm of edema in a child's airway may increase resistance to airflow greater than five times that of an adult with similar edema. Furthermore, the cross-sectional area is decreased by almost 75%. If postoperative croup is encountered, nebulized racemic epinephrine should be used. Observation should be maintained until symptoms have abated and pulse oximetry is mandatory. When stable for at least 4 hours, discharge can be considered.

HEAT LOSS

Heat loss is a serious concern in the very young child because of the increased surface area. The operating room should be warmed, the child should remain covered, and warmed or humidified gases can be used.

OCULOCARDIAC REFLEX

The oculocardiac reflex has its afferent limb in the trigeminal system and its efferent limb in the vagal system. It is believed to be triggered by pressure on the globe, a tight-fitting speculum, and traction on the extraocular muscles, especially the medial rectus muscle, as well as on other orbital tissues. The oculocardiac reflex is associated with bradycardia and may cause hypotension, asystole, and ventricular dysrhythmias. The reported incidence of this reflex ranges from 10 to 82%. Strabismus patients not pretreated with atropine have a reported 90% incidence.[4, 9] The use of atropine for premedication has no effect on the incidence of this complication because much higher doses are required to guard against it. The afferent limb of the reflex can be blocked by a retrobulbar anesthetic. Retrobulbar injection, however, has inherent risks and is not advocated. Tetracaine drops may be applied to the surgical field in an attempt to decrease the afferent limb of the reflex. Deep anesthesia may be of help in patients prone to the oculocardiac reflex. Adequate oxygenation should be carefully maintained in the face of this reflex. Some sources recommend routine preoperative atropine, .02 mg/kg.[9]

Intraoperative management depends on the severity of the reflex. The most important element of management is early recognition by the surgeon. An audible pulse tone from the pulse oximeter allows the surgeon to sense bradycardia rapidly. If bradycardia is encountered, the surgeon must release tension on the extraocular muscles. Muscle hooks should be relaxed and not removed because removing them may increase tension on the muscle.[1] Small amounts of bradycardia without hypotension may be tolerated. Bradycardia associated with hypotension or an irregular rhythm requires cessation of surgery, and the heart rate should be allowed to return to normal. Atropine, .01 mg/kg IV may be given, and one should observe for tachycardia before surgery resumes. One should note that intravenous atropine has been associated with asystole in the presence of the oculocardiac reflex; therefore, a normal rhythm should be present before injection of atropine. Ventricular arrhythmia may require intravenous lidocaine, 1 to 2 mg/kg. If the reflex is persistent or recurrent, a parabulbar infusion of 1 to 3 mL of 2% lidocaine via a sub-Tenon's infusion cannula, such as the Greenbaum cannula, or a retrobulbar injection may block the afferent limb of this reflex. The reflex has been observed to fatigue with each successive event. Younger patients are more susceptible to this event. Hertle and colleagues[19] suggested that patients with a positive intraoperative oculocardiac reflex are more likely to suffer a similar reflex if sutures are adjusted postoperatively. Perioperative fatalities have been attributed to the oculocardiac reflex, and the potential seriousness of this reflex must be considered.

NAUSEA AND VOMITING

Postoperative nausea is the most common reason for admission to the hospital after ambulatory strabismus surgery.[6] Patients with a preoperative history of motion sickness may be at increased risk for this complication. Postoperative nausea complicates 40 to 85% of cases without attempt at prophylaxis. Some studies have shown that preoperative droperidol, .075 mg/kg, or metoclopramide, .25 mg/kg, given before any manipulation of tissues dramatically reduces the incidence of emesis compared to controls.[12] This treatment did not delay the time to recovery, and no extrapyramidal side effects were noted. Controversy exists over the use of lidocaine for emesis control. Propofol, an intravenous general anesthetic, is associated with less postoperative emesis and faster recovery and may have inherent antiemetic properties.[13]

Factors that may contribute to postoperative nausea, such as pain, intraoperative muscle manipulation, narcotics, and postoperative movement, should be kept to a minimum. The oculogastric reflex has been implicated by some researchers as a possible cause.[9] It has been suggested that patients not be forced to consume fluids because this may increase nausea.

Trimethobenzamide hydrochloride (Tigan) suppositories may be used postoperatively to control nausea. The dose of trimethobenzamide hydrochloride is 100 mg rectally for children weighing less than 30 pounds and 100 to 200 mg rectally for children weighing 30 to 90 pounds. Parents can be given a prescription for this medication at the time of discharge.

PAIN CONTROL

Pain control is often underemphasized in pediatric patients. They often cannot verbalize pain, and physicians are reluctant to treat pain aggressively in children for fear of overdosage. Pain can contribute to nausea, vomiting, and airway irritation from crying. Narcotics should be avoided, and acetaminophen, orally or rectally, should be used for mild to moderate pain. Elixer of acetaminophen and codeine is also useful. For more severe pain, intramuscular or intravenous fentanyl may be given.

MALIGNANT HYPERTHERMIA

Malignant hyperthermia is a potentially fatal complication of anesthesia. It is often triggered by inhalational agents such as halothane and depolarizing agents such as succinylcholine. Exposure to these agents causes the sarcoplasmic reticulum of skeletal muscle to release calcium to the intracellular space. This may cascade into a fatal metabolic derangement.

The mortality rate from malignant hyperthermia has dropped from approximately 70% before the introduction of dantrolene to about 10% since its introduction. The incidence of malignant hyperthermia ranges from 1 in 5000 to 1 in 260,000 and is dependent on the criteria used to define malignant hyperthermia.[4, 9] A family history of unexplained perioperative death should raise suspicion about familial malignant hyperthermia. The inheritance pattern has been classified as autosomal dominant, autosomal recessive, and sporadic.

There may be an increased incidence of malignant hyperthermia in patients with strabismus, blepharoptosis, inguinal hernia, increased muscle bulk, focal muscle weakness, and muscle cramps.[4] It is advisable to avoid anesthetics that may potentiate malignant hyperthermia in patients with generalized muscle disorders such as Duchenne's muscular dystrophy and others. Because sensitization is required in many cases, a previous uneventful episode of anesthesia does not rule out the possibility of malignant hyperthermia.

Classic malignant hyperthermia is characterized by a rapid increase in body temperature, associated with muscle rigidity, tachycardia, dysrhythmias, rhabdomyolysis, acidosis (pH <7.25), increased end-tidal partial pressure of carbon dioxide (>60 mm Hg), hyperkalemia (potassium >6 mmol/L), and eventually disseminated intravascular coagulation. Successful treatment is dependent on early diagnosis. If treated, the patient should be observed and monitored for at least 24 hours after the event.

MASSETER MUSCLE RIGIDITY

Masseter muscle rigidity is often encountered after succinylcholine administration and is believed to be an exaggerated normal response to the medication. Masseter muscle rigidity has been associated with malignant hyperthermia, especially in severe cases in which the jaws cannot be separated. In cases of severe masseter muscle rigidity, the prudent action is to discontinue anesthesia and observe the patient for clinical and laboratory signs of malignant hyperthermia as described previously. Urine myoglobin and blood creatine kinase (CK) levels should be followed in recovery. CK levels greater than 15,000 IU portend a high probability of susceptibility to malignant hyperthermia. A patient who experiences masseter muscle rigidity of a severe degree should probably undergo muscle biopsy.[9]

Less severe episodes of masseter muscle rigidity may allow continuation of anesthesia with careful detail to biochemical indicators of malignant hyperthermia. End-tidal carbon dioxide levels are most valuable in the early detection of malignant hyperthermia. Tachycardia is also valuable in early detection. Temperature elevation is a late sign, and muscle rigidity may not be observed.

In summary, general anesthesia is used in the majority of pediatric strabismus cases performed. Outpatient management of the patients now predominates. It is the surgeon's responsibility to ensure that proper communication among him- or herself, the pediatrician, and the anesthesiologist is coordinated. Morbidity and mortality rates for this surgery under general anesthesia are reassuringly low. It is imperative that the surgeon be familiar with the anesthetic procedures performed on his or her patients and the potential risks involved. This understanding produces a team approach to patient care that will ultimately benefit the patient.

GENERAL ANESTHESIA FOR ADULT STRABISMUS PATIENTS

The approach to anesthesia for the adult strabismus patient is determined primarily by the procedure proposed. This decision is modified by the experience of the surgeon and the customs of the institution. Cases involving adult and mature adolescent patients allow more variation in the choice of anesthesia for strabismus surgery because of the improved techniques. Traditionally, complex adult strabismus cases involving re-operation, endocrine myopathy, restrictive disease, postscleral buckle surgery, oblique surgery, and paretic syndromes have been designated as indicating general anesthesia.[3] These situations require extensive dissection, which frequently results in extended surgical time and potentially greater orbital pain, which may prevent the use of local anesthesia.

General anesthesia should also be considered for the mature patient with a history of labile anxiety or mental retardation.

The psychological aspects of general anesthesia in the adult population may be less complex than with children. It is imperative, nonetheless, to be attentive to patients' anesthesia concerns, and an ample opportunity for patients to ask questions of the surgeon and the anesthesiologist should be provided. A coordinated approach to the adult strabismus patient encompasses the surgeon, the anesthesiologist, and, in cases involving systemic disease, the internist.

As with children, general anesthesia in adults is relatively safe. It has been found[2] that myocardial oxygen demand is increased more by local anesthesia than general anesthesia. Systemic medical conditions often are present in adult patients, which may be exacerbated by stress such as surgery. The ASA Physical Status Ranking for adult patients should be determined by a thorough history and physical examination. A history of any anesthesia complications is a vital element in the adult patient. Concurrent medical conditions should be recorded and evaluated thoroughly preoperatively if they pose a risk to general anesthesia. The physical examination should focus on the cardiopulmonary system and upper airway. Medications should be reviewed. Antihypertensive and antiarrhythmic medications can alter the amount of anesthetic required. Glaucoma patients taking echothiophate iodide (Phospholine Iodide) are at significant risk for an exaggerated and prolonged response to depolarizing neuromuscular agents. This medication must be discontinued at least 4 to 6 weeks before surgery. Smoking and alcohol use are known to affect the amount of anesthesia required and should be discouraged before surgery.

PREOPERATIVE LABORATORY TESTING

The majority of preoperative laboratory tests required for general anesthesia have been found to be unnecessary. Currently, general screening tests are recommended in addition to a tailored laboratory evaluation when associated medical conditions are present. In the past, a preoperative hemoglobin concentration of 10 g/dL was considered a requirement for surgery, and transfusions were recommended to reach this level if preoperative anemia was detected. The risks associated with blood transfusion are similar to those of general anesthesia; therefore, transfusions before elective surgery such as strabismus surgery are not advised. In the elective surgery setting, it is preferred to determine the underlying cause for anemia and institute therapy before surgery. Most medical problems and laboratory abnormalities discovered preoperatively for elective surgery should be handled in this fashion. Patients with concurrent medical problems require the internist's or medical subspecialist's involvement before ambulatory strabismus surgery. Decisions to postpone surgery are more often based on the patient's medical condition than the results of laboratory tests.

PREMEDICATION

Premedication protocols vary with the customs of the particular institutions, physicians, and patients involved. Because of the ambulatory nature of most strabismus surgery, premedication is frequently omitted. Benzodiazepines such as diazepam or midazolam are very effective for the particularly anxious patient and may be given orally or intramuscularly. Atropine should be used on a selective basis. Narcotics should be avoided because of their association with postoperative nausea and vomiting.

INDUCTION

A combined intravenous-inhalation induction technique is appropriate for strabismus patients undergoing general anesthesia. A short-acting intravenous anesthetic medication such as thiopental, 3 to 6 mg/kg, or midazolam is used to induce unconsciousness. Inhalational agents can then be administered via mask when the patient is unaware of the discomfort associated with the anesthesia mask and the disagreeable odor of the gas. Narcotic use is associated with increased postoperative nausea and vomiting and should be kept to a minimum, especially in the ambulatory surgery setting.

After induction, the patient is intubated with or without neuromuscular blockade. As discussed, depolarizing agents such as succinylcholine have been linked to masseter muscle rigidity and malignant hyperthermia. Furthermore, spurious results may be encountered on forced duction testing[9] when succinylcholine is used. Maintenance and emergence are similar to those described previously.

OCULOCARDIAC REFLEX

The oculocardiac reflex may complicate strabismus surgery in adults and should be prevented or corrected rapidly should it develop. Surgery should cease, and all traction on the extraocular muscles must be relaxed if bradycardia is observed.[1] Atropine should be administered as necessary. Restoration of a normal heart rate and rhythm is essential before injecting atropine because asystole has been associated with atropine use in the face of the oculocardiac reflex. If atropine fails to correct the problem or recurrent bradycardia occurs, either a retrobulbar or parabulbar infusion of 1 to 3 mL of 2% lidocaine can block the afferent loop of this reflex. A rebound tachycardia must be documented before continuing surgery.

PROPOFOL

Propofol (Diprivan) is a relatively new medication that is used for intravenous induction and maintenance of general anesthesia. A sedative-hypnotic agent, propofol has a rapid onset of action of less than 1 minute. Induction is accomplished with a bolus of 2.0 to 2.5 mg/kg. A neuromuscular blocking agent may not be necessary for intubation when propofol is used.[13] Maintenance of anesthesia is accomplished by intermittent bolus injections (25–50 mg) or continuous intravenous infusion (100–200 µg/kg/min) along with inhalational nitrous oxide and oxygen.

The depth of anesthesia is readily adjusted by titrating the rate of infusion on the basis of patient response to the medication. Patient age and preoperative medications influence the dose required. Very few adverse reactions to this medication have been encountered. Systemic clearance of propofol is rapid. Plasma levels fall below the awakening threshold approximately 5 minutes after cessation of a 1-hour infusion and 7 minutes after a 10-hour infusion. Rapid recovery along with minimal side effects has made propofol the intravenous anesthetic of choice for outpatient anesthesia.[13] Propofol has been described for use in adjustable suture cases, allowing immediate adjustment of sutures.[14]

OPERATIVE COMPLICATIONS

The complications of general anesthesia in the adult strabismus population are similar to those observed in pediatric patients. Each patient should spend an adequate amount of time in the recovery room to allow the staff to identify and manage any complications that may develop. Postoperative hypothermia is often present in adults, and efforts should be made to rewarm the patient. Postoperative pain relief should be managed as needed. One should keep in mind that strabismus surgery has been associated with an increased incidence of postoperative nausea and vomiting compared with other general anesthesia surgeries. This has been linked to a proposed oculogastric reflex. One should make an effort to reduce nausea and vomiting, with measures including the use of intraoperative antiemetics such as droperidol or metoclopramide, especially if intraoperative narcotics are used. Decreased intraoperative and postoperative narcotics and possibly minimal muscle manipulation during surgery may reduce the incidence of postoperative nausea and vomiting.

Malignant hyperthermia should also be monitored for in adult patients. As mentioned, a previous episode of uncomplicated general anesthesia does not rule out the risk of malignant hyperthermia. An episode of sensitization has been proposed and the first exposure to anesthetics has been uncomplicated in a patient at risk.

Adults with a history of myocardial infarction should not have elective strabismus surgery any earlier than 6 months after the event. After 6 months the risk of recurrent myocardial infarction drops to approximately 5%, which is still 50 times the normal risk.

ADJUSTABLE SUTURES AND GENERAL ANESTHESIA

Adjustable suture techniques have aided in the treatment of complex strabismus. They are often reserved for the adult patient or the extremely cooperative child or adolescent. Preoperative discussion of the procedure with the patient is necessary to prepare the patient for the technique and to determine whether the patient will tolerate adjustment.

Controversy exists over when and where suture adjustment should be performed. Suture adjustment must wait until the patient no longer manifests effects of anesthesia. If no complications of anesthesia such as nausea, vomiting, or pain are noted, same-day adjustment is typically performed 5 to 6 hours after surgery.[20] Avoidance of perioperative narcotics may facilitate recovery from anesthesia and same-day adjustment. Adjustment can be performed in the office or in the operating room depending on the surgeon's preference. Topical anesthesia such as tetracaine 0.5% or topical lidocaine 4% may be applied to the conjunctiva. Suture adjustment is often postponed until the morning after surgery to allow for full cooperation. However, it is sometimes difficult to mobilize the muscle on the eye after several hours have elapsed. Topical anesthesia is again used for these adjustments.

Hertle and colleagues[19] emphasized that patients who manifest the oculocardiac reflex during general anesthesia have a significantly increased incidence of vasovagal symptoms during adjustment. They also pointed out that younger patients are at increased risk for vasovagal complications during adjustment. It is important that the ophthalmologist take this finding into consideration when determining where suture adjustment will be performed. Patients with a significant intraoperative oculocardiac reflex should probably undergo suture adjustment in a setting equipped to provide cardiopulmonary resuscitation if it is needed.

McKeown and associates[14] supported the utility of propofol intravenous general anesthesia for adjustable suture strabismus surgery. Because of the rapid induction and rapid recovery profile of propofol, they have found that patients are awake enough 5 to 10 minutes after extubation to cooperate with suture adjustment on the operating room table. Patients are helped to a sitting position after extubation and are asked to fixate on a target, and prism cover testing is performed. Proparacaine hydrochloride .5% is used for adjustment. A rehearsal of cover testing is performed in the operating room before induction so the patient would be prepared for the adjustment experience. This technique allows for adjustment to be performed in the sterile environment of the operating room. Vasovagal complications of adjustment can be more efficiently managed in the operating room. Patients have a very low incidence of postoperative nausea, vomiting, or pain, and adjustment is not dependent on the patient's recovery room time. McKeown and others reported that the majority of patients are ambulatory and symptom free within 1 hour after surgery.

The authors used propofol without intubation for cases that do not require long periods of anesthesia, less than 40 minutes, and found it to be a very useful technique. Small doses of fentanyl are used to provide analgesia during this technique. This technique of propofol without intubation allows for suture adjustment within minutes in the operating room.

With the development of new short-acting inhalational anesthetics for the maintenance of general anesthesia, such as desflurane (Suprane), it is now possible to use intubation agents that afford rapid emergence from anesthesia. This allows for adjustment of sutures within a few hours of surgery.

Propofol and short-acting inhalational agents provide the anesthesiologist and surgeon increased flexibility in the choice of a preferred method for each individual case. This often affords the patient a more pleasant surgical experience.

LOCAL ANESTHESIA FOR STRABISMUS SURGERY

Local anesthesia for strabismus surgery has gained popularity because of an increased use of adjustable sutures and a shift toward outpatient surgery. Local anesthesia techniques used today include retrobulbar, peribulbar, sub-Tenon's, and topical anesthesia. Patients should be provided with a thorough explanation of the local anesthesia experience preoperatively. It is paramount to assess a patient's willingness to undergo local anesthesia before use. The surgeon's experience is a significant consideration in choosing to use local anesthesia and for determining the types of strabismus surgery for which it is appropriate. Some strabismologists use local anesthesia techniques as their primary choice for all cooperative patients. Local anesthesia techniques are used for both adjustable and nonadjustable strabismus cases. The authors suggest that adjustable suture cases are best performed with a local anesthesia technique that does not block the optic nerve and alter vision in the operated eye. Thus, topical anesthesia or sub-Tenon's infiltration of the muscle tendon insertion is recommended. In addition, local anesthesia techniques allow strabismus surgery to be performed in patients with complicated medical conditions that may preclude general anesthesia.

PREOPERATIVE EVALUATION

It may become necessary to convert from local anesthesia to general anesthesia because of patient anxiety or discomfort. Intraoperative findings may also necessitate conversion to general anesthesia. As a result, the preoperative considerations in patients undergoing local anesthesia are similar to those for patients undergoing general anesthesia. A preoperative evaluation by an internist is required in the face of any concomitant medical condition. Myocardial oxygen demand is greater during local anesthesia than general anesthesia,[2] possibly because of increased patient anxiety or pain. A CBC to rule out anemia and an electrocardiogram are mandatory. Preoperative chemistry profiles will screen for renal or hepatic disease, which may complicate intravenous monitored sedation used during strabismus surgery. It should be emphasized that postponement of elective strabismus surgery is usually due to a patient's medical condition as opposed to abnormal preoperative laboratory tests.

PREMEDICATION

Premedication is often not necessary for ambulatory strabismus surgery performed under local anesthesia. A preoperative discussion of local anesthesia techniques and strabismus surgery with the patient will help to reduce the need for premedication. If necessary, oral or intramuscular diazepam or midazolam can be used in anxious patients.

OPERATIVE SEDATION CONSIDERATIONS

A pulse oximeter with an audible pulse tracing, cardiac monitoring, and oxygen via nasal cannula should be in place before administering local anesthesia. Monitored intravenous sedation should be provided on the basis of the customs of the anesthesiologist. Deep sedation may reduce the anxiety and discomfort associated with retrobulbar and peribulbar injections. Methohexital sodium (Brevital), 1.0 to 1.5 mg/kg, is often used before these techniques. This medication is known to cause reflex sneezing in some patients, and needles should be withdrawn if a prodrome of a sneeze is detected.

Fentanyl, 1.0 to 2.0 µg/kg, is a relatively short-acting narcotic that provides both analgesia and sedation for procedures performed under local anesthesia. This medication produces respiratory depression, which may prohibit its use in patients with chronic obstructive pulmonary disease. Diazepam (Valium) has largely been replaced by midazolam (Versed) for intraoperative sedation. The sedative and amnestic response from midazolam is superb.

Propofol (Diprivan) is well suited for sedation during strabismus surgery because of its rapid onset and recovery profiles. Propofol can be given as a bolus or continuous infusion, which is readily titratable to the desired level of sedation. Furthermore, it has been reported that propofol has inherent antiemetic qualities.[13]

OCULOCARDIAC REFLEX

As with general anesthesia, the surgeon and anesthesiologist need to be aware of the oculocardiac reflex and the possibility of associated bradycardia, hypotension, and dysrhythmias. All tension on the extraocular muscles should be relaxed if bradycardia is noted. The excessive vagal tone induced by traction on the extraocular muscles can be very distressing to the patient. Excessive traction on orbital tissues should be kept to a minimum during all strabismus surgery because it may provoke this reflex. In addition, excessive manipulation of tissues may induce deep orbital pain not blocked by local anesthesia.

LID BLOCK

Lid blocks usually are not essential for performing strabismus surgery under local anesthesia. Normal orbicularis tone usually does not hinder strabismus surgery, especially under the influence of intravenous sedation. Peribulbar anesthesia often will produce significant lid akinesia. In the rare patient who squeezes against the lid speculum, a van Lint–type injection of 2% lidocaine with or without epinephrine may be indicated.

LOCAL ANESTHETIC AGENTS

Various anesthetic agents are used in retrobulbar, peribulbar, and sub-Tenon's anesthesia. These agents differ in their chemical nature and duration of effect. Amide anesthetic agents are preferred for local anesthesia. Amide anesthetic agents are metabolized by the hepatic system. Ester-based anesthetics may be locally deactivated by plasma pseudocholinesterase. No local deactivation of amide anesthetics occurs, and the duration of effect is limited by diffusion away from the site of injection. Systemic toxicity is also decreased with amide anesthetic agents. Ester-based agents are associated with more systemic toxicity and are affected by decreased levels of pseudocholinesterase inhibitors such as echothiophate. Epinephrine, 1:100,000, is often mixed with local anesthetics to cause local vasoconstriction to reduce diffusion.

Lidocaine (Xylocaine), an amide anesthetic, in concentrations of 2 to 4% takes effect rapidly and lasts approximately 1 to 2 hours. The maximal safe dose of lidocaine in an adult patient is 15 mL of a 2% solution. Doses in excess of this can result in cardiac conduction abnormalities. Mepivacaine (Carbocaine) is also an amide in strengths of 1 to 3%. Mepivacaine is rapid acting and lasts about 2 to 3 hours. The maximum recommended dose of mepivacaine is 25 mL of the 2% solution. Bupivacaine (Marcaine) is also an amide agent with a slower onset of action, but it may be effective for up to 8 hours. It is available from 0.25 to 0.75% solutions, and the maximum dose is 25 mL of a 0.75% solution. Bupivacaine is often mixed with lidocaine or mepivacaine. Etidocaine (Duranest) is a rapid-acting derivative of lidocaine and has an effect for up to 5 hours. The safe dose of etidocaine is the same as for lidocaine. Chloroprocaine (Nesacaine) 3% has been used by some researchers to achieve local anesthesia of between 2 and 3 hours' duration.[21] These differences in onset and duration of effect allow a surgeon to select an agent on the basis of the anticipated duration of a case. This is especially important when same-day suture adjustment is planned. Measurements during adjustment may be altered by residual anesthetic agent. Adequate time for cessation of effect is important. Mepivacaine seems to be a reasonable choice for most strabismus surgery cases.[22]

Wydase, a highly purified bovine testicular hyaluronidase, is often mixed with local anesthetic agents before injection. This enzyme improves the diffusion of the anesthetic agent through the orbital tissues. Because the metabolism of amide local anesthetics is dependent on diffusion away from the area, the use of hyaluronidase will decrease the duration of effect of the chosen local anesthetic agent.

RETROBULBAR ANESTHESIA

Retrobulbar anesthesia is in common use, but, because of its potential for complications, it is not recommended for strabismus surgery. This technique does provide deep orbital anesthesia and akinesia and blocks the potential oculocardiac reflex with a minimal amount of anesthetic agent. A long 25-gauge retrobulbar needle is used to inject 2 to 4 mL of the anesthetic agent of choice, with or without hyaluronidase, into the muscle cone. The block is usually effective approximately 5 minutes after injection. Adjustment of sutures after a retrobulbar anesthetic should not be performed until full extraocular motility, visual acuity, and cooperation of the patient have returned to preoperative levels.[20, 22]

Retrobulbar anesthesia, however, is not without associated morbidity. The most common complication of retrobulbar anesthesia is retrobulbar hemorrhage.[21, 22] This may lead to central retinal artery occlusion and optic atrophy if not treated properly. The nerve or its blood supply may be violated by the procedure, which may result in permanent vision loss.

Perforation of the globe has been documented and may be associated with vitreous hemorrhage and retinal detachment. Direct injection into the cranial cavity has been documented as has intravascular injection. This associated morbidity precludes the use of retrobulbar anesthesia for bilateral strabismus surgery. Safer local anesthesia techniques such as parabulbar or topical anesthesia are recommended by the authors.

PERIBULBAR ANESTHESIA

Peribulbar anesthesia does not require the muscle cone to be violated. Therefore, the direct ocular morbidity associated with this procedure may be reduced. However, this may not be the case with extraocular muscle trauma (see Chapter 1). Mepivacaine is commonly used for peribulbar anesthesia in strabismus surgery. Hyaluronidase is usually required to allow the anesthetic to diffuse posteriorly. The anesthetic is injected through the skin of the lower lid into the periocular space. The 25-gauge .5 in (1.6 cm) needle enters the skin at the junction of the middle and lateral thirds of the lower lid, and 3 mL is injected. The needle is then inserted between the superior orbital rim and the globe at the superior orbital notch, and a similar injection is performed. Ocular massage helps to diffuse the agent posteriorly. Anesthesia and akinesia require approximately 10 minutes to develop. Therefore, this block is often performed in the holding area. Pupillary dilation indicates that the anesthetic has diffused to the level of the ciliary ganglion, and adequate anesthesia is most likely present. Our experience has shown that patients who have had previous surgery under peribulbar anesthetic demonstrate a markedly decreased duration of anesthesia from subsequent peribulbar blocks.

The peribulbar technique avoids the possibility of injection into the optic nerve, the central retinal artery, and the central nervous system. The risk of globe perforation exists; however, it is much less than with retrobulbar techniques. Again, a return to preoperative levels of visual acuity and ocular motility is required before suture adjustment can be performed.[23]

SUB-TENON'S INFUSION (PARABULBAR)

Sub-Tenon's infusion of anesthetic has been successfully used for strabismus surgery under local anesthesia. The fact that optic nerve function is not compromised by this technique is a unique advantage over retrobulbar and peribulbar anesthesia. This allows more rapid visual recovery for the patient and earlier adjustment of adjustable sutures.

After the patient has been prepared and draped, topical tetracaine .5% is placed on the conjunctiva of the lower cul-de-sac of the operated eye. The conjunctival and Tenon's incisions are then performed in the fornix or at the limbus to expose bare sclera. This may be the same incision for the intended strabismus surgery or a separate incision. An irrigation syringe is used to infuse anesthetic into the sub-Tenon's space in the quadrant to be operated on. A mixture of bupivacaine and lidocaine is often used. In adjustable suture cases, lidocaine alone is used because it is short acting, and a minimal amount of agent is infused in proximity to the muscle tendon to be operated on. A disposable flexible infusion catheter has been developed by Greenbaum that can be introduced through a small conjunctiva and Tenon's incision. Once in the sub-Tenon's space, anesthetic agent can be infused and a block as effective as that of retrobulbar can be achieved. This avoids the risk of placing a needle behind the globe.[24] With the full parabulbar block, the onset of anesthesia and akinesia is rapid, and the block is usually performed in the course of surgery. The time between infusion and adjustment of sutures is dependent on the particular anesthetic agent used.

SUBCONJUNCTIVAL ANESTHESIA

Subconjunctival injections of local anesthetic agents can be performed at any site around the limbus. Topical tetracaine drops are instilled before the subconjunctival injection. Lidocaine 1 to 2% with or without epinephrine is injected just posterior to the limbus for a volume of 2 to 3 mL using a 27-gauge needle. The lids are then closed and massaged for 1 minute to allow the anesthetic to diffuse through the area.[1] A cotton-tipped applicator can be used to diffuse the anesthetic. This technique affords constant observation of the needle tip, thus avoiding untoward orbital complications. The anterior aspect of the globe is anesthetized, which is adequate for most strabismus surgery. The effects on motility are minimal, and adjustment usually can be performed immediately in the sterile and controlled operating room environment. The conjunctival incisions can also be closed in the operating room after adjustment. This technique is more useful for rectus muscle surgery than for obliques because of patient discomfort. The primary complication encountered with subconjunctival anesthesia is patient discomfort and the need for additional anesthesia; however, this occurrence is rare.

TOPICAL ANESTHESIA

Some strabismus surgeons perform surgery with topical anesthesia only. This requires a most cooperative patient. The patient who tolerates forced duction testing under topical anesthesia may be considered for topical strabismus surgery.[24] Additional time is required preoperatively to inform the patient of all the possible sensations and discomforts that may be experienced. Care must be taken by the surgeon to manipulate gently ocular tissues to ensure patient comfort.[25] Tetracaine .5%, cocaine 4%, and lidocaine 4% have been used in this technique. The anesthetic is applied before incising the conjunctiva, when the sutures are passed, and when discomfort is reported by the patient. Gonzales reported using slightly reduced illumination during adjustment to reduce glare and improve patient comfort.[26]

Ideally, topical anesthesia avoids the majority of the complications associated with more invasive local anesthesia methods. The surgeon must rely on judicious use of sedatives such as midazolam or propofol to maintain patient comfort and cooperation. The main advantage of this technique is that sutures can be adjusted immediately in the operating room.[1] This technique may be performed in bilateral cases. Cocaine is very effective as a topical agent; however, idiosyncratic reactions have occurred with its use. In rare cases syncope may occur. The authors do not recommend cocaine for topical anesthesia during strabismus surgery.

In summary, local anesthesia techniques are returning to the forefront of strabismus surgery after an almost 75-year hiatus. This change in approach to the strabismus patient is due in large part to a shift to outpatient strabismus surgery, the increased use of adjustable sutures, and the efficacy of new sedative and anesthetic agents. The selection of local anesthesia for strabismus surgery must be made jointly between the surgeon and the patient so that both parties will have a satisfying surgical experience. Once chosen, intimate involvement of the anesthesiologist is vital. These new local techniques will greatly reduce the use of general anesthesia in the mature patient population and may afford patients with medical contraindications to general anesthesia the opportunity to undergo treatment of ocular misalignment.

REFERENCES

1. Helveston EM. Surgical management of strabismus: an atlas of strabismus surgery. St. Louis, MO: Mosby Year-Book, 1993, p 1.
2. Blodi FC. Surgical ophthalmology. Berlin: Springer-Verlag, 1991.
3. Von Noorden GK. Binocular vision and ocular motility: theory and management of strabismus. St. Louis, MO: CV Mosby, 1985.
4. Tasman W, Jaeger EA. Duane's clinical ophthalmology: physical and psychological preparation of children for anesthesia and surgery. Philadelphia: JB Lippincott, 1994.
5. Cohen MM, Cameron CB. Should you cancel the operation when a child has an upper respiratory tract infection? Anesth Analg 1991;72:266.
6. Isenber SJ, Apt L. Overnight admission of outpatient strabismus patients. Ophthalmic Surg 1990;21:540.
7. Christensen S, Farrow-Gillespie A. Incidence of emesis and postanesthetic recovery after strabismus surgery in children: a comparison of droperidol and lidocaine. Anesthesiology 1989;70:251.
8. Watcha MF, White PF. Postoperative nausea and vomiting: a review article. Anesthesiology 1992;77:162.
9. McGoldrick KF. Anesthesia for ophthalmic and otolaryngologic surgery. Philadelphia: WB Saunders, 1992.
10. Dajani AS, Bisno AL, Chung KJ, et al. Prevention of bacterial endocarditis: a statement for health professionals from the Committee on Rheumatic Fever, Endocarditis, and Kawasaki Disease of the Council on Cardiovascular Disease in the Young, the American Heart Association. JAMA 1990;264:2919.
11. Burr ML. Changes in asthma prevalence: two surveys 15 years apart. Arch Dis Child 1989;64:1452.
12. Lin DM, Furst SR. A double-blind comparison of metoclopramide and droperidol for prevention of emesis following strabismus surgery. Anesthesiology 1992;76:357.
13. White PF. Patient management, ambulatory surgery. Open Airways 1994;7:4.
14. Ward JB, Niffenegger AS, McKeown CA. The use of propofol and mivacurium anesthetic technique for the immediate postoperative adjustment of sutures in strabismus surgery. Ophthalmology 1995;102:122.
15. Watcha JF, Simeon RM. Effects of propofol on the incidence of postoperative vomiting after strabismus surgery in pediatric outpatients. Anesthesiology 1991;75:204.
16. Professional information brochure: Diprivan (propofol). Wilmington, DE: Stuart Pharmaceuticals, 1994.
17. Patel RI, Hannallah RS, Norden J: Emergence airway complications in children: a comparison of tracheal extubation in awake and deeply anesthetized patients. Anesth Analg 1991;73:266.
18. Romano PE, Robinson JA. General anesthesia morbidity and mortality in eye surgery at a children's hospital. J Pediatr Ophthalmol Strabismus 1981;18:17.
19. Hertle RW, Granet DB, Zylan S. The intraoperative oculocardiac reflex as a predictor of postoperative vaso-vagal responses during adjustable suture surgery. J Pediatr Ophthalmol Strabismus 1993;30:306.
20. Brown DR, Pacheco EM, Repka MX. Recovery of extraocular muscle function after

adjustable suture strabismus surgery under local anesthesia. J Pediatr Ophthalmol Strabismus 1992;29:16.

21. Szmyd SM, Nelson LB, Calhoun JH, Harley RD. Retrobulbar anesthesia in strabismus surgery: use of a short-acting anesthetic agent. Arch Ophthalmology 1985;103:809.

22. Cheng KP, Larson CE, Biglan AW. A prospective, randomized, controlled comparison of retrobulbar and general anesthesia for strabismus surgery. Ophthalmic Surg 1992;23:585.

23. Sanders RJ, Nelson LB, Deutsch JA. Peribulbar anesthesia for strabismus surgery. Am J Ophthalmol 1990;109:705.

24. Steele MA, Lavrich JB, Nelson LB, Koller HP. Sub-Tenon's infusion of local anesthetic for strabismus surgery. Ophthalmic Surg 1992;23:40.

25. Klyve P, Nicolaissen B. Topical anesthesia and adjustable sutures in strabismus surgery. Acta Ophthalmol 1992;70:637.

26. Diamond GR. Topical anesthesia for strabismus surgery. J Pediatr Ophthalmol Strabismus 1989;26:86.

CHAPTER 6

NEURO-OPHTHALMOLOGIC AND NEUROLOGIC COMPLICATIONS OF OPHTHALMIC ANESTHESIA

MARK J. KUPERSMITH, MD

Supported by R L Kohns Foundation and Research to Prevent Blindness, Inc.

In general, anesthesia for ophthalmic procedures is safe, and neurologic or neuro-ophthalmologic complications are so rare that they are reportable usually as single cases or small clusters of cases. Although general anesthesia is occasionally used, most procedures can and are performed with some form of regional anesthesia. Careful patient selection and detailed medical evaluation are helpful in avoiding use of general anesthesia in patients with significant risk factors that could lead to complications. Because regional anesthesia is used in most ophthalmic surgeries, the principal focus of this chapter is on the potential complications associated with some of these techniques. Although some of the agents administered can be neurotoxic, the vast majority of complications are related to the actual method of delivery and the site of injection. Traditionally, for intraocular surgery, this includes retrobulbar or peribulbar needle placement and a block of the extracranial seventh nerve innervation of the orbicularis oculi. The complications are typically local, but adverse reactions at sites distant from the needle placement have been described. Most of the problems occur immediately, but some are delayed, developing within hours of the injection or procedure. Even when the problem has a rapid onset, it may not be noticed by the patient or surgeon. An example is the loss of vision from arterial occlusion or optic neuropathy that develops in association with anesthesia and an intraocular procedure. The surgically induced blurring, cloudy media, normal blocking effects of the anesthesia, and the patching of the operated eye all contribute to obscure any appreciation of an underlying problem.

RETROBULBAR ANESTHESIA

ANATOMIC CONSIDERATIONS OF RETROBULBAR INJECTION

The tip of the retrobulbar needle is directed toward the orbital apex within the muscle cone to effect akinesia and anesthesia of the sensory nerves. The intraconal space is not a discrete compartment, and it is bound by the extraocular muscles and the septum between the superior and lateral recti. The normal effects of retrobulbar anesthesia are determined by the diffusion of the anesthetic, which is dependent on the location of the needle tip, the septae separating compartments, the health of the orbital tissues, and the volume and characteristics of the injected agent. Sensory innervation to the eye is via the long and short posterior ciliary nerves, which pass through the ciliary ganglion behind the globe within the muscle cone. The sensory innervation of the conjunctiva is via the supratrochlear, supraorbital, and infraorbital nerves. Sensory innervation to the upper lid is from the supraorbital, supratrochlear, and lacrimal nerves and the zygomaticotemporal branch of the maxillary nerve. Lower lid sensory innervation is from the infraorbital nerve. Oculomotor innervation (from the third and sixth nerves but not the fourth nerve) courses in the muscle cone and enters the extraocular muscles from the inner surface. Because the dura of the optic nerve sheath is continuous at the globe with Tenon's capsule and is reflected at the orbital apex to the periorbital, the retrobulbar space is epidural. The position of the optic nerve varies with movement of the globe. The traditional method of having the patient look supranasally to avoid penetrating the globe with a retrobulbar injection rotates the optic nerve inferiorly and laterally where the nerve sheath or nerve may be more susceptible to penetration by the needle.[1] In fact, when the eye is rotated supranasally, the optic nerve becomes stretched taut and appears to be in the path of the usual retrobulbar injection, whereas with the eye in primary gaze the optic nerve is loose with bends and nasally positioned.[2, 3]

The distance from the inferior temporal rim to the nasal entrance of the optic foramen ranges from 42 to 54 mm.[4] Because of the shorter distance to the orbital apex from the posterior surface of the globe, shallow, low-volume orbits may be more prone to injury of the optic nerve or extraocular muscles or possibly have an injection into the subarachnoid space with the use of retrobulbar needles of conventional length. In fact, in these patients, when the needle is directed toward the orbital apex (Fig. 6–1), the optic nerve or sheath may be impaled in the midorbit. The optic sheath has been entered as close as 5 to 8 mm behind the eye when a curved needle was used.[5] In contrast to the axial length of the globe, the volume of the orbit is generally unknown before instillation of anesthetic. Nevertheless, it has been suggested that to avoid injury to orbital vessels or the optic nerve in the orbital apex, the tip of the retrobulbar needle should probably not be inserted deeper than 31 mm for either retrobulbar or peribulbar injections, and a needle less than 32 mm should be routinely used.[4] This seems reasonable, particularly when the needle is inserted medial to the globe and positioned parallel to the medial orbital wall. Also, the injector should avoid advancing the needle point by pushing the hub of the needle deeper so that it significantly depresses the lid or conjunctiva.

As the needle passes the equator of the globe, if it is angled 10 degrees toward the orbital apex, one of the rectus muscles is likely to be encountered. This is not dependent on the position of the eye because

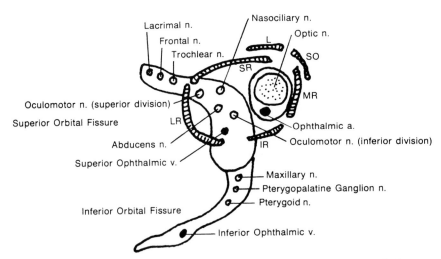

Figure 6–1. Orbital apex, superior and inferior orbital fissures. (MR, medial rectus; IR, inferior rectus; LR, lateral rectus; SR, superior rectus; L, levator; SO, superior oblique.) Note that the trochlear nerve lies outside the muscle cone. From Feldon SE, Beck RW, Cox TA, et al. Neuro-ophthalmology, section 5. San Francisco: American Academy of Ophthalmology, 1990, p 79. Used with permission.

the rectus locations vary only slightly with ocular movement. The needle must pass between these muscles to avoid needle or anesthetic injury.[6-8]

NORMAL TIME COURSE AND EFFECTS OF RETROBULBAR ANESTHESIA ON LID, PUPIL, OPTIC NERVE, AND EXTRAOCULAR MUSCLE FUNCTION

Depending on the anticipated duration of a given ophthalmic surgical procedure, most retrobulbar blocks are performed with a combination of medium-acting (e.g., lidocaine 2% or 4%) and long-acting (bupivacaine 0.75%) anesthetic agents as well as hyaluronidase to facilitate diffusion in the orbit. With this mixture, vision is blocked, ranging from no light perception (10%), light perception (8%), and hand motion perception (42%) to counting fingers (40%) within 10 minutes of injection. Complete akinesia is most common when the visual loss is no light perception, but the degree of akinesia does not correlate with other levels of vision.[9] The conduction block in the optic nerve can be verified by the amplitude reduction and delayed latency of the visual evoked potential.[10] As expected, a reverse relative afferent pupillary defect is associated with the optic nerve block (cannot evaluate direct response because of anesthetic-induced pupillary dilation secondary to parasympathetic innervation inhibition). However, a relative afferent pupillary defect cannot be demonstrated in all individuals.[11] The larger the afferent pupillary defect as measured by neutral density filters, the more complete the extraocular motility paresis.[12] When the saline-hyaluronidase mixture is injected alone, minor oculomotor weakness rarely develops but visual loss never occurs.[13] Not infrequently, the oculomotor akinesia is incomplete, and incyclotorsion remains.[11] Although retrobulbar anesthesia causes corneal and uveal sensory anesthesia and oculomotor akinesia, mild ptosis, if any, is seen.

Visual recovery develops in approximately 120 to 140 minutes. After lidocaine or prilocaine retrobulbar anesthesia, recovery of ocular motility follows return of corneal sensation; both occur within approximately 220 to 290 minutes.[14, 15] When mepivacaine is used, the visual, motor, and somatosensory blockades last for a slightly longer duration.

COMPLICATIONS

Visual Loss

Retrobulbar hemorrhage occurs in up to 3% of retrobulbar injections.[16] The risk of this complication increases with disorders that cause venous hypertension, that dilate the ophthalmic veins (arteriovenous shunt, dysthyroid ophthalmopathy, orbital apex lesions), and that pathologically increase arterial blood flow to the orbit (arteriovenous shunt, vascular orbital tumor). Fortunately, most retrobulbar bleeds are minor, secondary to puncture of an ophthalmic vein tributary. Slight proptosis and swelling of the conjunctiva and a rise in intraocular pressure do not lead to any permanent sequelae, but recognition of this complication before the eye is opened can avoid a catastrophe. In contrast, massive hemorrhage, possibly from rupture of an ophthalmic artery branch or a large vein, causes marked proptosis, orbital congestion, and severe restriction of eye movement. Visual loss results from dysfunction at different levels of the visual pathway. Immediate awareness of the problem with prompt treatment of the hemorrhage may prevent permanent, severe visual loss. Lateral canthotomy, medications to reduce intraocular pressure (e.g., an osmotic diuretic such as mannitol), and if necessary surgical decompression of the hematoma from the orbit are potential therapies. However, concomitant traumatic damage, vasospasm, and severe compression of the arterial supply to the retina, choroid, or optic nerve can cause irreversible visual loss despite immediate intervention (Figs. 6–2 and 6–3).

Central retinal artery occlusion from direct trauma or local hematoma compression can complicate a hemorrhage.[17] A marked elevation of intraocular pressure seems to increase the predisposition for retinal ischemia after a retrobulbar bleed. Additionally, direct injection of lidocaine and hyaluronidase into the central retinal artery can lead to retinal ischemia with the appearance of particulate emboli in the retinal arteries.[16]

Even without a retrobulbar bleed, retrobulbar anesthesia can be associated with visual loss. In patients with an underlying retinal arterial disorder, retrobulbar anesthesia (even without epinephrine) can be associated with a central retinal artery occlusion, retinal ischemia, and temporary (lasting minutes or hours) or permanent visual loss.[18–20] Vasospasm or direct trauma of the central artery where it enters the optic nerve sheath, from 10 to 15 mm behind the globe, may be the pathologic mechanism. Central retinal artery occlusion is more common with periocular or retrobulbar injections of agents in suspension, such as corticosteroids. When an optic nerve sheath hemorrhage develops, a combined central retinal artery and vein occlusion can cause visual loss that is permanent or only partially recovered.[1, 21]

Although an optic neuropathy can be seen with a massive retrobulbar hemorrhage, optic nerve dysfunction with varying degrees of visual loss, including no light perception, rarely occurs without signs of an orbital

---

Figure 6–2. *A,* The blood supply to the proximal optic nerve and choroid arises from branches of the medial (MPCA) and lateral (LPCA) posterior ciliary arteries, the incomplete circle of Haller-Zinn, the pial network, and the recurrent choroidal arteries. The posterior ciliary arteries send branches to the circle of Haller-Zinn and the pial network. The central retinal artery (CRA) provides minute branches to the optic nerve capillaries as it passes anteriorly to supply the retina. The central retinal vein (CRV) parallels the course of the CRA. *B,* Superior view of the intraorbital branches of the ophthalmic artery (Oph). The ophthalmic artery passes over the optic nerve in more than 80% of individuals. The vascular pattern differs if the ophthalmic artery passes beneath the optic nerve (inset on right). Ophthalmic branches include the following: medial muscular (MM), superior oblique (SO), posterior ethmoidal (PEth), anterior ethmoidal (AEth), falcine (Fal), medial palpebral (MP), dorsal nasal (DN), supratrochlear (ST), medial posterior ciliary (MPCA), lateral posterior ciliary (LPCA), central retinal (CRA), and lacrimal (Lac). In this orbit, the middle meningeal artery (MMA) provides a collateral branch, the meningolacrimal branch (MLB), through the supraorbital fissure to the lacrimal artery. (LG, lacrimal gland; ICA, internal carotid artery; ON, optic nerve.) From Kupersmith MJ. Neurovascular neuro-ophthalmology. Heidelberg: Springer-Verlag, 1993, pp 203–204. Used with permission.

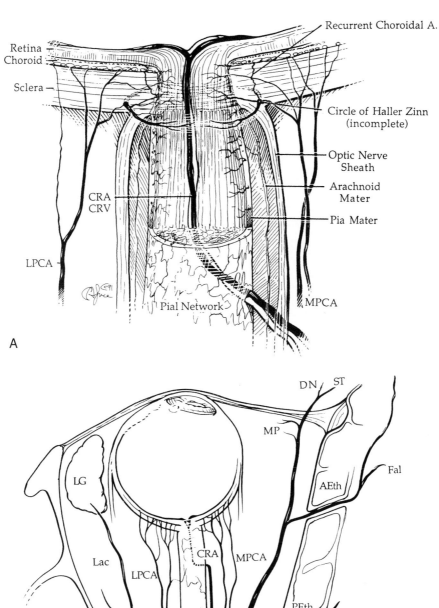

A

B

Figure 6–2. *See legend on opposite page*

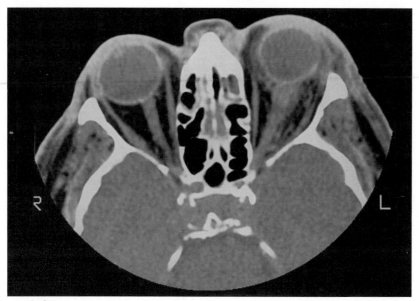

Figure 6–3. Axial computed tomography 1 day after methohexital retrobulbar anesthesia–related mild retrobulbar hemorrhage. When the anesthesia had worn off, the patient noted poorer vision in the left eye, and a relative afferent pupillary defect with a normal fundus was found. A slight increase in density of the retrobulbar space and swelling of the optic nerve are seen. Despite an immediate optic nerve sheath fenestration, the vision remained at finger counting.

bleed. If severe, the visual loss is noted by the first postoperative day. A mild degree of visual disturbance may not be noted for weeks and may be indistinguishable from the perioperative anterior ischemic optic neuropathy typically noted after cataract surgery. The latter complication of intraocular surgery seems to be unrelated to whether regional or general anesthesia is used.[22] Unless there is a concomitant central retinal artery occlusion, permanent visual loss is rare even after the retrobulbar needle has punctured the optic nerve.

Central Nervous System Toxicity

Experimental investigation in human cadavers has demonstrated that material injected into the optic nerve sheath can be recovered in the suprasellar cistern and middle cranial fossa.[23] This provides the functional anatomic evidence that explains why retrobulbar injection of a significant volume of anesthetic, delivered into the subdural space of the optic nerve, can diffuse into the intracranial subarachnoid space as far posteriorly as the brain stem[24] (Fig. 6–4). It may not be necessary to actually perforate the optic nerve sheath to introduce anesthetic intracranially because the sheath does not prevent the optic nerve from being blocked by retrobulbar anesthetics, and the cases of brain stem anesthesia are not associated with signs of optic nerve trauma. However, when the needle is located in the optic nerve sheath, it may be apparent because the injection requires twice as much pressure as injection into the retrobulbar orbital fat. Anesthetizing the brain stem, particularly

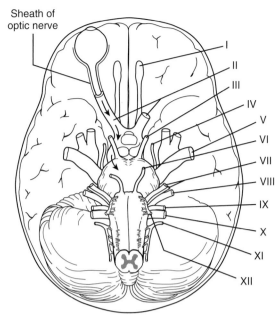

Figure 6–4. Via a base view, the route for injection of anesthesia into the intraorbital optic nerve sheath to the intracranial subarachnoid space. From Javitt JC, Addiego R, Friedberg HL, et al. Brain stem anesthesia after retrobulbar block. Ophthalmology 1987; 94:718–724. Used with permission.

the medulla, can depress the level of consciousness and respiration, leading to coma and apnea. These patients require immediate ventilatory support, are unresponsive to all stimuli, and are areflexic. Immediately recognizing this complication is life saving because the brain stem dysfunction and respiratory failure remit as the anesthesia wears off, which can be as short as 15 minutes or as long as several hours.[25–29] This type of complication occurs in approximately 0.2 to 0.79% of retrobulbar blocks.[29–32]

Brain stem dysfunction occurs with injection of bupivacaine, and extremely rarely only lidocaine is used.[27] Respiratory arrest appears to be less common (0.09%) when lidocaine 2% rather than lidocaine 4% is used with bupivacaine.[33] The pattern of neurologic dysfunction is dependent on the level of brain stem blocked by the anesthetic agent. The reticular activating system in the medulla and the pons and medullary nuclei—the nucleus ambiguus, dorsal motor nucleus of the 10th cranial nerve, and nucleus solitarius—are particularly susceptible to the effects of the anesthetic agents. The first signs are drowsiness, disorientation, and frank confusion, which develop within minutes of the retrobulbar injection. Although the respiratory depression can develop within 2 minutes, the onset can be delayed for 20 minutes. The surgeon must be observant and the operating room personnel prepared to give respiratory support if this complication occurs. Systemic hypotension and momentary cardiac asystole, in addition to respiratory depression, results from medullary anesthesia.[30, 34] This can be followed by a supraventricular tachycardia and pulmonary edema.[35] However, prolonged bradycardia or asystole can occur without other signs and probably results from a retrobulbar hemorrhage and exaggeration of the oculocardiac reflex.[36]

Uncontrolled, marked shivering is another sign, but this is also seen in patients in a cold operating room.[37] Motor extremity weakness, ranging from monoparesis to quadriplegia, has rarely been described.[38]

Other signs of intracranial anesthetic toxicity, possibly resulting from intra-arterial anesthetic (can occur with lidocaine alone) in the carotid circulation via injection into the ophthalmic artery,[39] include confusion or single, brief, generalized motor seizures.[38] An early sign of abnormal intracranial subarachnoid spread of anesthetic, which has been described with lidocaine alone, is the block of the contralateral optic nerve or any combination of ocular motor paresis or paralysis, leading to contralateral transient visual loss or ophthalmoparesis.[40–42] The contralateral ophthalmoparesis and visual loss usually last for 20 to 120 minutes. Particularly when bupivacaine is used, brain stem depression can, but does not always, follow the contralateral orbital dysfunction.[31]

Pupillary Dysfunction

Permanent pupillary dysfunction is infrequent. Pupil sphincter paralysis is probably more common when there is underlying ocular ischemia. An atonic pupil has been rarely described, with minimal responsiveness to pilocarpine and a normal dilatation response to mydriatic drops.[43]

Oculocardiac Reflex

Retrobulbar anesthesia usually adequately inhibits the oculocardiac reflex, but when a hematoma occurs the adverse effect may be severe. Vasovagal activity develops in less than 0.85% of all retrobulbar blocks.[44] (See General Anesthesia Complications, p. 165.)

Extraocular Muscle Disorders

Extraocular muscle paresis or contracture after retrobulbar or periocular injection of anesthesia has been described in numerous reports. Oculomotor dysfunction and diplopia are typically noted immediately after recovery from the anesthesia. The diplopia usually remits within weeks, but the paresis of a rectus muscle is more likely to be permanent if the muscle has been directly injected with 0.75% bupivacaine.[8] However, restriction has occurred with lidocaine use alone.[45] Direct injection into a muscle can also cause a local hematoma, needle-induced denervation, and myofiber injury. Because most retrobulbar injections are given through the inferior orbit, inferior rectus weakness and restriction are the most commonly encountered oculomotor problems. The presence of hypotropia in primary gaze that is worse in upgaze and positive forced duction on rotating the globe upward are diagnostic for restriction. When the diplopia persists, magnetic resonance imaging reveals the inferior rectus to be segmentally enlarged, however, without evidence of a prior hemorrhage.[45, 46] In the latter problem, recession of the affected inferior rectus may be required for persistent diplopia.[47] Inferior rectus paresis and superior rectus overaction are less common causes of vertical diplopia.[48–50] However, immediate postoperative inferior paresis followed by recovery of inferior rectus function and secondary overaction of the superior rectus can occur.[51]

Inferior oblique injuries are more rare despite the long course of the innervation to this muscle, which is exposed to a needle placed in the muscle cone. After retrobulbar bupivacaine and lidocaine, a delayed onset of several weeks of vertical diplopia with image tilt has been described because of inferior oblique overaction or contraction.[52] One theoretical, but unproven, mechanism for the overaction of the inferior oblique might be that supranormal reinnervation of the muscle occurred after an injury.[53]

Experimental investigations in monkeys and humans have not demonstrated significant myotoxicity from retrobulbar infusion of the commonly used anesthetics. Injection of bupivacaine, mepivacaine, or lidocaine with epinephrine into the retrobulbar space, and not into the extraocular muscle, of monkeys results in a minor loss of muscle fibers, areas of slight degeneration, and regeneration of fibers on the surface of the muscle exposed to anesthetic.[54] The myopathic response induced experimentally by retrobulbar injection of bupivacaine is a mild reaction in the exposed surface area of the muscle without significant myofibril necrosis.[55] The myopathic response resolves within 27 days. This is contrasted with the development of areas of significant muscle destruction and regeneration seen after direct injection into the extraocular muscle.[54]

Orbital Inflammation

There is one report of a pseudotumor of the orbit in five patients after retrobulbar anesthesia with hyaluronidase. Allergy tests revealed hypersensitivity to hyaluronidase in these patients, which suggested an immunologic or allergic mechanism for the orbital inflammation.[56]

Ptosis

This complication is explored in detail in the following section.

PERIORBITAL ANESTHESIA

To reduce the risk of retrobulbar hemorrhage, optic nerve injury, or globe perforation, periorbital and periocular anesthesia is used as an alternative to injections in which the needle is placed within the muscle cone. There are several types of approaches for this method of anesthesia. Again, the location of the needle tip seems to be the important factor, such that a periocular injection should be extraconal and anesthetize the sensory nerves to the lid and the preseptal motor seventh nerve fibers to the orbicularis oculi. In contrast, although a periorbital injection is extraconal, when the needle is inserted deeper, the anesthetic inhibits the sensory frontal nerves, and akinesia of the ocular muscles occurs because of diffusion or spread into the retrobulbar space posteriorly. A larger volume of anesthetic is typically used than for a retrobulbar injection.

ANATOMIC CONSIDERATIONS OF PERIOCULAR INJECTION

The needle tip with a medial periorbital injection is often located nearer to deeper orbital structures than injection via a lateral approach. Recalling that the orbital apex is posteromedial to the globe, a needle inserted in the nasal orbit and directed in the sagittal plane will anesthetize the optic nerve and oculomotor and parasympathetic nerves more easily than that inserted via a lateral approach. Thus, the akinesia may be less complete with a laterally placed injection, particularly if the orbital wall is hugged. Because there is less orbital fat in the posterior orbit, the nerves are more readily exposed to the anesthetic agents injected directly in this region, and a smaller volume is required to block the oculomotor and optic nerves. Inferior injection into the preseptal space anesthetizes the motor fibers of the lower lid portion of the orbicularis oculi and the sensory nerves to the conjunctiva and the temporal lower lid. A preseptal injection at the medial canthus will anesthetize the medial lids and conjunctiva, the medial orbicularis oculi, the lacrimal sac, canaliculi, and puncta. Injection into the supratemporal compartment anesthetizes the sensory lacrimal and frontal nerves, the conjunctiva, the lateral superior but not the lower lid, and the superior but not the inferior orbicularis oculi.

When the needle is placed directly posteriorly from the medial canthal area, the needle should not be longer than 15 mm, and the hub should not be pushed posteriorly to the level of the iris, to avoid the medial rectus. If the needle remains close to the orbital floor, the inferior oblique can be injured. A medially placed needle can injure the trochlear nerve or superior oblique muscle.

A needle that reaches the posterior orbit, particularly in the supranasal quadrant, is more likely to cause injury because of the compactness of the tissues surrounding the optic nerve in this region. Specifically, the rectus muscles are closer together and the ophthalmic artery (nasal) and superior division of the ophthalmic vein (nasal) have little space or orbital fat between them.

The superior division of the ophthalmic vein can be avoided if the needle is placed more anteriorly, 10 to 15 mm behind the globe. Needle penetration as deep as the supraorbital fissure could injure the sensory and motor nerves as they enter the orbit and the ophthalmic vein as it exits the orbit, or the needle can enter the subarachnoid space through the dura or the anterior cavernous sinus.

The superior ophthalmic vein, superior oblique tendon, and ethmoidal arteries are potential hazards; the levator, superior rectus, superior oblique, and medial rectus muscles are made akinetic; and the superior lid and forehead are anesthetized with injection into the supranasal compartment. Injection into the infranasal region gives akinesia of the inferior rectus and inferior oblique muscles, but the inferior oblique muscle, palpebral artery, and angular vein can be injured. No matter where the needle is placed, the presence of incomplete akinesia or sensory block is used to determine where additional anesthetic is required.

NORMAL TIME COURSE AND EFFECTS OF PERIBULBAR ANESTHESIA ON LID, PUPIL, OPTIC NERVE, AND EXTRAOCULAR MUSCLE FUNCTION

Diffusion of anesthetic into the retrobulbar space and orbital apex region has an effect similar to that of a retrobulbar injection on optic nerve and pupil function. The degree of akinesia is related to the location (see prior discussion) of the injection and volume of anesthetic. After injection of periocular anesthetic, akinesia is obtained within 10 minutes in 60 to 80% of patients, and visual depression to no light perception is achieved in 50% of patients.[57]

COMPLICATIONS

Visual Loss

Although rarer than after retrobulbar injections, peribulbar anesthesia can cause a retrobulbar hemorrhage and permanent blindness.[58] This can occur with injection through the skin of the upper and lower lids with a needle as short as 25 mm.

Extraocular Muscle Disorders

Oculomotor dysfunction with peribulbar injections is uncommon but can occur with direct muscle injection of anesthetic. Even with an injection 2.5 cm deep, trauma to the superior oblique tendon or trochlea has also been reported as a cause of an acquired Brown's syndrome.[59] Inferior oblique paresis, which required inferior oblique recession and superior oblique tenotomy, has been reported once from a peribulbar injection of 0.75% bupivacaine, lidocaine 2%, epinephrine, and hyaluronidase.[52] A medial orbital injection rarely injures the medial rectus.

Ptosis

Ptosis is noted on postoperative day 1 in 74% of cases but infrequently persists for more than 6 weeks.[57] The upper eyelid margin unusually covers the pupil except when dehiscence or disinsertion of the aponeurosis develops. This may occur in patients with pre-existing degeneration. Ptosis may be more common when supranasal placement of the anesthetic needle rather than a lower lid or inferior transconjunctival injection site of entry is used. However, most cases of ptosis are unrelated to the method of anesthesia. Ptosis is less common when a superior rectus bridle suture is not used.[60] Particularly in elderly patients, the ptosis can progress over months after ophthalmic surgery because of a disinsertion of the aponeurosis of the levator palpebrae.[61] This type of ptosis may be partially related to the use of a lid speculum.

FACIAL NERVE ANESTHESIA

Lid akinesia can be obtained with injection of anesthetic into the region of the facial nerve in a variety of locations, from the exit of the nerve from the base of the skull to the terminal branches to the orbicularis oculi. An optimal block is obtained within 20 minutes for both medium- and long-acting anesthetics.[62]

COMPLICATIONS

Respiratory-Swallowing Dysfunction

As with retrobulbar anesthesia, the complications associated with injections designed to inhibit seventh nerve akinesia depend on the location of the needle and the amount of dysfunction created in the adjacent local tissues. When a needle 16 mm or longer is used, injection around the seventh nerve as it exits the stylomastoid foramen (Nadbath block) can damage or anesthetize the ipsilateral vagus, glossopharyngeal, or spinal accessory nerves. Block of these nerves is more likely to occur when large volumes (>3 mL) are infused. Even though the block is unilateral, this can lead to swallowing and respiratory difficulties, which develop immediately or within 5 minutes of injection.[63, 64] The respiratory problem is worse in the supine position, and saliva aspiration can occur. Anesthetizing the vagus nerve blocks the motor innervation to the pharynx and larynx and sensation to the larynx. When the vagal branch, the recurrent laryngeal nerve, is affected, unilateral vocal cord paralysis develops.[65] Glossopharyngeal nerve anesthesia blocks sensation to the pharynx and contributes to pooling of oral secretions. The risk of respiratory complications is even greater if the opposite vocal cord is dysfunctional. Sitting the patient up usually relieves the problem, but intubation or a tracheotomy could be necessary if persistent laryngospasm develops. The dysfunction usually lasts from 30 to 75 minutes. This complication probably will not occur when the injecting needle is 5/8 inch or smaller.[60]

Even when a long needle is used (O'Brien block) and the main trunk of the facial nerve is punctured, persistent facial paralysis (up to 9 months) rarely occurs.[66] Injections (van Lint block) that deliver anesthetic to the small terminal motor fibers to the orbicularis oculi do not cause a cranial neuropathy. However, because this technique requires multiple infusions, the volume of anesthetic must be monitored to prevent systemic toxicity.

Visual Loss

Loss of vision is extremely rare with an anesthesia injection into the lids or orbicularis oculi. The mechanism for visual dysfunction is unknown, although it has been postulated that retinal arterial occlusion develops because of anesthesia injected into the ophthalmic arterial circulation via a collateral or branch artery at the site of injection.[67] This can occur without epinephrine in the infusate, so that a vasospastic mechanism is also unlikely. In contrast, the injection of other substances in suspension, such as corticosteroids, into this region has been demonstrated to cause particulate emboli in the retinal arteries.[22]

Oculomotor Dysfunction

Anesthetic agents subcutaneously injected into the periocular or preseptal regions infrequently diffuse into the orbit. This can result in several hours of mydriasis, paralysis of pupillary response to either light or accommodation, and ophthalmoplegia.[68]

GENERAL ANESTHESIA COMPLICATIONS

General anesthesia is much less commonly used than regional anesthesia in the treatment of ophthalmologic disorders.

COMPLICATIONS

Oculocardiac Reflex

Vagolytic agents such as atropine are typically given to inhibit the oculocardiac reflex that commonly occurs with a variety of ocular surgeries. Bradycardia or frank asystole can develop from traction on the extraocular muscles, particularly the medial rectus, or from pressure on the globe such as occurs with an intraocular injection or scleral depression.

Neurologic and Hyperthermia Disorders

Elderly patients may be slow to awake and become oriented after general anesthesia. This may be accentuated in the confused or demented patient, the type of patient who cannot cooperate for regional anesthesia. Judicious selection of patients with dementia to include only those who absolutely need ophthalmic surgery is mandatory before the use of general anesthesia. Patients deemed suitable include those with bilateral visual impairment for whom surgery could correct the vision; the return of vision might increase sensory input to the brain and help with patient orientation and cognitive function.

Rarely, other types of central nervous dysfunction occur as complications of general anesthesia. In patients given a phenothiazine (antiemetic) or a butyrophenone (droperidol), the malignant hyperpyrexia syndrome, including dyskinesia, rigidity, hyperthermia, and rhabdomyolysis, can develop in 1 in 200,000 cases.[69] Seizures, particularly with the use of enflurane, have been described. In patients with clinically apparent or subclinical underlying neurologic disorders, such as myasthenia gravis, Parkinson's disease, myotonic muscular dystrophy, or Alzheimer's disease, temporary decompensation can follow general anesthesia.

Cerebral or bilateral optic nerve infarcts can result from general anesthesia–induced profound hypotension, particularly when the patient has an underlying poor cardiac output, severe hypertension or atherosclerosis, or significant anemia.[70, 71] Persistent respiratory depression or delayed respiratory depression during or immediately after the procedure may also be encountered when systemic sedatives are used to reduce anxiety or augment the affects of regional anesthesia.

Neuromuscular Disorders

Neuromuscular blocking agents, commonly used to facilitate endotracheal intubation, temporarily paralyze extraocular muscles and the systemic voluntary muscles either by depolarization (suxamethonium) or blocking (d-tubocurarine) of neuromuscular receptors. Suxamethonium breakdown requires plasma pseudocholinesterase. Patients with a congenital defect of this enzyme or those taking anticholinesterase agents, such as Phospholine Iodide, to lower intraocular pressure will have prolonged paralysis of all voluntary muscles, which can result in respiratory failure after extubation.

Ptosis

Ptosis is almost as common after general anesthesia as it is with retrobulbar or periocular anesthesia. Approximately 50% of patients who have had cataract surgery experience postoperative ptosis on the first day, but it rarely lasts more than a week.[72] This suggests that the ptosis is less likely a result of myotoxicity with regional anesthesia and more likely a result of superior rectus bridle suture and lid speculum use in intraocular surgery. Ptosis related to aponeurosis disinsertion can also occur after general anesthesia, but it is half as frequent as the disinsertion after local anesthesia.[73, 74]

REFERENCES

1. Pautler SE, Grizzard WS, Thompson LN, Wing GL. Blindness from retrobulbar injection into the optic nerve. Ophthalmic Surg 1986;17:334.
2. Unsold R, Stanley JA, DeGroot J. The CT-topography of retrobulbar anesthesia: anatomic-clinical correlation of complications and suggestions of a modified technique. Graefe's Arch Ophthalmol 1981;217:125.
3. Smiddy WE, Michels RG, Kumar AJ. Magnetic resonance imaging of retrobulbar changes in optic nerve position with eye movement. Am J Ophthalmol 1989;107:82.
4. Katsev DA, Drews RC, Rose BT. An anatomic study of retrobulbar needle path length. Ophthalmology 1989;96:1221.
5. Drysdale DB. Experimental subdural retrobulbar injection of anesthetic. Ann Ophthalmol 1984;16:527.
6. Foster AH, Carlson BM. Myotoxicity of local anesthetics and regeneration of the damaged muscle fibres. Anesth Analg 1980;59:727.
7. Rao V, Kawatra V. Ocular myotoxic effects of local anesthetics. Can J Ophthalmol 1988;23:171.
8. Rainin EA, Carlson BM. Postoperative diplopia and ptosis: a clinical hypothesis based on the myotoxicity of local anesthetics. Arch Ophthalmol 1985;103:1337.
9. Griffiths JD, Pillai S, Lustbader JM. The effect of retrobulbar anesthesia on optic nerve function. Invest Ophthalmol Vis Sci 1994;35:1544.
10. Verma L, Arora R, Kumar A. Temporary conduction block of optic nerve after retrobulbar anesthesia. Ophthalmic Surg 1990;21:109.
11. Levin ML, O'Connor PS. Visual acuity after retrobulbar anesthesia. Ann Ophthalmol 1989;11:337.
12. Chaffin DB, Mannis MJ, Keltner JL. The effect of retrobulbar anesthesia on pupillary response. Invest Ophthalmol Vis Sci 1994;35:886.
13. Carroll FD, de Roeth A. The effect of retrobulbar injections of procaine on the optic nerve. Trans Am Acad Ophthalmol Otolaryngol 1955;59:356.
14. Boberg-Ans J. Experience in clinical examination of corneal sensitivity: corneal sensitivity and the nasolacrimal reflex after retrobulbar anesthesia. Br J Ophthalmol 1955;39:705.
15. Schimek F, Steuhl KP, Fahle M. Retrobulbar blockade of somatic, motor, and visual nerves by local anesthetics. Ophthalmic Surg 1993;24:171.
16. Morgan CM, Schatz H, Vine AK, et al. Ocular complications associated with retrobulbar injections. Ophthalmology 1988;95:660.
17. Kraushar MF, Seelenfreund MD, Freilich DB. Central retinal artery closure during orbital hemorrhage from retrobulbar injection. Trans Am Acad Ophthalmol Otolaryngol 1974;78:65.
18. Klein ML, Jampol LM, Condon PJ, et al. Central retinal artery occlusion without retrobulbar hemorrhage after bulbar anesthesia. Am J Ophthalmol 1982;93:573.
19. Cowley M, Campochiaro PA, Newman SA, Fogle JA. Retinal vascular occlusion without retrobulbar or optic nerve sheath hemorrhage after retrobulbar injection of lidocaine. Ophthalmic Surg 1988;19:859.

20. Lemagne JM, Michiels X, van Causenbroech S, Snyers B. Purtscher-like retinopathy after retrobulbar anesthesia. Ophthalmology 1990;97:859.
21. Sullivan KL, Brown GC, Forman AR, et al. Retrobulbar anesthesia and retinal vascular obstruction. Ophthalmology 1983;90:373.
22. Kupersmith MJ. Neurovascular neuro-ophthalmology. Heidelberg: Springer-Verlag, 1993, pp 203–204.
23. Wang BC, Bogart B, Hillman DE, Turndorf H. Subarachnoid injection—a potential complication of retrobulbar block. Anesthesiology 1989;71:845.
24. Kobet KA. Cerebral spinal fluid recovery of lidocaine and bupivacaine following respiratory arrest subsequent to retrobulbar block. Ophthalmic Surg 1987;18:11.
25. Chang JL, Gonzalez-Abola E, Larson CE, Lobes L. Brainstem anesthesia following retrobulbar anesthesia. Anesthesiology 1984;61:789.
26. Beltranean HP, Vega MJ, Kirk N, Blankenship G. Inadvertent intravascular bupivacaine injection following retrobulbar block. Reg Anesth 1981;6:149–151.
27. Mercereau DA. Brain-stem anesthesia complicating retrobulbar block. Can J Ophthalmol 1989;24:159.
28. Smith JL. Retobulbar Marcaine can cause respiratory arrest. J Clin Neuro-Ophthalmol 1981;1:171.
29. Castillo A, Lopez-Abad C, Macias JM, Diaz D. Respiratory arrest after 0.75% bupivacaine retrobulbar block. Ophthalmic Surg 1994;25:828.
30. Hamilton RC. Brainstem anesthesia following retrobulbar blockade. Anesthesiology 1985;63:688.
31. Javitt JC, Addiego R, Friedberg HL, et al. Brain stem anesthesia after retrobulbar block. Ophthalmology 1987;94:718.
32. Nicoll JM, Acharya PA, Ahlen K, et al. Central nervous system complications after 6000 retrobulbar blocks. Anesth Analg 1987;66:1298.
33. Wittpenn JR, Rapoza P, Sternberg P, et al. Respiratory arrest following retrobulbar anesthesia. Ophthalmology 1986;93:867.
34. Rosenblatt RM, May DR, Barsoumian K. Cardiopulmonary arrest after retrobulbar block. Am J Ophthalmol 1980;90:425.
35. Elk JR, Wood J, Holladay JT. Pulmonary edema following retrobulbar block. J Cataract Refract Surg 1988;14:216.
36. Cardan E, Pop R, Negrutiu S. Prolonged haemodynamic disturbance following attempted retrobulbar block. Anaesthesia 1987;42:668.
37. Lee DS, Kwon NJ. Shivering following retrobulbar block. Can J Anaesth 1988;35:294.
38. Ahn JC, Stanley JA. Subarachnoid injection as a complication of retrobulbar anesthesia. Am J Ophthalmol 1987;103:225.
39. Meyers EF, Ramirez RC, Boniuk I. Grand mal seizures after retrobulbar block. Arch Ophthalmol 1978;96:847.
40. Friedberg HL, Kline OR. Contralateral amaurosis after retrobulbar injection. Am J Ophthalmol 1986;101:668.
41. Antoszyk AN, Buckley EG. Contralateral decreased visual acuity and extraocular muscle palsies following retrobulbar anesthesia. Ophthalmology 1986;93:462.
42. Rogers R, Orellana J. Cranial nerve palsy following retrobulbar anesthesia. Br J Ophthalmol 1988;72:78.
43. Lam S, Beck RW, Hall D, Creighton JB. Atonic pupil after cataract surgery. Ophthalmology 1989;96:589.
44. Hamilton RC, Gimbel EV, Strunin L. Regional anesthesia for 12,000 cataract extraction and intraocular lens implantation procedures. Can J Anesth 1988;35:615.
45. Hamilton SM, Elsas FJ, Dawson TL. A cluster of patients with inferior rectus restriction following local anesthesia for cataract surgery. J Pediatr Ophthalmol Strabismus 1993;30:288.
46. Hamed LM, Mancuso A. Inferior rectus muscle contracture syndrome after retrobulbar anesthesia. Ophthalmology 1991;98:1506.
47. Ont-Tone L, Pearce WG. Inferior rectus muscle restriction after retrobulbar anesthesia for cataract extraction. Can J Ophthalmol 1989;24:162.
48. De Faber JHN, von Noorden GK. Inferior rectus muscle palsy after retrobulbar anesthesia for cataract extraction. Am J Ophthalmol 1991;112:209.
49. Grimmett MR, Lambert SR. Superior rectus muscle overaction after cataract extraction. Am J Ophthalmol 1992;114:72.
50. Esswein MB, von Noorden GK. Paresis of a vertical rectus muscle after cataract extraction. Am J Ophthalmol 1993;116:424.
51. Capo H. Ipsilateral hypertropia following cataract surgery. Invest Ophthalmol Vis Sci 1995;36:S955.
52. Hunter DG, Lam GC, Guyton DL. Inferior oblique muscle injury from local anesthesia for cataract surgery. Ophthalmology 1995;102:501.
53. Gonzalez C. Denervation of the inferior oblique: current status and long-term results. Trans Am Acad Ophthalmol Otolaryngol 1976;81:OP899.

54. Carlson BM, Emerick S, Komorowski TE, Rainin EA. Extraocular muscle regeneration in primates: local anesthesia-induced lesions. Ophthalmology 1992:99:582.
55. Porter JD, Edney DP, McMahon EJ, Burns LA. Extraocular myotoxicity of the retrobulbar anesthetic bupivacaine hydrochloride. Invest Ophthalmol Vis Sci 1988; 29:163.
56. Kempeneers A, Dralands L, Ceuppens J. Hyaluronidase induced orbital pseudotumor as complication of retrobulbar anesthesia. Bull Soc Belge Ophtalmol 1992;242:158.
57. Ropo A, Ruusuvaara P, Paloheimo M, et al. Periocular anaesthesia: technique, effectiveness and complications with special reference to postoperative ptosis. Acta Ophthalmol 1990;68:728.
58. Puustjarvi T, Purhonen S. Permanent blindness following retrobulbar hemorrhage after peribulbar anesthesia for cataract surgery. Ophthalmic Surg 1992;23:450.
59. Erie JC. Acquired Brown's syndrome after peribulbar anesthesia. Am J Ophthalmol 1990;109:349.
60. Kaplan LJ, Jaffe NS, Clayman HM. Ptosis and cataract surgery. Ophthalmology 1985;92:237.
61. Paris GL, Quickert MH. Disinsertion of the aponeurosis of the levator palpebrae superioris muscle after cataract extraction. Am J Ophthalmol 1976;81:337.
62. Schimek F, Steuhl KP, Thiel HJ, Fahle M. Lid akinesia after facial nerve blockade with local anesthetics. Invest Ophthalmol Vis Sci 1994;35:886.
63. Koenig SB, Snyder RW, Kay J. Respiratory distress after a Nadbath block. Ophthalmology 1988;95:1285.
64. Ruusuvaara P, Setala K, Tarkkanen A. Respiratory arrest after retrobulbar block. Acta Ophthalmol 1988;66:223.
65. Lindquist TD, Kopietz LA, Spigelman AV, et al. Complications of Nadbath facial nerve block and review of literature. Ophthalmic Surg 1988;19:271.
66. Spaeth GL. Total facial nerve palsy following modified O'Brien facial nerve block. Ophthalmic Surg 1987;18:518.
67. Brancato R, Pece A, Carassa R. Central retinal artery occlusion after local anesthesia for blepharoplasty. Graefes Arch Clin Exp Ophthalmol 1991;229:593.
68. Perlman JP, Conn H. Transient internal ophthalmoplegia during blepharoplasty: a report of three cases. Ophthalmic Plast Reconstr Surg 1991;7:141.
69. Ellis FR. Malignant hyperpyrexia. In: Inherited disease and anesthesia. Amsterdam: Elsevier, 1981, pp 163–169.
70. Sweeney PJ, Breuer AC, Selhorst JB, et al. Ischemic optic neuropathy: a complication of cardiopulmonary bypass surgery. Neurology 1982;32:560.
71. Rizzo JF, Lessel S. Posterior optic neuropathy. Am J Ophthalmol 1987;103:808.
72. Ropo A, Ruusuvaara P, Nikki P. Ptosis following periocular or general anesthesia in cataract surgery. Acta Ophthalmol 1992;70:262.
73. Deady JP, Price NJ, Sutton GA. Ptosis following cataract and trabeculotomy surgery. Br J Ophthalmol 1989;73:283.
74. Feldon SE, Beck RW, Cox TA, et al. Neuro-ophthalmology, section 5. San Francisco: American Academy of Ophthalmology, 1990, p 79.

CHAPTER 7

NEURO-OPHTHALMOLOGIC SURGERY

FLOYD WARREN, MD

The scope of surgery for neuro-ophthalmology includes muscle surgery and eyelid and orbital surgery. These, however, are covered in other chapters.

TEMPORAL ARTERY BIOPSY

Temporal arteritis is an inflammatory vasculitis occurring in the older (>60 years) population; the incidence markedly increases with increasing patient age up to the 80s. The diagnosis rests on a combination of clinical symptoms, signs, and laboratory evidence (erythrocyte sedimentation rate, biopsy). The symptoms include headache, scalp tenderness, jaw claudication, polymyalgia rheumatica, fever, anorexia, and weight loss. The most common presenting ophthalmic deficit is ischemic optic neuropathy; however, temporal arteritis may manifest as central retinal artery occlusion, ophthalmic artery occlusion, amaurosis fugax, and diplopia resulting from either cranial neuropathy or ischemic myopathy. If the diagnosis can be made before visual loss, devastating visual consequences may be avoided.

BIOPSY PROCEDURE

Generally, the temporal artery biopsy can easily be performed using only a local anesthetic agent; however, given the population in whom biopsy specimens are being examined, concomitant medical problems, such as hypertension and heart disease, frequently coexist; thus, consideration should be given to anesthesia monitoring.

The temporal artery should be palpated and marked with a marking pen. If the pulse cannot be located or is only faint, Doppler ultrasonography can be used to define better the course of the artery, and this is marked on the skin. If this proves unsuccessful, a "blind biopsy," making an incision 1 cm anterosuperior to the tragus, can be performed.

After the artery is marked, any hair in the field is shaved, and local anesthetic is infiltrated subcutaneously parallel to the artery using a long 25-gauge needle. Generally, 3 to 5 mL of anesthetic are used. I prefer 2% lidocaine (Xylocaine) with epinephrine for hemostasis if not medically contraindicated. Some authors prefer not using epinephrine to avoid vessel constriction. However, because the vessel is localized and marked before injection, I have not found this to be a problem.

The skin is incised to the level of the superficial temporalis fascia. Blunt dissection within the fascia isolates the vessel. A segment of vessel 3 to 6 cm in length is isolated; 4-0 chromic ties are placed proximally and distally. These are tied, the artery is cleared of fascial attachments, and small branches are coagulated with bipolar cautery. The segment between the ties is excised. The wound is irrigated to ensure that hemostasis is present. The wound is closed with interrupted 6-0 nylon sutures.

OPTIC NERVE SHEATH FENESTRATION

Optic nerve sheath fenestration may be the one true neuro-ophthalmic procedure. Its main indications include papilledema with pseudotumor cerebri and progressive visual loss with traumatic optic nerve sheath hemorrhage. It can also be used with visual loss resulting from papilledema from intracranial tumors when shunting is contraindicated. Other possible although less clear indications include progressive central retinal vein occlusion, low-tension glaucoma, and progressive anterior ischemic optic neuropathy. The rationale for the procedure (main indications) is to reduce increased pressure within the confines of the restrictive nerve sheath by allowing egress of cerebrospinal fluid or blood with traumatic neuropathy.

PROCEDURE

The fenestration is performed under general anesthesia. Although it can be performed with retrobulbar anesthesia, I have found that discomfort may occur with extreme rotation of the globe. In addition, other possible considerations against retrobulbar injection include increasing the orbital pressure, decreasing nerve head perfusion, and thus potentially further exacerbating the visual problem. There could also be a possible increased risk of inadvertently penetrating the nerve sheath with the needle because of its distended state. The procedure itself should be almost bloodless. Blood pressure should be maintained; there is no reason for hypotension, and theoretically it is probably contraindicated.

The procedure is performed using a peritomy for 360 degrees with relaxing incisions nasally. The medial rectus is imbricated on 6-0 Vicryl double locked at either end, and the muscle is disinserted from the globe and gently pulled medially. Traction sutures are then either placed through the stump of the medial rectus muscle or passed beneath the vertical recti (surgeon's preference), and the globe is rotated laterally. Traction will cause a ridge to form, which leads directly to the optic nerve. Malleable retractors are placed to isolate the nerve from reflected posterior Tenon's and any orbital fat. With a super sharp blade, an avascular portion of the sheath is incised; a tenotomy hook is placed in the opening to make a tent of the sheath, and the incision is extended with microscissors or the blade. Adhesions are lysed by gently manipulating the hook within the subarachnoid space. Additional fenestrations can then be made. The muscle is reattached with the Vicryl suture, and the conjunctiva is closed with 6-0 plain suture. A light patch is applied. It is important for the patient to avoid retching and vomiting postoperatively because hemorrhage along the sheath with visual loss can occur. Antiemetics (Tigan suppository, 200 mg [adult] or 100 mg [pediatric] three times a day as needed) should be used if necessary.

Rizzuto and colleagues reported on the use of sub-Tenon's anesthesia for optic nerve sheath fenestration. They found this technique to be highly safe and effective.

REFERENCE

1. Rizzuto PR, Spoor TC, Ramocki JM, McHenry JG. SubTenon's local anesthesia for optic nerve sheath fenestration. Am J Ophthalmol 1996; 121:326.

CHAPTER 8

ANESTHESIA IN VITREORETINAL SURGERY

BENJAMIN CHANG, MD
YALE L. FISHER, MD

The primary goals of anesthesia in ophthalmic surgery are to induce akinesia and analgesia during the operation, with additional considerations for amnesia and postoperative comfort. These are particularly important in vitreoretinal surgery, in which delicate intraocular maneuvers demand near to total absence of eye movement, and placement of a scleral buckle entails repeated traction on extraocular muscles and ocular manipulation, which can engender a great deal of pain. In the past, these anesthetic goals had been achieved with inhalational general anesthesia and endotracheal intubation, fraught with potential associated perioperative morbidity, including postoperative nausea and vomiting, sore throat, as well as delayed ambulation and difficulty with immediate postoperative positioning. However, the strict need for immobility as well as consideration of patient comfort, especially during lengthy cases, had resulted in general anesthesia being the traditionally preferred technique for vitreoretinal surgery,[1-3] usually in conjunction with extended inpatient hospitalization. In contrast, local anesthesia has long been used in many other types of ophthalmic surgery, with the advantages of reduced cost as well as greater patient convenience, postoperative comfort, and compliance with instructions. More recently, local anesthesia has been successfully used in vitreoretinal surgery with demonstrated safety and efficacy equivalent to that of general anesthesia.[4-7] Modern instrumentation and surgical techniques, enhanced by improved understanding of the pathophysiology of ocular diseases, have greatly improved surgical outcomes, expanded the indications for surgical intervention, and decreased operating time. Evidence also exists that early ambulation and discharge from the hospital with rapid resumption of full physical activity had little to no effect on outcome of retinal reattachment surgery.[8] With increasing financial and medical motivation toward shifting vitreoretinal surgery from an inpatient, extended hospitalization modality to the outpatient ambulatory setting, local anesthesia has now become the preferred technique for many vitreoretinal surgeons.

In choosing between local versus general anesthesia for vitreoretinal surgery, several factors must be weighed. General anesthesia remains the procedure of choice in children, the mentally retarded, and demented patients and in suspected or apparent open globe injuries. Relative contraindications for local anesthesia include claustrophobia, deafness, and language barrier. The anticipated length of the procedure must necessarily be considered because few patients can remain comfortable on the table under local anesthesia for procedures exceeding 2 hours. However, increased patient age along with other systemic comorbidity (e.g., diabetes mellitus, atherosclerotic cardiovascular disease, inadequately controlled hypertension, and recent food ingestion) argues for the use of local as opposed to general anesthesia. Frequently, intraocular gas or silicone oil tamponade is used, and compliance with immediate postoperative head positioning can best be achieved in the awake and alert patient after local anesthesia. Although not a medical consideration per se, the greater cost of general anesthesia and hospitalization for control of postoperative nausea, vomiting, and pain must also be factored in. The patient's experience with similar surgery will often influence the choice of anesthesia. Ultimately, advantages and disadvantages of both anesthetic options should be explained to the patient and the final decision arrived at after thoughtful discussion among patient, surgeon, and anesthesiologist.

The use of general anesthesia during vitreoretinal surgery does not differ significantly in principle from its use in other forms of ophthalmic surgery. One notable consideration is the insufflation of air or inert gas as a retinal tamponade agent concomitant with use of nitrous oxide. In some instances, a patient must return to the operating room for further surgery under general anesthesia while intravitreal gas is still present from prior surgery. The physical interactions of nitrous oxide with intracameral gas as well as the ocular implications are discussed further later.

Retrobulbar injection of anesthetic has been the traditional means of achieving local anesthesia for ophthalmic surgery. Although several variations exist for the technique of introducing the needle into the orbit as well as the type of needle used (e.g., transcutaneous vs. transconjunctival, straight vs. curved needle, short-bevel vs. long-bevel needle tip), all share in common placement of the needle tip into the intraconal space. A thorough discussion of retrobulbar anesthesia can be found elsewhere in this text. This technique allows the use of a small volume of anesthetic to achieve ocular akinesia and analgesia rapidly, usually through a single injection site. However, orbicularis akinesia is rarely effected, and an adjunctive block of the orbicularis muscle or facial nerve is necessary to prevent lid squeezing and closure. Nonetheless, the efficacy and relative safety of retrobulbar anesthesia over the decades for cataract surgery attest to its effectiveness. It has been successfully adopted for vitreoretinal surgery and has been used for such extensively. In one variation, a 50:50 mixture of 4% lidocaine hydrochloride without epinephrine and 0.75% bupivacaine hydrochloride with 150 IU of hyaluronidase, to a total volume of 5 mL, is drawn up into a syringe. The combination of lidocaine and bupivacaine has the advantages of rapid onset (from the lidocaine), prolonged anesthesia (bupivacaine has up to three times the duration of action as lidocaine), and safe systemic toxicity profile, which are all necessary in vitreoretinal surgery.[5] A small skin wheal is made with a short 30-gauge 1.6-cm (⅔ inch) needle in the lower eyelid skin at the junction of the inner two thirds and outer one third of the inferior orbital rim. Using the same syringe and anesthetic, the 30-gauge needle is switched for a long 25-gauge 3.8-cm (1½ inch) retrobulbar needle. Without any intravenous sedation to ensure patient cooperation, the patient is instructed to maintain eye position in primary gaze, and the retrobulbar needle is introduced transcutaneously through the anesthetized skin parallel to the orbital floor until the needle tip is past the equator of the globe, at which point the needle is redirected toward the orbital apex. Approximately 3 to 4 mL of the anesthetic mixture is slowly injected into the intraconal space, usually without any patient discomfort after the initial 0.5 mL has been introduced. This is followed by a facial nerve block with or without short-acting intravenous sedation. This has been the preferred technique of one of us for nearly 15 years.

Although retrobulbar injection is relatively safe in experienced hands, the potential for serious ocular as well as systemic morbidity, including ocular perforation, subarachnoid injection, optic nerve injury, retrobulbar hemorrhage, grand mal seizures, and retinal vascular obstruction, is a real and well-recognized concern. Peribulbar anesthesia was introduced by Davis and Mandel in 1986 as an alternative to retrobulbar injections in anterior segment surgery.[9] The deliberate avoidance of advancing a sharp needle near the globe and into the intraconal space is believed by many to constitute a safer technique, and diffusion of the anesthetic anteriorly into the lids often results in effective orbicularis akinesia without the need for an additional facial nerve block. This approach has been successfully adopted in scleral buckling and pars plana vitrectomy procedures.[10–12] A prospective, randomized, double-blind study compared retrobulbar with peribulbar anesthesia in vitreoretinal surgery and found the latter technique to be as effective as traditional retrobulbar anesthesia.[13] Because of the theoretical advantages of the peribulbar technique, one of us routinely uses it for vitreoretinal surgery when local anesthesia is selected. In his cases, a 10-mL syringe is filled with an equal mixture of 4% lidocaine hydrochloride and 0.75% bupivacaine hydrochloride, to which is added one vial (150 IU) of hyaluronidase. A short 25-gauge 1.6-cm sharp needle is used. The patient is given a short-acting intravenous sedative, followed by a two-site transcutaneous peribulbar injection, the first in the inferotemporal orbit delivering approximately 5 mL of the anesthetic mixture, and the second superiorly just below the supraorbital notch delivering approximately 3 to 4 mL of the anesthetic. At each site a small amount of anesthetic (approximately 0.5 to 1 mL) is injected as the needle is withdrawn to ensure adequate anterior diffusion of the mixture into the orbicularis and lids. Care is taken at each site to direct the needle purposefully away from the globe to avoid inadvertent ocular injury. The use of an oculocompression device (e.g., Honan balloon, Superpinky, Hustead's device) is optional but should be avoided in patients with glaucoma. Although the time to onset of peribulbar anesthesia is longer than for a direct retrobulbar block, the time taken for the surgeon to scrub and prepare and drape the patient usually is sufficient to achieve adequate anesthesia to start the case. Other variations of peribulbar anesthesia have been described and all are likely equally efficacious; the interested reader is directed to the pertinent sections of this text.

Despite theoretical advantages of peribulbar over retrobulbar sharp needle injections with regard to complications as noted previously, it is not free of risks, as evidenced by reports of similar complications during peribulbar anesthesia. This is likely attributable to an inability to visualize the sharp needle tip during its advancement into the orbit with either technique. In 1990 Mein and Woodcock reported a technique of blunt cannula sub-Tenon's retrobulbar infusion of local anesthetic for use in 58 consecutive vitreoretinal surgeries and found the technique effective while virtually eliminating the complications associated with sharp needle injections.[6] Since that initial report, several groups have also reported their modifications on the theme with high degrees of success.[14–16] All these variations share in common initial anesthesia of the conjunctiva by either topical anesthetic or anterior subconjunctival infiltration with direct visualization, followed by incising conjunctiva and Tenon's capsule down to bare sclera in one or more quadrants. A blunt irrigating cannula, usually 19-gauge and curved, is passed along the sub-Tenon's space, following the curvature of the globe until the cannula tip is positioned in the intraconal space. At this point, the desired anesthetic mixture can be directly infused and the procedure repeated in other quadrants if desired to effect retrobulbar anesthesia. An often-cited reason for preference of this technique over retrobulbar or peribulbar injections is the elimination of risk of ocular perforation, especially in eyes with long axial length, scleral thinning, or staphyloma, which are often the very eyes undergoing vitreoretinal surgery.

This is an overview of anesthetic options for vitreoretinal surgery. Interested readers are asked to consult standard texts on vitreoretinal surgery. What follow are, it is hoped, pertinent discussions related to specific topics in vitreoretinal surgery.

SCLERAL BUCKLING SURGERY

Scleral buckling surgery has been the standard procedure for repairing rhegmatogenous retinal detachments for several decades and still remains today the procedure of choice for the vast majority of retinal detachment cases. During the surgery, several or all four rectus muscles are isolated on traction sutures to allow manipulation of the globe. Frequent and extensive traction on extraocular muscles and placement of often bulky buckling material around the globe and under rectus muscles contribute to significant pain and discomfort for the patient with inadequate anesthesia. Therefore, scleral buckling surgery has been traditionally performed under general anesthesia, even by experienced surgeons who prefer local anesthesia for vitrectomy procedures. However, increased surgeon experience and comfort with local anesthesia have resulted in many surgeons relying on local anesthesia for scleral buckling surgery.[4–6, 10–16] One common problem associated with use of local anesthesia during this type of surgery is intraoperative loss of adequate anesthesia, in up to 72% of cases reported in one series.[11] These instances require supplementation of local anesthesia or intravenous sedation, or both, to allow safe continuation and completion of surgery. This can be easily accomplished in scleral buckling surgery because the sub-Tenon's space is always well exposed in several quadrants, permitting infusion of supplemental anesthetic directly into the intraconal space using a blunt irrigating cannula,[17] in much the same manner as described previously for initiation of retrobulbar anesthesia with a blunt cannula. This maneuver can be simply repeated as necessary during the operation to yield adequate anesthesia throughout the case and has allowed safe performance of scleral buckling surgery under local anesthesia in nearly 100% of cases reported in most series.[6, 10–17] A less frequently used technique to supplement anesthesia utilizes an indwelling retrobulbar catheter.[18] A thin-walled polyethylene catheter is advanced through a transcutaneous 19-gauge needle into the intraconal space, the needle is withdrawn, and the tube is secured to the lower eyelid skin. Additional anesthetic is given through the catheter as needed during the operation.

One additional problem encountered with scleral buckling surgery is postoperative pain secondary to extensive intraoperative manipulation of muscles, globe, and orbital tissue.[5] In one series of 200 patients evaluated for hospitalization needs after vitreoretinal surgery, some under general anesthesia and others under local anesthesia, 22% required inpatient management for control of postoperative pain.[19] Bupiva-caine hydrochloride is a common component of local anesthesia for ocular and nonocular surgery, with a duration of action up to 12 hours. Irrigation of bupivacaine into the retrobulbar space at the completion of surgery has the theoretical effect of achieving postoperative pain control. In a prospective study done at Wills Eye Hospital, retrobulbar irrigation with 0.75% bupivacaine at the end of scleral buckling surgery provided sufficient pain relief such that 85% of patients did not require parenteral pain medication after surgery.[20] Although this technique will not entirely eliminate the need for parenteral medication and hospitalization after scleral buckling procedures, it is safe, effective, and inexpensive and currently widely used by vitreoretinal surgeons.

Local anesthesia, by whichever technique the surgeon prefers, combined with intraoperative blunt cannula augmentation and retrobulbar bupivacaine irrigation at the completion of surgery is a satisfactory anesthetic technique and often preferable to general anesthesia. This is the current method of one of us for routine scleral buckling procedures.

OCULOCARDIAC REFLEX

The oculocardiac reflex, mediated by the afferent trigeminal nerve and the efferent vagal nerve, can be stimulated by pressure or traction exerted on the globe and orbital tissue, such as by pulling on extraocular muscles. This is most often encountered in pediatric strabismus surgery. It is also not uncommon to elicit this phenomenon during vitreoretinal surgery, especially when scleral buckling is involved requiring vigorous traction on muscles and manipulation of the globe. The reflex often manifests as sinus bradycardia but may present as any one of several dysrhythmias and is more common in children. Although the reflex may occur with general or local anesthesia, one means of suppressing it is by way of a retrobulbar injection to block the trigeminal afferent limb of the reflex arc. However, it can also be stimulated by the retrobulbar injection itself. Both the surgeon and the anesthesiologist must be alert to the first signs of the response and be prepared to treat it appropriately. A more complete discussion of the oculocardiac reflex can be found in Chapter 5.

PNEUMATIC RETINOPEXY

Selected cases of rhegmatogenous retinal detachments may be repaired by an outpatient office procedure first independently described by Dominguez in 1985[21] and by Hilton and Grizzard in 1986.[22] The procedure involves intravitreal injection of a small volume of an expansile, inert gas (such as sulfur hexafluoride, SF_6, or a perfluorocarbon gas), which with proper head positioning internally tamponades the retinal break and allows resorption of subretinal fluid, in conjunction with creation of a permanent chorioretinal adhesion by either cryoretinopexy or laser photocoagulation. Most surgeons elect to give a retrobulbar or peribulbar block because scleral depression, transconjunctival gas injection, ocular massage (to lower intraocular pressure), and transconjunctival cryoretinopexy can cause variable degrees of discomfort. In many instances, the sudden rise in intraocular pressure from the gas injection closes the central retinal artery, and anterior chamber paracentesis must also be performed. Because the entire procedure generally takes less than 30 minutes to complete, a short-acting agent such as 2% lidocaine is often sufficient. Some surgeons prefer only topical anesthesia (e.g., tetracaine), whereas others use a subconjunctival injection of a short-acting anesthetic instead of a retro- or peribulbar injection. Although general anesthesia has also been used for pneumatic retinopexy, this defeats the inherent advantages of the procedure and these instances are likely to be rare. The surgeon must be conscious of concurrent nitrous oxide use under these circumstances.

The convenience of the procedure for both surgeon and patient, coupled with the reduced cost compared with surgical repair in the operating room, has stimulated widespread use of this technique. The outcomes of this procedure compared favorably with those of conventional scleral buckling surgery in a multicenter randomized clinical trial, with initial reattachment rates of greater than 80%.[23] With increasing surgeon experience, appropriate patient selection, and greater economic pressures to reduce cost of health care, pneumatic retinopexy will play a significant role in ophthalmology in years to come.

Intravitreal air or gas injection, similar in principle to pneumatic retinopexy, is sometimes used during scleral buckling surgery. Usual indications are to tamponade a "fish-mouthed" retinal tear, a tear that is not adequately supported on a poorly positioned buckle, or intraocular volume restoration after drainage of subretinal fluid. If the surgery is being performed under local anesthesia, no additional anesthetic considerations need be made. However, as in the instance mentioned previously, if nitrous oxide is used with general anesthesia, then additional precautions to account for the gas–nitrous oxide interaction must be taken (see later discussion).

PARS PLANA VITRECTOMY SURGERY

Posterior segment vitreous surgery, most commonly performed via a three-port pars plana approach, is a relatively new and technologically demanding surgical endeavor. During the early years of its development, pars plana vitrectomy cases were often long and tedious procedures on account of primitive instrumentation and surgeon inexperience. For these and other reasons, vitrectomy cases were routinely performed under general anesthesia.[1–3] Subsequent improvements in microinstrumentation, coupled with increasing surgical skills, better appreciation of the pertinent pathophysiology, and greater experience, have led to improved outcomes and decreased operating time. The indications for pars plana vitreous surgery have also rapidly expanded to encompass a wide array of vitreoretinal diseases, including nonclearing vitreous hemorrhage, complicated retinal detachments with or without proliferative vitreoretinopathy, fibrovascular complications of proliferative diabetic retinopathy, endophthalmitis, macular pucker, trauma, intraocular foreign body, idiopathic macular hole, giant retinal tear, subretinal choroidal neovascularization and hemorrhage, and retinal detachments associated with viral retinitis, as well as for diagnostic purposes in non-Hodgkin's lymphoma, infectious chorioretinitis, and inflammatory conditions. Concurrent with the increase in vitrectomy procedures performed, there has been a shift from inpatient general anesthesia to outpatient surgery with local anesthesia. This latter approach has been repeatedly shown to be safe and effective[4, 6, 7, 11–16] and has become the preferred anesthetic technique of many vitreoretinal surgeons. However, for reasons alluded to earlier in this chapter, certain circumstances still mandate general anesthesia as the optimal means for accomplishing the surgical objectives. When local anesthesia is selected, any one of several techniques discussed previously may be used (i.e., retrobulbar injection, peribulbar injection, or sub-Tenon's cannula irrigation). This in conjunction with intraoperative anesthetic augmentation via retrobulbar cannula irrigation has allowed local anesthesia to be used successfully in the great majority of pars plana vitrectomy operations.

Brucker and colleagues described a new approach to anesthesia for these procedures.[24] In a series of 15 selected patients undergoing pars plana vitrectomy for various indications, anesthesia was effected using only perilimbal subconjunctival local anesthetic injections over the three intended sclerotomy sites. Eye immobilization was achieved by means of the two intraocular instruments, allowing performance of delicate maneuvers without incident. No intraoperative supplementation of anesthetic was necessary, and no patient reported any surgical discomfort, even with scleral depression and laser photocoagulation. These authors postulated that this technique may be suitable for select patients undergoing pars plana vitrectomy surgery, minimizing the dose of anesthetic used and eliminating the risks of needle perforation associated with other local injection techniques. However, in cases in which a scleral buckle is also placed or a pre-existing one is modified, anesthetic issues pertinent to scleral buckling surgery as discussed previously should be considered, and the latter technique may not be appropriate.

Historically, retinal detachments associated with giant retinal tears (tears of 90 degrees or greater in circumferential extent) were difficult to repair and usually required lengthy surgery with intraoperative prone positioning of the patient for intravitreal air-fluid exchange, often with the patient strapped to specially designed multipositional operating tables.[25, 26] This presented unusual challenges to the anesthesiologist, who must deal with positional cardiovascular changes as well as the logistics of adequate tubing length and potential dislodgement of the endotracheal tube. Although the use of local anesthesia facilitated many of the maneuvers, the surgery remained tedious and cumbersome for the entire surgical team. With the introduction of heavier-than-water perfluorocarbon liquids in vitreous surgery, the inverted retinal flap and retinal detachment could be repaired with the patient supine throughout the procedure.[27] This entirely eliminated the need to reposition the patient during surgery and greatly shortened operating time, simultaneous with increased surgeon control over ocular disease, and resulted in high levels of successful outcomes. In many centers this technique is currently the procedure of choice for repairing giant retinal tears, and its use will become widespread assuming U.S. Food and Drug Administration approval of perfluorocarbon liquids as a surgical adjunct.

INTRAOCULAR TAMPONADE

Vitreoretinal surgery often incorporates intraoperative infusion of sterile air, air-gas mixture, or silicone oil into the vitreous cavity for prolonged postoperative internal tamponade of retinal breaks. The choice of a gas mixture versus silicone oil is dictated by the desired duration of tamponade, need for additional surgery to remove silicone oil, specific indication of surgery (e.g., retinal detachment secondary to cytomegalovirus retinitis) as well as surgeon experience and preference. When silicone oil is used, no additional anesthetic considerations need to be made whether the procedure is performed under local or general anesthesia. The physical properties of intraocular gases introduce special issues with regard to inhalational anesthesia.

Commonly used gases for internal tamponade include air, xenon, sulfur hexafluoride (SF_6), and short-chain perfluorocarbons (usually C_2F_6 and C_3F_8). Air and xenon are nonexpansile gases, whereas the others are expansile. The latter can be admixed with air to yield nonexpansile concentrations. These gases share many properties that make them ideal for intraocular use: availability in highly purified form, inert, colorless, odorless, inflammable, high surface tension in an aqueous environment, and low water solubility.[28] Once introduced into the vitreous cavity, the gas forms a bubble, which, if larger than the retinal breaks, effectively tamponades the break, permitting subretinal fluid resorption to occur, while the surface tension of the gas prevents its passage through the break into the subretinal space. In addition, the lower specific gravity of gas relative to water allows a properly positioned gas bubble in the eye to rise and exert an upward buoyant force to push the retina against the retinal pigment epithelium as well as displace subretinal fluid through the retinal break back into the vitreous cavity.

The ability of intraocular gases to effect prolonged tamponade relies on the low water solubility of these gases. After introduction of gas into the eye, highly soluble oxygen and nitrogen in the blood and body tissue fluid rapidly diffuse into the gas bubble, resulting in initial gas expansion. The gas bubble's low solubility allows for equilibration and subsequent slow dissolution as it and accompanying oxygen and nitrogen diffuse out of the eye over days to weeks. Because of air's high water solubility (air being composed of 78% nitrogen and 21% oxygen), it is rapidly absorbed into the body from the eye, thus making it an ineffective long-term tamponade, but allows it to be mixed with other gases to yield nonexpansile mixtures.

Nitrous oxide (N_2O) is commonly used in inhalational general anesthesia, often at a ventilatory concentration of 50 to 70%. Nitrous oxide is also highly soluble, being 34 times that of nitrogen. The inhalation of nitrous oxide leads to rapid diffusion into intraocular gas bubbles with resultant increases in volume of the gas bubble. Using a computer simulation, Stinson and Donlon showed a threefold increase in intraocular gas bubble volume with concurrent nitrous oxide inhalation and up to 30% increase in bubble volume even when nitrous oxide is discontinued at the time of gas injection.[29] Their model suggests that nitrous oxide be discontinued at least 15 minutes before gas injection into the eye to prevent a rapid rise in intraocular volume. Others working with animal models have shown a dramatic increase in intraocular pressure, peaking approximately 15 to 20 minutes after initiation of nitrous oxide inhalation in the presence of an intravitreal gas bubble.[30, 31] Furthermore, if equilibrium pressure and volume are achieved in the presence of circulating nitrous oxide, there will be a rapid postoperative decrease in bubble size as intraocular nitrous oxide diffuses into the blood and is cleared in the lungs. Thus, it has been suggested that nitrous oxide not be used or be discontinued at least 15 minutes before intraocular gas injection and nitrous oxide be entirely omitted in patients with an intraocular gas bubble requiring reoperations under general anesthesia.[31]

SUMMARY

Anesthesia for vitreoretinal surgery may be successfully achieved through several safe and effective approaches. The options include general as well as local anesthesia, the latter via many different techniques. Factors that must be weighed into the choice of anesthesia delivery include the patient's systemic and ocular profile, intended surgical goals, and estimated length of procedure as well as surgeon's experience and comfort with the varying options. As such, no one technique is appropriate under all circumstances. Like other forms of surgery, adequate anesthesia must be achieved and sustained throughout the operation, with additional considerations for postoperative issues of comfort, pain control, and special positioning. The surgical plan, such as use of intravitreal gas tamponade during general anesthesia, should be made known to the anesthesiology staff as well as to the operating room personnel so that special needs may be anticipated to effect smooth and efficient completion of the operation. The surgeon and anesthesiologist alike must develop experience and comfort with alternative techniques as well as diagnosis and treatment of anesthesia-related complications. Ultimately, the decision for the type of anesthesia should be made after discussion between the physicians and an informed patient.

REFERENCES

1. Machemer R. Vitrectomy: a pars plana approach. New York: Grune & Stratton, 1975.
2. Michels RG. Vitreous surgery. St. Louis, MO: CV Mosby, 1981.
3. Charles S. Vitreous microsurgery, 2nd ed. Baltimore, MD: Williams & Wilkins, 1987.
4. Wilson D, Barr CC. Outpatient and abbreviated hospitalization for vitreoretinal surgery. Ophthalmic Surg 1990;21:119.
5. Holekamp TLR, Arribas NP, Boniuk I. Bupivaciane anesthesia in retinal detachment surgery. Arch Ophthalmol 1979;97:109.
6. Mein CE, Woodcock MG. Local anesthesia for vitreoretinal surgery. Retina 1990;10:47.
7. Gonçalves JCM, Turner L, Chang S. Monitored local anesthesia for pars plana vitrectomy. Ophthalmic Surg 1993;24:63.
8. Bovino JA, Marcus DF. Physical activity after retinal detachment surgery. Am J Ophthalmol 1984;98:171.
9. Davis DB II, Mandel RM. Posterior peribulbar anesthesia: an alternative to retrobulbar anesthesia. J Cataract Refract Surg 1986;12:182.
10. Arora R, Verma L, Kumar A, et al. Peribulbar anesthesia in retinal reattachment surgery. Ophthalmic Surg 1992;23:499.
11. Nicholson AD, Singh P, Badrinath SS, et al. Peribulbar anesthesia for primary vitreoretinal surgery. Ophthalmic Surg 1992;23:657.
12. Benedetti S, Agostini A. Peribulbar anesthesia in vitreoretinal surgery. Retina 1994;14:277.

13. Demediuk OM, Dhaliwal RS, Papworth DP, et al. A comparison of peribulbar and retrobulbar anesthesia for vitreoretinal surgical procedures. Arch Ophthalmol 1995;113:908.
14. Friedberg MA, Spellman FA, Pilkerton AR, et al. An alternative technique of local anesthesia for vitreoretinal surgery. Arch Ophthalmol 1991;109:1615.
15. Wald KJ, Weiter JJ. Modified technique of blunt cannula retrobulbar anesthesia for vitreoretinal surgery. Ophthalmic Surg 1993;24:336.
16. Simcock PR, Raymond GL, Lavin MJ, Whitley CL. Combined peribulbar injection and blunt cannula infiltration for vitreoretinal surgery. Ophthalmic Surg 1994;25:232.
17. Mein CE, Flynn HW. Augmentation of local anesthesia during retinal detachment surgery. Arch Ophthalmol 1989;107:1084.
18. Schepens CL. Retinal detachment and allied diseases, vol 1. Philadelphia: WB Saunders, 1983.
19. Isernhagen RD, Michels RG, Glaser BM, et al. Hospitalization requirements after vitreoretinal surgery. Arch Ophthalmol 1988;106:767.
20. Duker JA, Nielsen J, Vander JF, et al. Retrobulbar bupivacaine irrigation for postoperative pain after scleral buckling surgery: a prospective study. Ophthalmology 1991;98:514.
21. Dominguez A. Cirugia precoz y ambulatoria del desprendiemento do retina. Arch Soc Esp Oftalmol 1985;48:47.
22. Hilton GF, Grizzard WS. Pneumatic retinopexy: a two-step outpatient operation without conjunctival incision. Ophthalmology 1986;93:626.
23. Tornambe PE, Hilton GF, The Retinal Detachment Study Group. Pneumatic retinopexy: a multicenter randomized controlled clinical trial comparing pneumatic retinopexy with scleral buckling. Ophthalmology 1989;96:772.
24. Brucker AJ, Saran BR, Maguire AM. Perilimbal anesthesia for pars plana vitrectomy. Am J Ophthalmol 1994;117:599.
25. Schepens CL, Freeman HM, Thompson RF. A power driven multipositional operating table. Arch Ophthalmol 1965;73:671.
26. Peyman GA. A new operating table for the management of giant retinal breaks. Arch Ophthalmol 1981;99:498.
27. Chang S, Lincoff H, Zimmerman NJ, Fuchs W. Giant retinal tears: surgical techniques and results using perfluorocarbon liquids. Arch Ophthalmol 1989;107:761.
28. Chang S. Intraocular gases. In: Ryan SJ, ed. Retina, 2nd ed, vol 3. St. Louis: CV Mosby, 1994, p 2115.
29. Stinson TW, Donlon JV. Interaction of intraocular air and sulfur hexafluoride with nitrous oxide: a computer simulation. Anesthesiology 1982;56:385.
30. Smith RB, Carl B, Linn JG, Nemoto E. Effect of nitrous oxide on air in vitreous. Am J Ophthalmol 1974;78:314.
31. Wolf GL, Capuano C, Hartung J. Nitrous oxide increases intraocular pressure after intravitreal sulfur hexafluoride injection. Anesthesiology 1983;59:547.

CHAPTER 9

VITREORETINAL COMPLICATIONS OF OCULAR ANESTHESIA

BRIAN H. JEWART, MD
STEVE CHARLES, MD
SID BORIRAK-CHANYAVAT, MD

The majority of vitreoretinal complications from ocular anesthesia are secondary to the anesthetic needle penetrating the globe. The less common systemic complications are due to the anesthetic agents gaining access to the central nervous system or systemic circulatory system. In this chapter, we discuss the most common vitreoretinal complications associated with ocular anesthesia, including their diagnosis and management.

In discussion of these complications, it is important to remember that the best method of preventing vitreoretinal complications is adequate planning before beginning ocular anesthesia. The surgeon is responsible for ensuring that the patient is positioned properly, that sedation is under control, and that the personnel performing the anesthetic block are well trained in the procedure and have a thorough understanding of ocular anatomy. Once a complication has occurred, the surgeon must then be prepared to deal with this situation in a calm, efficient, and rational manner. Finally, potential complications can be minimized by matching the appropriate block technique (i.e., peribulbar, parabulbar, or retrobulbar) to the procedure that is to be performed while taking into account certain patient characteristics (i.e., high myopia, previous surgery, or inflamed orbit).

VITREORETINAL COMPLICATIONS AND THEIR MANAGEMENT

RETROBULBAR HEMORRHAGE

Retrobulbar hemorrhage is the most common complication from administration of ocular anesthesia. Studies currently quote an incidence rate of .1% to 1.7%[1-4] to 3%. These studies were done after monitoring both retrobulbar and peribulbar anesthetic injections. The incidence of retrobulbar hemorrhage after retrobulbar injection is higher than after peribulbar injection. Severe and permanent visual loss results from prolonged compromise of retinal perfusion secondary to the elevated intraocular and orbital pressure. In a primate model, Hayreh and coworkers reported irreversible cell injury following 90 minutes of central artery occlusion.[4a]

Retrobulbar bleeding may be venous or arteriolar in origin. With venous bleeding, the physician will typically notice a gradual spread of blood anteriorly toward the limbus. The intraocular pressure in these cases will show a much less dramatic rise with less pronounced proptosis of the globe.

Arteriolar retrobulbar hemorrhages progress more rapidly. There is rapid proptosis with the onset of globe immobility and subconjunctival engorgement with blood.

Immediate measures in the treatment of retrobulbar hemorrhage start with digital orbital pressure to tamponade the bleeding. Once the tamponade has been effective, attention must be directed to measurement of intraocular pressure and prevention of retinal vascular occlusion. If the intraocular pressure is very elevated, indirect ophthalmoscopy should be used to directly view the retinal vasculature. A solid blood column does not necessarily mean that a vessel is perfusing.

Osmotic diuresis and topical intraocular pressure–lowering agents may be used in the acute setting. In addition, a lateral canthotomy may be necessary to allow orbital compression in severe cases of retrobulbar hemorrhage. When acute occlusion of the retinal vessels can be visualized in the fundus, an anterior chamber paracentesis may be performed if other measures have not been effective. A small 30-gauge needle mounted on a tuberculin syringe (with the plunger still in) will permit a gradual and controlled decompression of the globe and decrease the likelihood of a secondary choroidal hemorrhage.

Once acute hemorrhaging has subsided and the retinal circulation is no longer compromised, the surgeon must then decide to cancel or proceed with the case.

Most anterior segment and elective posterior segment procedures should be postponed. A 1- to 2-week period should be allowed for the hemorrhage to clear. The surgery can then be rescheduled and consideration given to surgery under general or parabulbar anesthesia after obtaining bleeding studies.

If a trans–pars plana vitrectomy is scheduled and the procedure needs to be done without delay, the physician may elect to proceed with surgery on the day of retrobulbar hemorrhage. Once the infusion cannula is placed, the intraocular pressure can be artificially maintained at a certain level to ensure that there is no compromise of retinal circulation.

GLOBE PENETRATION AND PERFORATION

Globe penetration or perforation during administration of ophthalmic anesthesia is a rare complication. The rarity of this event frequently gives rise to overreaction on the part of the surgeon. It is not unusual for the referring ophthalmologist to demand immediate action from a vitreoretinal specialist. Although immediate vitreoretinal surgery is seldom indicated, the anxiety of the primary surgeon, coupled with an aggressive vitreoretinal surgeon, can result in unnecessary surgery.

In single ocular penetration, in which the needle is passed only through the sclera with a single perforation with or without anesthetic injection, the visual results are usually not severe.[5] The wounds from a retrobulbar needle are self-sealing and do not require exploration or suturing (Fig. 9–1). Retinopexy or scleral buckling is usually not necessary because rhegmatogenous retinal detachment formation after a traumatic retinal penetration is quite rare. If the needle is passed into the eye and anesthetic injection occurs, retinal toxicity, if any, will occur almost immediately. The pharmacologic agent diffuses from the vitreous cavity very rapidly. Studies have shown that fluorescein dye injected into the vitreous cavity diffuses from the eye within 10 minutes.[6] Immediate vitrectomy for removal of injected anesthetic mixture is probably unwarranted.

The rate of globe perforation during retrobulbar anesthesia has been reported ranging from zero incidence in 2000 consecutive peribulbar injections to 3 in a series of 4000 retrobulbar injections and 1 in a series of 1200 injections.[1–3]

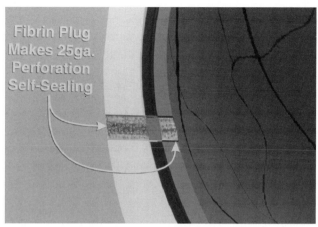

Figure 9–1. Single globe perforations are self-sealing and do not need emergent repair.

One must remember that certain eyes may be at an increased risk of ocular perforation during anesthetic injection. Although highly myopic eyes, especially associated with staphyloma formation, are at high risk, any eye is at risk for perforation if there is inadequate attention to technique.

There is concern over needle selection when performing retrobulbar injection. Atkinson's original report suggests using a blunted needle no longer than 35 mm in length.[7] Morgan and colleagues have documented that sharp 25-gauge needles can cause globe perforation more often than blunt-tip 23-gauge needles.[8] Rinkoff, Doft, and Lobes reported on a study involving 12 ocular perforations. Eleven of the 12 perforations occurred using sharp 25-gauge needles.[5]

A similar controversy exists regarding who should be performing ocular anesthesia. Rinkoff, Doft, and Lobes summarized 50 cases of known perforation that had existed in the literature at the time of their report.[5] They found that 60% of the injections were given by the surgeon and 40% by a nonophthalmologist. There are advantages and disadvantages of having either one perform the injection. Regardless of one's feelings on who is best suited to perform the injection, certain requirements exist. The person performing the injection must understand orbital anatomy in great detail. The personnel must completely understand the changing orbital dynamics of having the eye in primary gaze or having different versions occur during injection. Specifically, the relative position of the optic nerve and consideration of the axial length of the eye need to be taken into account.

We have found that the only way to ensure adequate anesthesia and akinesia without risk of ocular perforation is to use parabulbar anesthesia, the sub-Tenon's infusion of an anesthetic mixture via cannula. We first use a Weck cell soaked in sterile tetracaine placed over the inferotemporal conjunctiva near the inferior temporal fornix. After this area is adequately anesthetized, Wescott scissors and 0.12 forceps are used to make a small incision in the conjunctiva. Blunt dissection through the conjunctival opening is performed to dissect Tenon's capsule. Topical anesthetics should be avoided because of the frequency of punctate corneal keratopathy. A 10-mL syringe attached to a Greenbaum cannula is then passed through the conjunctival buttonhole under Tenon's capsule and directed around the curvature of the globe toward the muscle cone. Small-toothed forceps are used to pinch closed the conjunctival buttonhole to prevent the anesthetic mixture from escaping. In our experience, adequate anesthesia and akinesia are obtained within minutes. This technique allows supplementation to be performed at any time during the case. We have found that supplementation is necessary in approximately 25% of our patients, depending on the type of vitreoretinal surgery being performed and the surgeon's experience with the technique.

Ocular perforation may be first noted by the physician or anesthetic personnel performing the block. They may feel a sudden increase in resistance as the needle penetrates or perforates the globe (Fig. 9–2). The patient may first notice the perforation because of severe pain and sudden loss of vision. Clinical signs at the time of perforation or penetration may include hypotony, poor red reflex, and vitreous hemorrhage. If ocular penetration or perforation is suspected, the physician must attempt indirect ophthalmoscopy.

If a perforation or penetration is seen, globe exploration is not indicated. There is no need to search for the actual perforation site because of the self-sealing nature of the wounds. If a retinal hole is visualized, focal laser or cryotherapy may not be indicated.

Retinopexy increases the risk of vitreous hypocellular gel contraction, formation of epiretinal membranes, and subretinal scarring.

If a vitreous hemorrhage occurs, the case should be canceled and a vitreoretinal consultation obtained. Ultrasonography should be performed if the fundus cannot be visualized with indirect ophthalmoscopy. The referral need not be on an emergency basis and can be done once the patient leaves the hospital or surgical facility.

There is no indication for vitrectomy immediately after perforation. Immediate vitrectomy may increase the risk of rhegmatogenous retinal detachment as well as cataract formation. Emergency surgery is unnecessary and increases the risks and costs.

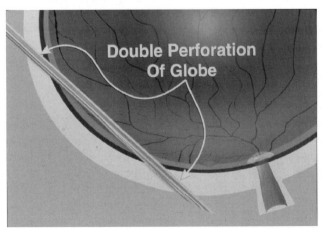

Figure 9–2. Double globe perforation. Globe exploration is unnecessary because of sealing wounds.

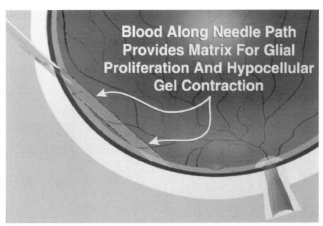

Figure 9–3. Intravitreal blood along needle path induces glial proliferation and hypocellular gel contraction.

The indications for vitrectomy after perforation are identical to those occurring after foreign body perforation of the globe during trauma. In both of these instances, the vitreous needs to be observed through the postinjury course. If hypocellular gel contraction is noted by the loss of vitreous mobility, vitrectomy is indicated (Fig. 9–3). If this occurs, there is a higher likelihood that a traction retinal detachment will occur because of retinal surface proliferation. Hypocellular gel contraction occurs over a 7- to 14-day period.

Scleral buckling is not indicated immediately after ocular penetration or perforation because there is minimal risk of rhegmatogenous retinal detachment after ocular penetration. Most detachments will be nonrhegmatogenous as a result of late hypocellular gel contraction. Scleral buckling with or without trans pars plana vitrectomy is then indicated.

Penetration of the needle within the globe, followed by injection of anesthetic mixture, can cause rupture of the globe. In an eye previously operated on, the most likely site of rupture is the previous incision site. In the eye without a history of ocular surgery, the most likely source of rupture is just posterior to the insertion of the rectus muscles where the sclera is the thinnest. If intraocular pressure is raised high enough without globe rupture, the critical closing pressure of the retinal vasculature may be exceeded.

The occurrence of an ocular perforation or penetration does not automatically mean the scheduled surgery must be canceled. Rinkoff, Doft, and Lobes reported that in their series of 12 ocular perforations, 9 of the cases proceeded with cataract extraction at the time of the perforation.[5] Seven of these 9 cases had a successful anatomic result. Poor final visual acuity after ocular perforation or penetration results in a final visual acuity of 20/50 or better in 50% of the cases.

PERFORATION OR PENETRATION OF THE GLOBE WITH INJECTION OF LOCAL ANESTHETIC

Retinal damage may also occur as a result of direct retinal toxicity caused by local anesthetic injected into the eye (Fig. 9–4). There is a

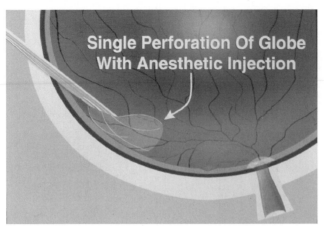

Figure 9–4. Injection of anesthetic directly into globe may cause immediate toxic damage to the retina.

well-documented myotoxic effect of local anesthetics on rat extraocular muscles that occurs within minutes of injection.[9–15] Researchers found that lidocaine caused an ischemic effect on the muscle cells, whereas bupivacaine caused a direct toxic effect to the muscle cells; however, no studies verify retinal toxicity from anesthetic agents.

Rinkoff, Doft, and Lobes reported good visual recovery in two patients who received intraocular injection of both .5 and 2% lidocaine with 1:100,000 epinephrine.[5] The same researchers also created an animal model to study the varying effects of changing volume and concentration of lidocaine, epinephrine, and hyaluronidase. After performing multiple variations with the just-mentioned medicine, they could find no retinal damage in the animal model. However, we have evaluated a young person who developed a permanent hemifield defect after receiving an inadvertent intraocular injection of lidocaine with epinephrine prior to chalazion excision. For this reason we avoid using epinephrine and hyaluronidase in our anesthetic technique.

Because there are no convincing studies that confirm permanent human retinal toxicity as a result of local anesthetics, we believe that immediate vitrectomy after injection of intraocular local anesthetic is unwarranted. However, until further studies clarify the true extent of hyaluronidase toxicity on the retina, an argument could be made for emergent vitrectomy in instances in which the anesthetic mixture injected contains hyaluronidase.

Local anesthetic can be injected directly into the optic nerve head. This may cause retrograde travel of the anesthetic agent through the brain stem. Brain stem anesthesia can cause respiratory arrest.

RETINAL VASCULAR OCCLUSION

Retinal vascular occlusion has been reported after retrobulbar injection.[16–18] Central retinal artery occlusion has been reported and is said to be more common in patients with a history of glaucoma or systemic vascular disease, including diabetes mellitus and sickle-cell anemia. The site of vascular obstruction can be at the optic nerve head. Central retinal artery occlusion can occur as a result of a large volume of retrobulbar anesthetic injected behind the eye. A retrobulbar hemorrhage could also result in optic nerve compression and vascular occlusion as well. Central retinal artery occlusion or branch retinal artery occlusion can also occur as a result of vasospasm.

A combined central retinal artery and central retinal vein occlusion has been reported.[19] This case was due to a retrobulbar hemorrhage compromising the retinal circulation.

A Purtscher's-like retinopathy has also been reported. Purtscher's retinopathy is known to be related to intravascular aggregation of white cells and complement fixation. Purtscher's retinopathy has been linked to a Valsalva maneuver, thoracic decompression, air and fat embolism, and acute pancreatitis. The article suggests that the increased retrobulbar pressure, induced by the anesthetic agents, caused the pressure within the retinal vasculature to increase, simulating a Valsalva maneuver. In this reported case, visual recovery was excellent.

Unfortunately, most of the retinal vascular complications of retrobulbar injections are not amenable to treatment. Simple precautions, such as backflushing before injecting, can be taken to decrease the frequency of these injuries. Remember, if the pressure required to inject the anesthetic mixture is more than usual, it may be prudent to redirect the needle so as to prevent direct injection into the optic nerve.

CONCLUSION

The vitreoretinal complications of ocular anesthesia are quite rare but can cause severe permanent loss of vision. Complications include retrobulbar hemorrhage, globe penetration and perforation, injection of ocular anesthetics after ocular perforation, and retinal vascular occlusion. With appropriate preoperative evaluation by the personnel performing the ocular anesthesia, many of these complications can be avoided. Aspects that need to be evaluated before performing ocular anesthesia include consideration of ocular position within the orbit, axial length of the eye, patient movement during procedure, and exquisite understanding of ocular anatomy.

Once a complication has occurred, the responsibility for management is the direct responsibility of the ophthalmologist. Immediate vitrectomy, scleral buckling, and retinopexy are rarely required. This is due primarily to the self-sealing nature of the ocular perforation. In most instances, the best plan of action is observation of the ocular perforation. It is certainly recommended that a vitreoretinal consultation be obtained early in the management course.

In modern ophthalmic surgery, the vast majority of procedures have shifted to an outpatient basis. These settings often feature rapid turnaround time, nonophthalmologists performing the ocular anesthesia, and often limited preoperative discussions between the patient anesthetist or anesthesiologist and the physician performing the surgery. This means that there must be constant communication among all parties involved in the surgery. With communication lines open, complications can be anticipated, recognized quickly, and managed in an appropriate manner that will maximize the patient's recovery.

Minimizing these complications still appears to be the best approach. With the recent advent of parabulbar anesthesia, it is possible to avoid the great majority of the complications associated with retrobulbar anesthesia without sacrificing any anesthetic efficacy. We have found parabulbar anesthesia to be as effective as retrobulbar anesthesia in all vitreoretinal cases.

REFERENCES

1. Hamilton RC, Gimbel HV, Strunin L. Regional anesthesia for 12,000 cataract extraction and intraocular lens implantation procedures, Can J Anaesth 1988;35:615.
2. Ramsay RC, Knobloch WH. Ocular perforation following retrobulbar anesthesia for retinal detachment surgery. Am J Ophthalmol 1978;86:61.
3. Davis DB, Mandel MR. Posterior peribulbar anesthesia: an alternative to retrobulbar anesthesia. Cataract Refract Surg 1986;12:182.
4. Cibis PA. Discussion. In: Schepens CL, Regan CDJ, eds. Controversial aspects of the management of retinal detachments. Boston: Little, Brown, 1965, p 251.
4a. Hayreh SS, Kolder HF, Weingeist TA. Central retinal artery occlusion and retinal tolerance time. Ophthalmology 1980;87:75.
5. Rinkoff JS, Doft BH, Lobes LA. Management of ocular penetration from injection of local anesthesia preceding cataract surgery. Arch Ophthalmol 1991;109:1421.
6. Maurice DM. Protein dynamics in the eye studied with labelled proteins. Am J Ophthalmol 1959;47:361.
7. Atkinson WS. Retrobulbar injection of anesthetic within the muscular cone. Arch Ophthalmol 1936;16;1936:494.
8. Morgan CM, Schatz H, Vine AKM, et al. Ocular complications associated with retrobulbar injections. Ophthalmology 1988;95:660.
9. Friedberg HL, Kline OR Jr. Contralateral amaurosis after retrobulbar injection. Am J Ophthalmol 1986;101:688.
10. Benoit PW, Belt WD. Destruction and regeneration of skeletal muscle after treatment with a local anaesthetic, bupivacaine (Marcaine). J Anat 1970;107:547.
11. Benoit PW, Belt WD. Some effects of local anesthetic agents on skeletal muscle. Exp Neurol 1972;34:264.
12. Basson MD, Carlson BM. Myotoxicity of single and repeated injection of mepivacaine (Carbocaine) in the rat. Anesth Analg 1980;59:275.
13. Carlson BM, Rainin EA. Rat extraocular muscle regeneration—repair of local anesthetic-induced damage. Arch Ophthalmol 1985;103:1373.
14. Yagiela JA, Benoit PW, Buoncristiani RD, et al. Comparison of myotoxic effects of lidocaine with epinephrine in rats and humans. Anesth Analg 1981;60:471.
15. Foster AH, Carlson BM. Myotoxicity of local anesthetics and regeneration of damaged muscle fibers. Anesth Analg 1980;58:727.
16. Brown GC. Complications of retrobulbar injection. In: Spaeth GL, Katz LJ, Parker KW, eds. Current therapy in ophthalmic surgery. Philadelphia: BC Decker, 1989, p 11.
17. Horven I. Ophthalmic artery pressure during retrobulbar anesthesia. Acta Ophthalmol 1978;56:574.
18. Kraushar MF, Seelenfreund MH, Freilich DB. Central retinal artery occlusion during orbital hemorrhage from retrobulbar injection. Trans Am Acad Ophthalmol Otol 1974;78:65.
19. Lemagne J-M, Michiels X, Van Causenbroech S, Snyers B. Purtscher-like retinopathy after retrobulbar anesthesia. Ophthalmology 1990;97:859.

CHAPTER 10

ANESTHESIA FOR OCULOPLASTIC SURGERY

BRIAN S. BIESMAN, MD
ALBERT HORNBLASS, MD

The goal of any oculoplastic procedure is to accomplish the desired surgical result while causing as little anxiety and disruption of the patient's life as possible. Each individual has unique fears, preconceptions, and misgivings before undergoing surgery, and it is imperative that the surgeon explore these feelings preoperatively. Failure to do so may produce an unnecessarily stressful or dissatisfying experience and an unhappy patient.

Concerns commonly expressed by patients include preprocedure anxiety; fear of discomfort from the injection of local anesthesia; intraoperative discomfort; amount of postoperative swelling and bruising; length of time away from work, which may be related to postoperative swelling and bruising; postoperative pain; requirements for postoperative care, including number and timing of office visits; discomfort associated with suture removal; and, of course, postoperative results. Whereas we as surgeons tend to focus on postoperative results, some patients may be equally concerned or perhaps even more concerned about some of these other issues. A complete understanding of each patient's fears and expectations can help the surgeon achieve more patient satisfaction and thus a better postoperative result. A knowledge of current techniques in anesthesia can help the surgeon plan the ideal procedure for each patient.

Most oculoplastic procedures fall into one of three categories: eyelid and adnexal, lacrimal, and orbital. Anesthesia for each of these categories is addressed separately after a review of the sensory innervation of the involved structures.

Sensory innervation of the eyelids and orbit is derived from the fifth cranial nerve. The fifth cranial nerve (trigeminal) has both sensory and motor components. It arises from several subnuclei within the brain stem and spinal cord and has three major branches: ophthalmic, maxillary, and mandibular. The first two of these divisions supply orbital and ocular structures. The ophthalmic division (V1) travels within the cavernous sinus, where it branches into the lacrimal, frontal, and nasociliary nerves. The lacrimal nerve enters the orbit through the supraorbital fissure above the annulus of Zinn and courses along the lateral orbital wall, where it is joined by fibers from the zygomatic nerve carrying parasympathetic innervation to the lacrimal gland. The lacrimal nerve then exits the orbit and provides sensory innervation to the skin of the lateral upper eyelid. The frontal nerve, the largest of V1's three branches, also enters the orbit through the supraorbital fissure above the annulus of Zinn. This nerve travels along the orbital roof between the levator and the periorbita. It divides into its two terminal branches, the supraorbital and supratrochlear nerves that exit the orbit, providing innervation to the remainder of the upper eyelid and brow. The third division of V1 is the nasociliary nerve. It also enters the orbit through the supraorbital fissure but, as opposed to the lacrimal and frontal nerves, passes through the annulus of Zinn. It then turns toward the medial orbital wall and gives off a branch to the ciliary ganglion. As the nasociliary nerve travels along the medial orbital wall, it gives rise to the long ciliary nerves, which provide sensation to the globe and carry sympathetic fibers to the dilator muscle of the iris. The nasociliary nerve continues anteriorly in the medial orbit, where it divides into the anterior and posterior ethmoidal and infratrochlear nerves. These nerves

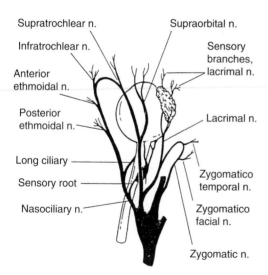

Supratrochlear n.

Infratrochlear n.

Anterior
ethmoidal n.

Posterior
ethmoidal n.

Long ciliary

Sensory root

Nasociliary n.

Supraorbital n.

Sensory
branches,
lacrimal n.

Lacrimal n.

Zygomatico
temporal n.

Zygomatico
facial n.

Zygomatic n.

Figure 10–1. The distribution of the ophthalmic division of the fifth cranial nerve within the right orbit.

supply the ethmoidal and nasal mucosa and may be anesthetized with local injections to allow performance of dacryocystorhinostomy (DCR) under local anesthesia. The infratrochlear nerve, the terminal branch of the nasociliary, exits the orbit to supply sensory innervation to the lacrimal sac, conjunctiva, and skin of the medial canthal region (Fig. 10–1).

The maxillary nerve (V2), the second branch of the trigeminal, travels briefly within the cavernous sinus before exiting to pass through the foramen rotundum to enter the pterygopalatine fossa. It is here that the zygomaticotemporal nerve branches off, carrying parasympathetic fibers that will join the lacrimal nerve before entering the lacrimal gland. The terminal branch of V2 is the infraorbital nerve, which runs anteriorly in the infraorbital groove before exiting the maxilla several millimeters below the infraorbital rim. In this location on the orbital floor, the infraorbital nerve is susceptible to injury when orbital floor fractures occur, as is common after blunt trauma. Symptoms of infraorbital nerve damage include numbness of the lower eyelid, side of the nose, upper lip, and upper teeth on the involved side. In some cases, these may be the only symptoms of an orbital fracture. As an additional clinical note, the varicella-zoster virus, a member of the herpesvirus family, has a latent phase in which it can remain dormant for many years within the trigeminal (semilunar) ganglion. In times of stress, extreme sunlight exposure, or immune suppression, the virus becomes active and herpes zoster ophthalmicus may occur. Ocular involvement is often seen when the tip of the nose (nasociliary nerve) is involved. The third division of the trigeminal nerve does not innervate orbital or adnexal structures and is not discussed[1] (Fig. 10–2).

LOCAL ANESTHETIC AGENTS

Local anesthetic agents are used extensively by oculoplastic surgeons, even in cases performed under general anesthesia. There are two major categories of local anesthetics: those that are applied topically and those

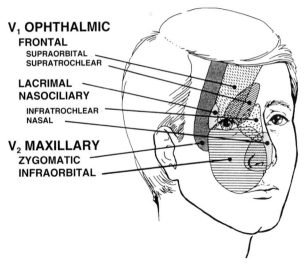

Figure 10–2. Sensory distribution of the trigeminal nerve to the facial skin. Most oculoplastic procedures involving soft tissues and the lacrimal system can be performed under local anesthesia if the appropriate branches of cranial nerve V1 and V2 are anesthetized.

that require injection. The injectable agents may be used either to produce a regional nerve block, in which the entire distribution of the affected nerve is anesthetized, or simply to anesthetize the area into which the agent is injected. Familiarity with local anesthetic agents and their potential complications and side effects is important for the oculoplastic surgeon.

All local anesthetic agents currently useful clinically are tertiary amines, which may be classified as esters or amides on the basis of the nature of the linkage between the aromatic lipophilic component with the hydrophilic amine. Commonly used esters include procaine (Novocain), cocaine, tetracaine, proparacaine, and benoxinate (Fluress). Some of the frequently used amide local anesthetics include lidocaine (Xylocaine), bupivacaine (Marcaine), mepivacaine (Carbocaine), and etidocaine (Duranest). The ester-based local anesthetics are broken down rapidly in the blood stream by plasma cholinesterase and more slowly in tissue by tissue cholinesterase. A by-product of the degradation of the ester anesthetics, with the exception of proparacaine, is para-aminobenzoic acid, a highly allergenic compound. This accounts for the greater incidence of allergic reactions to the ester anesthetics and severely limits the use of these agents in local injection. The amide group, in contrast, is degraded not in tissue or the blood stream but rather in the liver.[2]

Both the amide and ester groups of drugs are available commercially as organic salts because they are unstable in their base amine form. They are most potent over a pH range of 3 to 6.5 and with increasing alkalinization begin to precipitate. The addition of sodium bicarbonate to stock solutions of local anesthetics has been suggested to raise the pH and thus improve the patient's comfort level with injection, but caution is required because the pH of each solution may vary and addition of a standard amount of bicarbonate without pH control can result in the development of a precipitate. If this occurs, on injection the precipitate will be deposited in the tissue and appear as a tattoo.[3]

Local anesthetics are often supplied in a solution containing epinephrine in a ratio of 1:100,000 or 1:200,000 to the local anesthetic. The epinephrine additive prolongs the duration of anesthetic effect and decreases systemic toxicity by causing local vasoconstriction. Epinephrine should not be used in retrobulbar anesthetics unless the block is being administered before enucleation. Lidocaine and procaine are available in a 4% solution as well as in less potent strengths. Because of solubility issues, the 4% solutions are prepared in sterile water, whereas the preparations containing less than 4% anesthetic are applied in isotonic saline solution. This is a particularly important distinction to recognize because sterile water is extremely painful when injected.

Careful consideration must be given to the toxicity of local anesthetics, a topic often overlooked in surgical texts. Toxic reactions may occur in a dose-related fashion, in an idiosyncratic fashion, or as a hypersensitivity reaction and may be serious or fatal. An overdose of local anesthetic may affect the central nervous system (CNS), the cardiovascular system, or both. The CNS may become stimulated or depressed. Stimulation may manifest as restlessness, tremors, lightheadedness, nervousness, apprehension, euphoria, confusion, tinnitus, diplopia, twitching, or shivering and may progress to seizures. Coma and respiratory arrest may follow CNS stimulation or may present as the first sign of local anesthetic overdose. Cardiovascular effects may include depressed conduction, leading to heart block and severe bradycardia, ventricular arrhythmias, hypotension, and cardiovascular collapse. The management of systemic toxic reactions to local anesthetic agents begins with the establishment and maintenance of an airway and effective ventilation with 100% oxygen. If seizure activity occurs, hypoxia, hypercarbia, and acidosis will develop rapidly. Seizure activity may be controlled with intravenous benzodiazepines or other antiseizure agents. Succinylcholine may be administered to induce paralysis if necessary. The cardiovascular system must be addressed and supported with intravenous fluids or pressors as necessary. Hemodialysis is generally of little benefit in the management of local anesthetic overdose.[4, 5]

The local anesthetic agents most often used in oculoplastic surgery are bupivacaine and lidocaine. Although lidocaine is often used independently of bupivacaine, the latter agent is not usually used alone because of the prolonged delay in onset of its analgesic effects (30–45 minutes) compared with the nearly instantaneous onset of action of lidocaine. Conversely, lidocaine is metabolized relatively rapidly (half-life of 1.5–2 hours), whereas bupivacaine produces a more lasting analgesia (half-life of about 3.5 hours). For this reason, lidocaine and bupivacaine are sometimes administered as a mixture either to maintain analgesia for a lengthy case or to provide several hours of postoperative pain relief after a shorter procedure.

The maximum recommended total dose of bupivacaine administered to a healthy adult is approximately 175 mg, whereas that of lidocaine should not exceed 300 mg (or 4.5 mg/kg). If the anesthetic preparations contain epinephrine as an additive, the total dose of bupivacaine may be increased to approximately 225 mg and the total dose of lidocaine to about 500 mg (7.5 mg/kg). Dosages should be reduced for children, elderly patients, and those with liver disease. Although these dosages appear to offer a large safety zone given the usual requirements for a typical oculoplastic procedure, the surgeon is reminded that 1 mL of a 1% solution of anesthetic contains 10 mg of drug and that 1 mL of a 2% solution contains 20 mg of drug. The same vasoconstrictive effect that increases the safety margin of the local anesthetic from a dosing standpoint may be used to the surgeon's benefit by reducing the amount of intraoperative hemorrhage.[6] To take full advantage of this effect, a full 15 minutes should be allowed to pass before making an incision. To save time and expense in the operating room, if proper monitoring is available, the local anesthetic may be injected while the patient is in the holding area. It is generally wise to mark proposed eyelid incisions before injection of anesthetic to avoid distortion of the tissues. Injections should be subcutaneous and not intramuscular. Some surgeons prefer suborbicularis muscle injections before performing eyelid surgery.

Bupivacaine hydrochloride is available in concentrations of .25%, .5%, and .75%. All three concentrations are available with epinephrine added at a ratio of 1:200,000. Solutions containing epinephrine should not be autoclaved and should be protected from sunlight. Lidocaine is also supplied as the hydrochloride salt and is available in concentrations of .5%, 1.0%, 1.5%, and 2.0%. The 1% and 2% solutions are available with epinephrine diluted at 1:100,000, although all concentrations may be purchased without epinephrine or with epinephrine added at a 1:200,000 dilution.[6]

Allergic reactions to local anesthetics are rare and may occur as a result of sensitivity to the drug itself or to the antimicrobial preservatives such as methylparaben, which is added to most multidose vials. The symptoms and signs of a true hypersensitivity reaction to a local anesthetic agent are those of any type IV reaction and may include urticaria, pruritus, erythema, angioneurotic edema, tachycardia, sneezing, nausea, vomiting, dizziness, sweating, fever, and even hypotension. Most local anesthetic agents are available in methylparaben-free preparations. The treatment of an allergic reaction to a local anesthetic does not differ from the management of any other type IV reaction.[7]

ANESTHESIA FOR EYELID AND ADNEXAL SURGERY

GENERAL MEDICAL CONSIDERATIONS

Before performing any surgical procedure, a careful and complete medical history must be taken. Specific questions regarding cardiopulmonary symptoms must be asked because patients may be unable or unwilling to volunteer this information freely. Similarly, other systemic problems such as hypertension, diabetes mellitus, thyroid dysfunction, renal insufficiency, and systemic inflammatory diseases should be as stable as possible. The importance of a thorough preoperative evaluation cannot be overemphasized. Despite pressure and encouragement from patients to proceed with a procedure as soon as possible, elective procedures should be postponed until other medical conditions have been thoroughly assessed and determined to be stable. Communication with the patient's primary care physician is critical. Even "minor" procedures may evoke enough anxiety in an unstable patient to cause serious cardiovascular effects because of a surge in systemic catecholamine levels. The American Society of Anesthesiology (ASA) has developed a uniform system classifying each patient into one of five categories on the basis of overall health. The ASA class should be determined for each patient as part of the routine preoperative evaluation so as to assess the *relative* risk of the proposed procedure. The ASA classifies patients as follows:

Class I: A normal, healthy patient
Class II: A patient with mild systemic disease
Class III: A patient with severe systemic disease that limits activity but is not incapacitating
Class IV: A patient with an incapacitating systemic disease that is a threat to life
Class V: A moribund patient not expected to survive more than 24 hours with or without surgery

Although there is no *direct* correlation between ASA class and operative morbidity, overall morbidity is four to five times greater in Class III and IV patients than in Class I patients. The surgeon should never choose to perform an elective procedure against the wishes of the anesthesiologist if he or she believes that additional medical evaluation is necessary to assess a patient's medical status properly. For urgent cases, the relative risk of not performing surgery must be weighed relative to the risks of anesthesia. Although emergent cases obviously must be performed, careful consideration must be given to each case before it is determined to be a true emergency.[8, 9]

MEDICATIONS

Patients should be encouraged to continue taking as many of their usual medications as possible on the day of surgery. Medications may be taken at home with a sip of water, and nonessential products (e.g., vitamins) may be withheld. Careful inquiry into the use of aspirin or other nonsteroidal anti-inflammatory medications must be made because many patients do not consider these over-the-counter products to be "medicine."

The antiplatelet activity associated with use of nonsteroidal anti-inflammatory medications can have a profound effect on any eyelid, adnexal, lacrimal, or orbital procedure. At the very least, nonsteroidal use within 7 to 10 days of surgery will cause increased intraoperative bleeding, swelling, and tissue distortion, leading to unpredictable effects of some procedures, especially ptosis repair, and a longer postoperative recovery period. In a more extreme but well-recognized scenario, blindness caused by orbital hemorrhage can occur.[10] We recommend postponing all elective eyelid, lacrimal, and orbital procedures if patients have taken any nonsteroidal anti-inflammatory agent within 10 days before surgery. In urgent cases, such procedures may be performed with caution. Any orbital procedure performed in patients who have taken nonsteroidal drugs should include placement of a drain to be kept in place until all drainage has resolved for at least 24 hours. Although some surgeons routinely obtain prothrombin and partial thromboplastin times preoperatively, these studies will fail to disclose a bleeding diathesis caused by impaired platelet function. The function of the entire coagulation system may be easily assessed by obtaining a bleeding time, a simple and underused test that is performed by inflating a blood pressure cuff to 40 mm Hg and making a 1-mm deep cut with a blade in the forearm. Every 30 seconds, the excess blood is absorbed onto a piece of filter paper without touching the lesion. The bleeding should stop in 5 to 7 minutes. The bleeding test may also be accomplished with a device known as the Thrombostat 4000.[11]

Other general medical considerations that may affect the administration of anesthesia include the patient's age; the ability to lie flat for the duration of the operation; presence of arthritis, which may affect the cervical spine; airway abnormalities such as acute rhinitis, nasal tumors, or deformity; acute respiratory disease; psychiatric disorders; and pregnancy.

GENERAL VERSUS LOCAL ANESTHESIA

The anesthetic state is characterized by an induced state of unconsciousness during which surgical stimulation elicits only autonomic reflex responses. The patient should not exhibit any voluntary movements, but changes in vital signs may be monitored. This definition differs from that of the analgesic state, in which there is no sensibility to pain. The analgesic state may be produced by narcotics in much smaller doses than are required to produce unconsciousness. General anesthetic agents are usually administered by inhalation through a nasotracheal or endotracheal tube but may also be given intravenously. Although many eyelid and adnexal procedures can be performed under local or regional anesthesia, general anesthesia may be appropriate for the treatment of infants and children, for orbital procedures, for some lacrimal procedures, for extensive or long procedures, and for the treatment of patients who may be unable to lie still because of neurologic or mental disorders.[12]

Inhalational general anesthetic agents commonly used include halothane, enflurane (Ethrane), and nitrous oxide. Care must be taken to avoid the use of nitrous oxide in patients who may have had intraocular gas injections after repair of a retinal break or detachment. In such cases, the nitrous oxide will fill the eye and may raise the intraocular pressure high enough to cause a central retinal artery occlusion. Good communication with the anesthesiologist will ensure the ideal choice of a general anesthetic agent for a given patient and procedure.

General anesthetics may be supplemented with injections of local anesthesia to help control postoperative pain and to take advantage of the epinephrine additive to improve intraoperative hemostasis. We generally inject 1% lidocaine containing epinephrine added in a ratio of 1:100,000 after general anesthesia has been induced. For cases in which postoperative pain control is a concern (e.g., enucleation surgery), we inject a 1:1 mixture of 2% lidocaine with epinephrine at a concentration of 1:100,000 and .75% bupivacaine.

Most eyelid and adnexal surgery may be performed under local or regional anesthesia. As discussed, the anesthetic agents most often used by oculoplastic surgeons are lidocaine and bupivacaine. For performing relatively short eyelid procedures, we recommend using 2% lidocaine with epinephrine added in a ratio of 1:100,000. For longer cases and DCRs, we generally use a combination of .75% bupivacaine and 2% lidocaine containing epinephrine 1:100,000 mixed in a 1:2 ratio. Local anesthesia for most eyelid procedures is administered via direct subcutaneous injection in the area where the surgery is to be performed. In preparation for adult ptosis surgery, care should be taken to minimize the amount of anesthetic injected because an excessive volume can result in partial or complete akinesia of the levator muscle, making intraoperative assessment of appropriate eyelid position very difficult. In most cases 1 mL of 2% lidocaine administered subcutaneously into the central upper eyelid in the region of the eyelid crease is adequate. A 27- or 30-gauge needle is used to decrease patient discomfort and to minimize trauma to the eyelid tissues. Whether injecting the upper or lower eyelid, a protective scleral shield should be in place, and the needle should always be directed away from the globe so that an unanticipated movement by the patient will not result in penetration or perforation of the sclera. An alternative approach to anesthetizing the upper eyelid is a regional blockade of the frontal nerve. A 30-gauge long needle is advanced along the roof of the orbit, and approximately .5 mL of anesthetic is injected after gently withdrawing on the plunger to ensure extravascular placement of the needle. If surgery is to be performed in the medial or lateral aspect of the upper lid as well, supplemental blockade of the supratrochlear or lacrimal nerve, respectively, may be required. Some surgeons prefer a retrobulbar needle to administer the frontal nerve block. The lacrimal nerve block is administered by sliding the needle along the roof of the lateral orbit, whereas the supratrochlear nerve is anesthetized by entering the medial orbit above the level of the medial canthal tendon. All three blocks should be given on the orbital aspect of the periosteum. To avoid akinesia of the extraocular muscles or the levator palpebrae superioris muscle, injection should be given external to the intermuscular septum.

To perform lower eyelid surgery such as external blepharoplasty, entropion repair (external approach), or tumor excision with reconstruction, lidocaine 2% with epinephrine diluted 1:100,000 is injected subcutaneously and allowed to diffuse with gentle massage. An alternative to this approach is an infraorbital nerve block. The course and distribution of the infraorbital nerve are described previously in Chapter 1 (Figs. 1–1 and 1–2). The infraorbital nerve may be approached transconjunctivally, percutaneously, or via the gingival buccal mucosa. The transconjunctival infraorbital nerve block is given by pulling the lower lid inferiorly, thus exposing the inferior fornix. A 30-gauge short ⅝ inch (1.6-cm) needle is then introduced through the fornix until it lies anterior to the infraorbital rim and is then advanced down the anterior surface of the maxilla along a vertical line drawn inferiorly from the supraorbital notch, a structure that can be easily palpated along the supraorbital rim. The infraorbital nerve block may be administered percutaneously by placing the needle adjacent to the lateral alae of the nose along the same line dropped vertically from the supraorbital notch. The infraorbital nerve is approached through the gingival buccal mucosa just lateral to the canine tooth by advancing a 27- or 30-gauge dental needle along the anterior surface of the maxilla, directing the needle toward the infraorbital foramen, which may be readily palpated in this fashion. The transconjunctival and transoral approaches avoid bleeding, which may occur when passing a needle through the facial musculature in a percutaneous approach. If transconjunctival blepharoplasty is to be performed, the inferior fornix is exposed and the 30-gauge short needle is directed slightly posterior to the infraorbital rim into the orbital fat, where 1 mL of local anesthetic is injected. If lateral canthoplasty is to be performed in conjunction with lower eyelid surgery, the periosteum inside the lateral orbital rim must be anesthetized separately by advancing the needle until bone is encountered, withdrawing the plunger to avoid intravascular injection, and then administering about .5 mL of anesthetic solution.

Complications of local anesthetic injections in the eyelids are rare. A hematoma may form if the injection is given intramuscularly rather than subcutaneously. Patients should be warned before introduction of the needle to avoid inadvertent head movements that may endanger the eye itself. To help prevent accidental intraocular injection, the tip of the needle should always be directed away from the globe, and, if necessary, the patient's head and hands may be stabilized. Care should always be taken to confirm the contents of a syringe before injecting. Injection of the wrong agent has occurred and can have devastating consequences. All syringes and solutions on the sterile field must be clearly and properly marked. If there is any doubt as to the proper identification of a solution, it should be discarded.

SEDATION

Before the administration of a general or a local anesthetic, pharmacologic agents are often administered to promote relaxation and relief of anxiety before surgery and, in some instances, to induce the anesthetic state for a short period of time while a noxious stimulus such as a local anesthetic is applied. Sedative agents may be given orally, sublingually, or intravenously.

The benzodiazepines are anxiolytics whose effect is believed to be related to action on the limbic system, the thalamus, and the hypothalamus. The benzodiazepines commonly used by the oculoplastic surgeon include diazepam (Valium), lorazepam (Ativan), and midazolam (Versed). These drugs differ primarily in their half-lives and time to onset of action. They may be administered orally (diazepam, lorazepam), intravenously, intramuscularly, sublingually, or by inhalation (midazolam). Midazolam has the shortest half-life (1.2–12.3 hours) compared with lorazepam (16 hours) and diazepam (2–3 days). The clinical effects of midazolam generally last 2 to 6 hours. In addition to relief of anxiety, the benzodiazepines are also skeletal muscle relaxants and have an amnestic effect. Because of its relatively short half-life and duration of effect, midazolam is the benzodiazepine used most often as an adjunct to oculoplastic surgical procedures. When administered intravenously, sedation occurs within 3 to 5 minutes but may occur sooner if narcotic premedication has been given. It is thus beneficial for use preoperatively as well as intraoperatively. Before noxious stimuli such as the injection of local anesthesia, additional sedation may be required. Peak sedation occurs in about 30 minutes and lasts approximately 2 hours. The sedative effect of the benzodiazepines is accentuated by premedication with narcotics, and in these situations dosages should be decreased by at least one third.[13]

All benzodiazepines must be administered in a careful, patient-specific fashion. Because the respiratory depressant effects may not become manifest immediately, midazolam must be administered intravenously in small doses of 1 mg. There is some discomfort with the intravenous administration of the diazepam because it is supplied for injection in a solution of propylene, ethanol, and water. Diazepam is less potent than midazolam and is usually given in doses of 2.5 to 5 mg intravenously. Great care must be taken not to use diazepam when administering midazolam. This mistake was made frequently when midazolam was first introduced, leading to unexpected respiratory depression.[14]

The major adverse effects of the benzodiazepines include CNS and respiratory depression. Respiratory arrest and cardiovascular collapse can occur. For this reason, careful monitoring of respiration, pulse, and blood pressure is required when these drugs are administered. Excessive dosages are manifest clinically by snoring followed by airway obstruction, which usually responds to jaw lift maneuvers to maintain the airway. As opposed to narcotic overdosage, the patient overdosed with benzodiazepines will often make a respiratory effort. Ventilation is not usually required. When severe respiratory depression does occur, a benzodiazepine antagonist flumazenil may be administered. It is given intravenously in doses of .4 mg. Although the sedative and psychomotor effects of benzodiazepines may be reversed, the half-life of flumazenil is short and resedation may occur. Airway and cardiovascular support must be maintained even if flumazenil is used.[6]

Hiccups are a more minor adverse effect found in approximately 4% of patients receiving midazolam. This is insignificant unless hiccups occur intraoperatively when delicate maneuvers are being performed.[6]

Recently, a new ultra-short-acting sedative-hypnotic medication has become available that has proven extremely useful to the oculoplastic surgeon. Propofol is a sedative-hypnotic with minimal water solubility supplied in a white oil-in-water emulsion for intravenous administration. After injection, hypnosis is usually induced with one circulation through the CNS. After a single injection, peak hypnosis usually occurs within 2 minutes. Hypnosis is usually profound, and this drug is thus extremely useful before injection of local anesthetics. Patients will be fully awake several minutes after a single bolus. Apnea may occur and may be profound, although it usually resolves within 1 minute. Propofol may also be administered as a continuous drip to maintain sedation throughout a procedure. This is particularly useful when operating on extremely anxious patients or when performing lengthy procedures under local anesthesia. Propofol has also been used to perform postoperative adjustment of extraocular muscle position after strabismus surgery. After a 1-hour continuous infusion of propofol, serum levels are nearly zero 20 minutes after discontinuation of the drug. This makes propofol ideal for use in an outpatient surgery setting.

The usual dosage of propofol for induction of general anesthesia is 2.0 to 2.5 mg/kg in healthy adults and 1.0 to 2.0 mg/kg in elderly or debilitated adults every 10 seconds until induction onset occurs. Alternatively, to initiate monitored sedation and to avoid hypotension and apnea, slow infusion of .5 mg/kg may be given over 3 to 5 minutes. This may be followed immediately by an infusion of 1.5 to 4.5 mg/kg/h. Bolus dosing should be avoided in ASA Class III and IV patients.

The major adverse effects of propofol are related to cardiovascular and respiratory depression. Arterial hypotension is common, and this drug should be used with extreme caution in ASA Class III and IV patients. Respiratory depression may result in apnea, airway obstruction, and oxygen desaturation. Propofol should be given only by persons trained in the administration of general anesthesia and not by the surgeon performing the operation or procedure. Continuous monitoring of the airway, respiratory, and cardiovascular status is critical. Ventilatory and circulatory support should be immediately available.[15, 16]

Failure to observe careful aseptic technique during the preparation of propofol for injection has resulted in iatrogenic infection, including infectious endophthalmitis. Rapid growth of micro-organisms can occur in the propofol solution.[17, 18]

ANESTHESIA FOR LACRIMAL SURGERY

Lacrimal procedures may be performed under local or general anesthesia. If general anesthesia is not used, intravenous sedation should be administered in conjunction with the local anesthetic. Most lacrimal procedures, including DCR, conjunctivodacryocystorhinostomy (CDCR), canalicular intubation in adults, and dacryocystectomy, may be performed under local anesthesia. Most lacrimal procedures on infants and children are performed under the influence of general anesthetic agents, although some authors have advocated no anesthesia at all. Because most lacrimal procedures require intranasal manipulation, before surgery the nose should be packed with gauze or neurosurgical pads soaked in an agent to produce vasoconstriction and analgesia of the mucosa. Failure to decongest the mucosa will result in compromised visualization and increased intraoperative bleeding. Four percent cocaine is an excellent choice because it meets both needs. In some hospitals this agent may be difficult to obtain, and a 1:1 mixture of phenylephrine .25% (Neo-Synephrine) and 4% lidocaine may be used instead. If cocaine is applied, the drug may remain detectable in the serum for 1 week or more. The packing should be placed adjacent to the middle turbinate before DCR or CDCR surgery and should be placed beneath the inferior turbinate before canalicular intubation.

To perform lacrimal surgery under local anesthesia, regional blocks are administered to the supraorbital, supratrochlear, infratrochlear, and infraorbital nerves. When performing either a DCR or a CDCR, the local anesthetic is also injected in the proposed cutaneous incision site and directly into the nasal mucosa. The nasal mucosa may be injected intranasally before placement of the packing or, alternatively, may be injected from within the wound once the osteotomy has been completed. We generally inject a 2:1 mixture of .75% bupivacaine and 2% lidocaine containing epinephrine at a 1:100,000 dilution.

We believe that hemostasis is maximized when local anesthesia is used in DCR and CDCR procedures. This may be due to decreased vascular tone under general anesthesia, a well-recognized phenomenon that is sometimes taken advantage of when starting intravenous catheters in infants before surgery.

ANESTHESIA FOR ORBITAL SURGERY

The traditional approach to orbital surgery is to perform procedures under general anesthesia. In most cases in which bone removal and extensive intraorbital dissection are planned, general anesthesia is commonly used, whereas anterior orbital surgery may be comfortably performed under intravenous sedation and local anesthesia. If significant postoperative pain is anticipated, bupivacaine can be injected intraoperatively. Khan and Wegener performed orbital bone resection and orbital exploration under local anesthesia with intravenous sedation.[19] Although they have enjoyed good success with this approach, it should be attempted only by skilled orbital surgeons and anesthetists.

Before performing enucleation surgery, we give a retrobulbar block of two parts lidocaine 1% with epinephrine 1:100,000 to one part bupivacaine .75%. We prefer to perform enucleation surgery with the patient under general anesthesia because in our experience most patients prefer this from a psychological standpoint. The addition of a retrobulbar block at the beginning of the case not only improves hemostasis but also significantly reduces the requirement for general anesthetic agent and postoperative pain. We have not found that soaking an orbital implant (porous or solid) in local anesthetic agent before its insertion provides effective postoperative pain relief.

The decision as to which anesthetic agents to use and under which conditions surgery should be performed should be made with the best interest of the patient and surgeon in mind. A surgeon will be most comfortable with a relaxed, cooperative patient. The patient's wishes must also be considered. Although most patients will trust a surgeon's judgment, some will have had adverse experiences that will affect their approach to their care in the future. A relaxed, informative preoperative discussion allows the surgeon to explore these issues and to choose the best anesthetic for each patient on an individual basis.

REFERENCES

1. Miller NR, ed. *Walsh and Hoyt's clinical neuro ophthalmology,* vol 2, 4th ed. Baltimore, MD: Williams & Wilkins, 1983.
2. Gills JP, Hustead RF, Sanders DR. *Ophthalmic anesthesia.* New York: McGraw-Hill, 1993, p 75.
3. Hinshaw KD, Fiscella R, Sugar J. Preparation of pH adjusted local anesthetics. *Ophthal Surg* 1995;26:194.
4. Gilman AG, Rall TW, Nies AS, et al. *The pharmacological basis of therapeutics,* 8th ed. New York: Pergamon Press, 1990.
5. Baker TJ, Gordon HL, Stuzin JM. *Surgical rejuvenation of the face.* St. Louis, MO: CV Mosby, 1996.
6. *Physicians' desk reference,* 49th ed. Oradell, NJ: Medical Economics, 1995.
7. Jackson D, Chen AH, Bennett CA. Identifying true lidocaine allergy. *J Am Dent Assoc* 1994;125:1362.
8. Fagraeus L. Anesthesia. In: Sabiston DC, ed. *Essentials of surgery.* Philadelphia: WB Saunders, 1987, p 109.
9. Menke H, Klein A, John KD, Junginger T. Predictive value of ASA classification for the assessment of the perioperative risk. *Int Surg* 1993;78:266.

10. Goldberg RA, Markowitz B. Blindness after blepharoplasty. *Plast Reconstr Surg* 1992;90:929.
11. Alshameeri RS, Mamman EF. Clinical experience in the Thrombostat 4000. *Semin Thromb Hemost* 1995;21:1.
12. Epstein GA. Anesthesia in ophthalmic plastic surgery. In: Hornblass A, ed. *Oculoplastic, orbital and reconstructive surgery,* vol 1. Baltimore, MD: Williams & Wilkins, 1988, Chapter 4, pp 42–51.
13. Hustead RF, Hamilton RC. Pharmacology. In: Gills JP, Hustead RF, Sanders DR, eds. *Ophthalmic anesthesia.* New York: McGraw-Hill, 1993, pp 69–102.
14. White PF, Vasconez LO, Mathes SA, et al. Comparison of midazolam and diazepam for sedation during plastic surgery. *Plast Reconstr Surg* 1988;81:703.
15. Friedberg BL. Propofol-ketamine technique. *Aesth Plast Surg* 1993;17:297.
16. Davies BW, Pennington GA, Guyuron B. Clinical office anesthesia: the use of propofol for induction and maintenance of general anesthesia. *Aesth Plast Surg* 1993;17:125.
17. Bennett SN, McNeil MM, Bland LA, et al. Postoperative infections traced to contamination of an intravenous anesthetic, propofol. *N Engl J Med* 1995;333:184.
18. Daily MJ, Dickey JB, Packo KH. Endogenous *Candida* endophthalmitis after intravenous anesthesia with propofol. *Arch Ophthal* 1991;109:1081.
19. Khan J, Wegner P. Extensive orbital bone and soft tissue surgery under IV sedation with local anesthesia: a dynamic approach to intraoperative pain. Presented at 25th Annual Meeting of the American Society of Ophthalmic Plastic and Reconstructive Surgery, Atlanta, GA, November 1995.

CHAPTER 11

ANESTHESIOLOGIST'S VIEW OF OCULAR ANESTHESIA

JONATHAN W. KONOVITCH, MD

Few subspecialty practices demand the balance of medical knowledge, technical expertise, and physician-patient sensitivity required of the ophthalmic anesthesiologist. In addition, these skills must be applied across the entire gamut of anesthesia situations: pediatric, adult, and geriatric; ambulatory and hospitalized; elective and emergent; monitored anesthesia care (MAC) and general anesthesia.

The anesthesiologist's goal is to provide the surgeon with the best possible operating conditions and the patient with the safest and most pleasant experience.

PREOPERATIVE CONSIDERATIONS

The routine anesthesia preoperative visit is intended to gather information from the patient, impart information to the patient, and obtain an informed consent for the proposed treatment plan. Ideally the anesthesiologist should have the opportunity to meet with the patient and review the pertinent laboratory work approximately 2 to 7 days before the scheduled surgery. This is often accomplished in the preadmission processing environment and enables the exchange of information between the physician and patient to take place in a calm and unhurried manner. It also allows for the identification of potential problems with sufficient time to address, treat, and resolve them or to postpone the operation in a timely fashion so as not to cause undue disappointment and confusion to the patient and loss of time and resources to the surgeon and the operating facility.

Nevertheless, in the era of ambulatory surgery and managed care, the anesthesiologist will very often meet the patient on the day of surgery. The surgeon must be aware of this likelihood and recognize that he or she and the office staff must take an active role in the prehospital phase of the patient's preparation for anesthesia. It is extremely important that the surgeon and anesthesiologist have a clear and mutual understanding of the guidelines of their respective practices and their institution. If the surgeon's office questionnaire or interview yields anything that may be of concern, a discussion with the anesthesiologist may be advisable. This chapter relates to an elective patient scheduled to have a microscopic intraocular procedure, which will most commonly be an anterior segment operation. Other situations or contingencies are addressed under "Special Situations."

Each patient should be instructed and required to visit his or her personal physician and obtain a concise note, including a complete history and physical, a list of current medications, and any appropriate recommendations. User-friendly hospital forms can be provided for this purpose, thereby ensuring some standardization. As noted previously, this form along with pertinent laboratory reports should be available for review by the anesthesiologist a few days before the day of scheduled surgery.

The healthy, asymptomatic patient presenting for a relatively noninvasive elective procedure requires a minimum of laboratory tests. Although this varies from institution to institution, a representative regimen is shown in Table 11–1. Routine overtesting is unnecessarily costly; undertesting can result in delays or cancellations on the day of surgery,

Table 11–1. Sample of Letter That Patient Should Present to Personal Physician as Part of Preadmission Process

Dear Doctor:
   Attached please find the Preoperative Medical Evaluation form for your patient who is scheduled for surgery at _____ Hospital. Please fill out both sides completely. Please also complete the Preoperative Order sheet.
   • If the history and physical examination are unremarkable, just check the box for standard age-related preoperative testing.
   • If you believe any additional tests are indicated, please order them.
Thank you.

The following are the standard preoperative laboratory tests required for healthy asymptomatic patients scheduled for elective surgery at _____ Hospital.

	CBC	ECG	CXR	SMA-6
Patients younger than 40 years	+			
Patients older than 40 years	+	+		
Patients older than 60 years undergoing general anesthesia	+	+	+	

Certain medical conditions **require** additional tests to be ordered.

Patients with diabetes mellitus	FBS
Patients taking digoxin or diuretics	SMA-6
Menstruating women who have not had their period for >30 days	HCG

   All other laboratory tests should be ordered on the basis of the findings of the history and physical examination. Please note that although it is not our intention or responsibility to serve as a screening clinic for the patient's general health, it is our responsibility to ensure that the patient is suitably fit to undergo the proposed operation and anesthetic. Accordingly, any medical condition elicited by the history and physical examination should be evaluated with appropriate laboratory tests.
   Your judiciousness in not ordering unnecessary tests will help contain the cost of health care delivery.
   Your scrupulousness in ordering the appropriate tests will avoid delays on the day of surgery.

CBC = complete blood cell count; ECG = electrocardiogram; CXR = chest x-ray film; FBS = fasting blood sugar; HCG = human chorionic gonadotropin.

---

which can be costly and inconvenient. The key to the proper balance is a conscientious history and physical examination with judicious ordering of laboratory tests based on the findings.

   The preoperative assessment should address all current medical conditions. Chronic conditions should be diagnosed, optimally managed, and stable. The operative question is: Can the patient's condition be significantly improved by delaying the surgery? In making this decision, the nature of the surgery and the proposed anesthetic should be considered relative to the possible expected improvement.

   Two other important matters should be clearly provided for before the day of surgery. The first is instruction to the patient regarding "nothing by mouth" (NPO) status. This is one of those areas that now often fall to the surgeon's office staff because they are frequently the last people to speak with the patient before presentation to the surgical facility.

Table 11–2. A Representative "Nothing by Mouth" (NPO) Guideline Statement

NPO Guidelines

1. **No solid food on the day of surgery.** Ideally patients should be advised to eat a light dinner the evening before surgery and as sparingly as possible after dinner.
2. **Patients are permitted unrestricted clear liquids until 3 hours before scheduled surgery.** Clear liquids are water, tea, apple juice (preferably diluted), and coffee, although the latter should be kept to a minimum because it stimulates acid production and release in the stomach. Liquids such as milk and orange juice are *not* clear liquids. Patients should abstain from alcohol.
3. **In most cases, patients should be instructed to take their usual oral medications on the morning of surgery.**
4. **Infants: The last formula feeding should be 8 hours before scheduled surgery. Unrestricted clear liquids are permitted and should be encouraged up to 3 hours before surgery.**

These guidelines are designed to maximize the safety of the surgical-anesthetic experience for our patients. With the vast majority of our surgery being done on an ambulatory or same-day admission basis, often the final preoperative instructions are provided in your office. Please be sure that your office staff is familiar with these guidelines and instruct your patients appropriately.

   Thank you for your attention to this important matter. Compliance with these guidelines will directly contribute to reducing hospital expenses, making our hospital more efficient, and providing a more pleasant experience for our patients.

Again, this policy will vary with the institution (Table 11–2). The second issue is the time of arrival to the facility. The surgeon's office should be familiar with the time required by the facility to process and prepare a patient for surgery adequately. It is unnecessary and less than ideal care for a patient, particularly an elderly person, to be or feel rushed. It is also unnecessary and unpleasant for the patient to spend an excessive amount of time in the facility before the operation. The patient should be given the most accurate estimate possible of the expected time of surgery, and the NPO and arrival instructions should reflect that time.

   It cannot be emphasized enough that quality patient care is a collaborative effort. Should any question arise with respect to a patient's medical status, medication, or any other aspect of the preoperative assessment and preparation, the anesthesiologist will always welcome and appreciate a telephone call from the surgeon. The surgeon may want to convey information, ask a question, or request that the anesthesiologist speak with the patient's private medical physician. Any and all of these are welcome. The more information the anesthesiologist has, the better the care he or she can provide.

THE DAY OF SURGERY

PREOPERATIVE PERIOD

When the anesthesiologist meets with the patient on the day of surgery, he or she will have already reviewed the preadmission information and will seek to clarify particular items or gain additional information as necessary. He or she will then present the anesthetic options to the

Table 11–3. Special Considerations for Ophthalmic Surgery

Patient Requirements
  Elderly patients with concomitant disease
  Very anxious
Surgeon Requirements
  Still, cooperative patient
  "Soft" eye
  Anesthesia-akinesia of globe, orbital contents, and lids
Anesthesiologist Requirements
  Comfort level in giving anesthesia with an unsecured airway from the side of the table
  Zero tolerance for complications

patient, bearing in mind the need to meet the special requirements for ophthalmic surgery (Table 11–3).

It should be noted that the trend for most ophthalmic surgeries is toward the use of MAC techniques, that is, anesthesia monitoring with administration of appropriate intravenous medications in conjunction with local anesthetic drugs delivered by one of several techniques. This does not mean that the option of general anesthesia should be withheld from the patient; it is, however, especially important to document the thinking behind a decision that goes counter to the national and international norms. The surgeon and the anesthesiologist must be aware of the prevailing standards of care, and this is yet another example of a situation in which it is advantageous to have a close working relationship. It is often beneficial for the surgeon to communicate with the anesthesiologist in advance, thereby avoiding the possible confusion and loss of confidence the patient may face when presented with differing opinions of what is optimal care.

All patients having surgery are apprehensive; the anxiety of the patient scheduled for eye surgery is even more acute. An anesthesiologist familiar with ophthalmic surgery can provide the patient with an explanation of what will be done and what the patient's perception of the procedure will be; this will help allay the patient's preoperative concerns as well as prepare the way for a smoother intraoperative course.

General Anesthesia

All of the surgical criteria presented in Table 11–3 are easily met with general anesthesia. The guarantee of a still patient and the additional

Table 11–4. Commonly Used Ophthalmic Drugs with Anesthetic Implications

Drug	Comment
Propranolol, timolol	When administered as ophthalmic drops, they can cause systemic β-blockade (i.e., bradycardia, diminished cardiac response to increased demand, and bronchoconstriction).
Acetazolamide	Chronic use can result in hypokalemia and metabolic acidosis. This should be corrected preoperatively, particularly in patients taking digitalis preparations.
Echothiophate iodide	Its anticholinesterase activity results in prolonged blockade from neuromuscular blocking agents metabolized by pseudocholinesterase.
Phenylephrine hydrochloride mydriatics and vasoconstrictors	Drops can cause a marked rise in blood pressure. The 10% solution should not be used, and the 2.5% solution should be used with caution in patients with cardiac and hypertensive histories.

Table 11–5. Advantages to Blocking in a Separate Area

Time to sedate properly	Time to supplement
Time to observe	Increased efficiency

requirement of a rapid recovery so desirable in view of the shortened surgical times and the ambulatory setting have been greatly facilitated by the advent of low-solubility inhalation agents and short-acting, non-depolarizing neuromuscular blocking agents. The specific choice of drugs is strictly an anesthetic determination as is the decision whether or not to premedicate the patient. It is understood that the anesthesiologist is familiar with the commonly used ophthalmic medications and their potential interactions with anesthesia (Table 11–4).

MAC

If MAC is the anesthetic plan selected, two questions should be addressed before the actual administration of the anesthetic: Where should the patient be blocked? Should the patient be sedated?

Traditionally, anesthetics have been administered with the patient on the operating table just before the operation begins. With shortened operating times, increased surgical volumes, increased operating room costs, and the widespread use of orbital decompression devices, many institutions have adopted the practice of blocking the patient before he or she enters the operating room (Table 11–5). This can easily be accomplished in a designated area in the operating suite. Standards of safety must be met (Table 11–6, Fig. 11–1), but if properly established and supported, this practice can contribute significantly to the efficiency of an ophthalmic surgical facility.

The administration of the blocks can be accomplished with or without sedating the patient. Ophthalmic surgery often provides its own "controlled" studies because patients frequently have at least two operations. Patients, surgeons, and anesthesiologists have learned that there are distinct advantages to providing sedation before the administration of the blocks (Table 11–7).

SPECIAL SITUATIONS

The special circumstances sections throughout this chapter are meant to discuss scenarios that present commonly in ophthalmic surgery. There are no absolutes as to how these situations should be handled; the comments herein are intended as considerations and guidelines.

In analyzing and resolving situations that present in the preoperative period, it is important to keep in mind several principles:

Table 11–6. Equipment Needed in the Blocking Area

Oxygen (nasal)	Monitors
Suction (connected and ready)	Resuscitative equipment and drugs
Airways, Ambu bag, and laryngoscope	

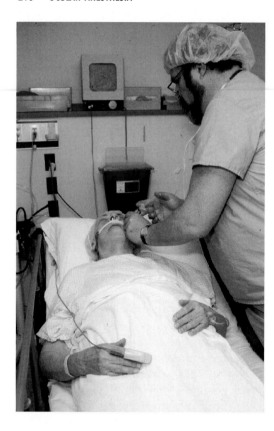

Figure 11–1. Patient being blocked. Note the intravenous catheter, nasal oxygen, and pulse oximeter.

- Do not become lulled by routine. Eye operations, in their simplest form, can be straightforward and repetitive. It is important to always be aware that each technical exercise called an eye operation is being performed on a whole patient, each with his or her own unique medical history and problems. As discussed, most issues should have been recognized and resolved during the preadmission processing phase of the patient's operative experience; nevertheless, problems will arise on the day of surgery. Each patient needs to be evaluated and prepared individually, including the possibility of having the operation delayed or postponed, if indicated. It is sometimes too easy to lose this focus when performing a repetitive series of relatively noninvasive operations.
- Do not be intimidated by a high-volume environment. Even an experienced anesthesiologist can be caught up in the pressure attendant with a high-volume, rapid-turnover practice. In evaluating medical issues, one must be aware and not allow oneself to be unduly swayed by facts such as the patient has waited a long time for the operation; the family has arranged their schedule to bring the patient to the facility and care for him or her postoperatively, and the surgeon does

Table 11–7. Advantages of Sedation

Patient cooperation	Decreased sympathetic response
Increased patient acceptance of procedure	Little downside risk

not like snags, delays, or cancellations because his or her schedule is too busy to accommodate rescheduling the patient.

- Most anesthesiologists will make every reasonable effort to enable an operation to proceed. There will, however, be circumstances under which an operation should be canceled. It is important that both the anesthesiologist and the surgeon speak with the patient and the family to ensure that they understand exactly why the procedure is being canceled. It should be explained to them that you understand that this is a disappointment and an inconvenience, but that the physician's primary responsibility is to the well-being of the patient. If there is any doubt that the patient is not in optimal condition for surgery, especially an elective procedure, the physician will always choose to err on the side of caution.

- Assess emergencies. The declaration of the urgency with which an operation must be undertaken is a surgical decision. The medical readiness of the patient to undergo surgery and anesthesia is usually best determined by the anesthesiologist, often with the assistance of a medical consultant. In the rare circumstances when there is a potential risk-to-organ versus risk-to-life situation, the surgeon and anesthesiologist working together can modify the timing and surgical or anesthetic plans so as to provide the best care for the patient.

- Do not overreach a facility's ability. Ophthalmology procedures are performed in multiple settings with very different levels of care available. Not every venue is appropriate for every patient. An honest assessment must be made as to whether a facility has the necessary support services that may be reasonably required for a particular patient before undertaking the case there.

As discussed, most preoperative issues should have been identified and resolved during the preadmission processing phase of the patient's operative experience. Nevertheless, situations will present that need to be addressed:

- The patient presents for surgery with an upper respiratory tract infection (URI) or cough.

  In the face of the onset of new symptoms or an active URI it is often best to postpone surgery, depending on the nature and severity of the symptoms. Patients who are clearly in the convalescent phase can frequently proceed without problems.

  A cough presents a particular problem for open eye surgery. The significance of a cough during the operation must be explained to the patient, and both the patient and the symptoms should be evaluated by the surgeon and the anesthesiologist. Medication with hydrocodone bitartrate, 5 mL orally, or lidocaine hydrochloride with or without a narcotic intravenously will often be of physiologic as well as psychological benefit.

  Children will usually require endotracheal intubation for their procedure. In view of the histopathologic changes resulting from a URI, the delicacy of the pediatric airway, and the possibility of postintubation laryngotracheal bronchitis, these operations should almost always be postponed until 2 to 3 weeks after the child is symptom free. The use of the laryngeal mask airway (LMA) may provide somewhat more leeway in this area, but, in general, surgery involving children with an active intercurrent disease process should be postponed.

- The patient reports having had chest pain or wheezing on the morning of surgery.

In this patient population, many of whom give a history of long-standing angina, asthma, or chronic bronchitis, the key is distinguishing the patient's baseline from a new or more acute presentation. Episodes that fall within the patient's chronic stable pattern and respond and resolve with the customary treatment regimen usually do not preclude proceeding with surgery. New symptoms or a change in pattern or severity deserves an evaluation and workup before surgery.

- The patient presents with previously undiagnosed disease.

As indicated, new findings usually deserve a workup. Certain laboratory findings, especially in the absence of symptoms, can sometimes safely be followed up after surgery.

- The patient is hypertensive in the ambulatory unit or in the holding area.

Eye surgery is an anxiety-provoking experience, which can often be manifested by increases in blood pressure. Although all anesthesiologists have their own cutoff points, many use 200/100 mm Hg as a guideline. Known, treated hypertensives who are judged to be on an adequate regimen will often benefit from any or all of a combination of nitroglycerin ointment, sedation (orally or intravenously), and a mixed α- and β-blocker labetalol or esmolol. "White coat hypertension" is a diagnosis of exclusion and requires careful documentation.

- The patient is taking anticoagulants.

This area requires specific communication and coordination among the surgeon, anesthesiologist, and internist. The overriding consideration is often the identification of the original indication for the patient to have been placed on this therapy. The internist must determine whether the cessation or diminution of anticoagulation, with its potential resultant hypercoagulable state, can safely be undertaken for the perioperative period. If so, this is, of course, preferable. If it is not possible, both anesthesiologist and surgeon must adjust their techniques to proceed in the manner least likely to cause bleeding.

- Prepare children for surgery.

There is nothing unique about ophthalmic surgery in the management of the pediatric patient. Good practice includes establishing rapport with the child, teaching and reassuring (showing the child the mask, for example), and considering the use of a topical anesthetic cream (lidocaine, 2.5%, prilocaine, 2.5% = EMLA) if an intravenous induction is contemplated (Fig. 11–2). Depending on the degree of separation anxiety of the patient and parent, the parent may want to come into the operating room for the induction, and this should almost always be permitted. If premedication is desired, a simple and satisfactory oral cocktail to remember is 2.0 mg/kg of meperidine, 0.2 mg/kg of diazepam, and 0.02 mg/kg of atropine sulfate.

The surgeon and the anesthesiologist should be aware that there is a higher incidence of malignant hyperthermia in strabismus patients. As always, a careful family history should be taken. A heightened state of attentiveness and preparedness is appropriate (see Malignant Hyperthermia).

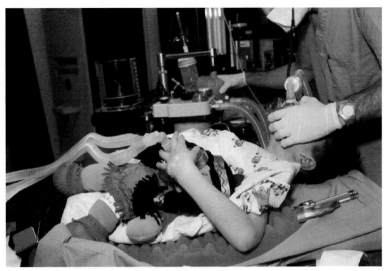

Figure 11-2. A gentle pediatric inhalation induction.

When caring for congenital conditions such as cataracts or glaucoma, it must be borne in mind that infants born prematurely are at higher risk for postanesthesia apnea. This situation persists until at least 46 and possibly up to 60 weeks of postconceptual age. When possible, surgery should be delayed. If delay is deemed inadvisable, an overnight stay in a facility with appropriate monitoring and support services is recommended.

• The patient presents for surgery with an open eye and a full stomach.

This is a classic problem about which much has been written. Some of the newer nondepolarizing neuromuscular blocking agents (and the potential use of parabulbar anesthesia [see Chapter 1]) have made this somewhat less of a problem, but succinylcholine (with its attendant increase in intraocular pressure) remains the fastest way to secure and protect an airway. "Precurarization" is indicated. It should also be noted that there is abundant anecdotal information among experienced ophthalmic anesthesiologists reporting the safe use of succinylcholine without untoward ophthalmic results despite the theoretical and published considerations. In making choices, it is important to remember that occurrences such as crying and struggling also raise the intraocular pressure, as does bucking on an endotracheal tube placed before adequate neuromuscular blockade. Although we would always like to achieve all our goals, the priority is clear: ABC before IOP, that is, *A*irway, *B*reathing, and *C*irculation before *I*ntra*O*cular *P*ressure.

ADMINISTRATION OF ANESTHESIA

General Anesthesia

It is, of course, beyond the scope of this text to provide detailed instruction as to how to plan and conduct a general anesthetic. An experienced anesthesiologist will be able to formulate a satisfactory plan for the typical elderly patient with several concurrent medical problems.

Induction is most frequently accomplished with an ultra-short-acting barbiturate (thiopental sodium [Pentothal] or methohexital sodium), and intubation is facilitated with a short-acting neuromuscular blocking agent. The endotracheal tube is positioned and taped so as to be unobtrusive to the surgeon (a preformed angled tube is particularly good for this purpose), and the anesthesiologist will be positioned at the side of the table to allow free access to the head for the surgical team (Fig. 11–3).

The challenge at this juncture lies in the recognition that the operation begins very shortly after the induction, it is stimulating and the patient must be perfectly still, and then the operation can often be finished quickly. A satisfactory level of anesthesia must, therefore, be established rapidly, but the pharmacokinetic profile of the agents used must be such as to also allow for a rapid recovery. Furthermore, in today's ambulatory surgery environment, the patient is expected to be ready to go home 2 to 3 hours after the operation has ended. This can be achieved with either a nitrous oxide–narcotic–relaxant technique or a potent inhalation agent, a choice best left to the individual anesthesiologist. Particular attention must be given to avoid bucking or coughing during the procedure and on emergence. "Deep extubation," when possible, should be considered.

MAC

The object of the block is to provide a pain-free experience for the patient and optimal conditions for the surgeon. Surgical requirements will vary greatly among surgeons. Lid block, extraocular muscle block, and even degrees of anesthesia are of relative importance to different surgeons,

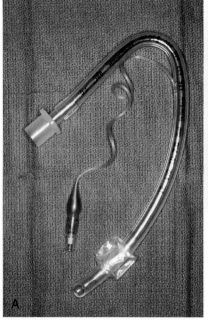

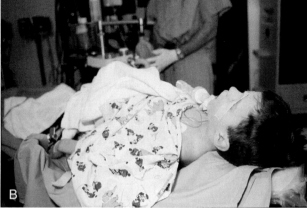

Figure 11–3. *A,* Use of a preformed angled endotracheal tube keeps anesthesia equipment out of the surgeon's way. *B,* Anesthesia machine and anesthesiologist are positioned at patient's side.

depending on their operative techniques, personal emotional demeanor, and surgical time. It is always important and advantageous for the anesthesiologist to be aware of each surgeon's preferences and needs and strive to provide for them.

Blocks of cranial nerves II (vision), V (anesthesia to the globe), III, IV, and VI (extraocular muscle akinesia) can be accomplished with a midorbit or posterior orbit extraconal block or an intraconal block. Because of fenestrations in the intraorbital and intermuscular septa, this same block will provide motor anesthesia to the lids (orbicularis oculi muscle, cranial nerve VII), especially with the use of orbital decompression devices. The experienced ophthalmic anesthesiologist will have several supplemental cranial nerve VII blocks available should they be required.

In view of the bony anatomy and the desire to enter the orbit by the most avascular route possible (adipose tissue channels), the inferotemporal approach is most preferred. Although there are many choices as to anesthetic agents and equipment, a favored technique involves the administration of 6 to 10 mL of a mixture of 4% lidocaine, .75% bupivacaine, and 150 U hyaluronidase via a 25-gauge 1½ inch (3.75-cm) blunt Atkinson needle to a peribulbar or retrobulbar site. Intraconal injections should be limited to 2 to 3 mL. Specific details of anesthetic drugs and injection techniques are discussed elsewhere as are parabulbar and topical anesthesia, two approaches that have gained favor with the advent of newer surgical techniques.

As the literature will bear out, there are many ways to provide satisfactory anesthesia for ophthalmic surgery, and there are ardent proponents and supporters of each. The important thing is that each practitioner be familiar with at least one of them and become intimate with it. One must achieve a high level of proficiency while knowing its advantages, disadvantages, and limitations. The more experienced physician will have not only a preferred technique but also one or more options to turn to with reliable results should it be necessary. There is no substitute for experience. An anesthesiologist who provides blocks for all the surgeons in an institution will certainly acquire and maintain that experience and skill more easily than one who services only a single surgical practice of normal volume.

Monitoring for anesthesia for ophthalmic surgery involves an electrocardiogram, blood pressure, and pulse oximetry. Supplemental oxygen should be used routinely. A precordial stethoscope may be used, and temperature monitoring should be available. General anesthesia requires the use of end-tidal gas monitoring as well.

During the preoperative conversation, the patient will have been prepared for what to expect in the operating room itself. If a general anesthetic is to be administered, the patient will have been made aware of the monitors to be used and what will most likely be experienced during the induction. A MAC technique will require more instruction and reassurance for the patient. While being positioned on the operating table, the patient will be reminded that even though conversations among the surgeons and nurses or sounds from some of the surgical equipment may be heard, it is very important that every effort be made to keep the head as still as possible. If there is a problem, the patient should certainly speak up and it will be taken care of, but the patient should be reassured that the anesthesiologist will be able to provide a safe and comfortable procedure.

SPECIAL SITUATIONS

- Claustrophobia

  This is an example of the type of problem that is best identified before the onset of surgery. Either an anesthesiologist experienced with ophthalmic surgery will have inquired directly of the patient with regard to this condition, or it will have been expressed by the patient in response to the anesthesiologist's explanation of the procedures that the patient will experience in the operating room. Often patients with less severe symptoms can be managed with reassurance, sedatives, draping as openly as the surgeon feels comfortable, and constant communication and contact throughout the procedure. This situation requires sensitivity and patience on the part of all concerned. It is wise to proceed with the preparations for surgery in a deliberate manner, allowing time to be certain that the patient can tolerate each stage. It is important that the anesthesiologist be familiar with the surgeon's ability to deal with a patient's needs during the operation as well as the surgeon's realistic expected surgical time and to take these into account when formulating an anesthetic plan. Unless absolutely contraindicated, general anesthesia should always be given consideration. Having to convert from a MAC technique to general anesthesia in the middle of an operation is the least desired situation, but it can be safely accomplished by experienced personnel and good communication.

- Complications of the block

  As with all other anesthetic techniques, it is, of course, imperative that the anesthesiologist be familiar with the potential complications of the blocks used. The anesthesiologist must be able to diagnose and treat them. Of particular concern are retrobulbar hemorrhage, intravenous or intra-arterial injections of local anesthetic, and the late (5–10 minutes after the block) occurrence of respiratory arrest. Appropriate monitoring and contingencies for assistance when required should be in place in any location where patients are being blocked.

- Inadequate block

  The surgeon should not begin the procedure if he or she is not comfortable with the level of akinesia or if there is evidence that the level of anesthesia may not be satisfactory. The block can be supplemented by either the anesthesiologist or the surgeon through one of several techniques, but it must be understood that intravenous sedation cannot compensate for a poor block (or, under other circumstances, a block that has worn off because the surgeon has greatly exceeded the time usually required for a particular operation and the anesthesia provided by a particular agent). Again, a close working relationship and understanding between the surgeon and anesthesiologist will help determine how best to handle these situations. A confident, capable surgeon who is sensitive to the situation, gentle with tissues, and economical in maneuvers is an asset.

- Patients with organic mental syndrome or patients who exhibit "sundowning"

  Patients who manifest signs of senility require careful preoperative evaluation as to their ability to cooperate with a MAC technique. General anesthesia should be avoided if possible because gerontology experience has shown that there are, at times, unpredictable postoperative deteriorations in mental status after well-conducted, uneventful general anesthetics. Despite preoperative assessment and preparation, loss of patient cooperation may still arise in the operating room and may result in the cancellation or abortion of the procedure or the conversion to general anesthesia. Early reports with propofol seem to offer a satisfactory and perhaps superior option in these circumstances. All other causes of restlessness or disorientation must be ruled out, as discussed next.

- Restless or uncooperative intraoperatively

  Often this situation can be anticipated. Certain elderly patients simply may not be able to tolerate the necessary position on the operating table for very long. Every effort should be made to make the patient comfortable before the start of surgery. Appropriate positioning of the table (a "beach chair" position) and the placement of pillows or padding under the knees, neck, and so on are important, particularly for arthritic patients. The surgeon should be attentive to having the patient be on the operating table for as short a time as possible. This includes promptly beginning the operation when the patient is placed on the table as well as efficient surgical technique.

  Obese patients, those with a history of congestive heart failure, and those with hiatus hernia or gastroesophageal reflux may not tolerate the Trendelenburg position many surgeons favor, and a compromise may be necessary. Preoperative teaching and preparation help a patient psychologically but cannot overcome real physical discomfort.

  The entire differential diagnosis of restlessness must be rapidly explored whenever this situation occurs. Drug reactions, airway obstruction with hypoxia, and carbon dioxide retention under the drapes are all considerations. Occasionally, a patient may be assessed to be in an intermediate state of disinhibition without tranquilization. This will require additional sedation or, perhaps preferably, allowing the sedation to wear off (or even reversing some of the medication) so that meaningful communication can occur and cooperation be restored.

- Malignant hyperthermia

  Inquiry as to a family history of this rare but serious complication is always made during the preoperative evaluation. A negative history and, indeed, even a history of the patient's having had uneventful previous anesthetics do not ensure that this phenomenon will not occur. Any facility in which patients are anesthetized must be prepared for this event.

  As with any potential complication, diagnosis is based on knowledge of the entity (one cannot diagnose something one does not know) and maintaining a high index of suspicion (one cannot diagnose something one does not think of). The earliest signs are often tightness of the jaw (masseter spasm) and unexplained, excessive, persistent tachycardia and tachypnea (manifestations of a hypermetabolic state). These signs usually precede the detectable rise in temperature. If this syndrome is suspected, the standard malignant hyperthermia protocol should be followed immediately.

• The use of nitrous oxide when a gas-fluid exchange is anticipated

An anesthesiologist experienced with vitreoretinal surgery will understand and anticipate the physics involved in the relative diffusion properties of nitrous oxide and the various gases used for tamponade. The anesthesiologist will either select a technique that does not require nitrous oxide or be prepared to turn it off at the appropriate juncture in the operation and have provided for an adequate continued level of anesthesia (see Chapter 8).

POSTOPERATIVE PERIOD

Every effort should be made to achieve as smooth and undisturbed a postoperative period as possible. In the case of general anesthesia, "deep"

POST OPERATIVE TRIAGE
AND EVALUATION

AMBULATORY SURGERY PATIENTS

☐   Patient transferred to Post Anesthesia Care Unit.
Standard P.A.C.U. monitoring initiated.
Report given to P.A.C.U. RN.

BP_____   P_____   R _____   SaO$_2$ _____

_____   M.D./C.R.N.A.

DATE_____   TIME_____

☐   Vital signs stable. Emergence and recovery from anesthesia proceeding satisfactorily. No anesthetic related complaints. Patient may proceed to post-operative ambulatory care area. Would expect patient to be ready for discharge in ____ to ____ hours.

_____   M.D./C.R.N.A.

DATE_____   TIME_____

☐ Patient's status changed to hospital inpatient. (see below)

Figure 11–4. Sample of a form filled out by anesthesia personnel on completion of surgery.

extubation, coupled with some of the newer inhalation agents, provides for a calm, yet rapid emergence.

Patients who have had MAC with little or no additional sedation after the block are almost always able to leave the operating room in a lounge-type chair rather than a stretcher. Most often, in fact, they will not require the services of the traditional recovery room. Policies should be in place allowing these patients to proceed directly to a more appropriate and comfortable setting (Fig. 11–4).

A patient's progress through the postoperative phase is individualized. It is always a good practice to observe a patient for at least one-half hour and to ensure that he or she has returned close to baseline in most major areas of function. The discharge criteria to declare a patient "home ready" are necessarily more demanding than when a patient is being sent from the recovery area to a hospital bed. Postanesthesia discharge scores (Fig. 11–5) are in common use and facilitate patient flow. A reliable adult must always accept responsibility for the patient on discharge from the facility.

NOTE: *R.N.'s may discharge patients when all of the following criteria are satisfied:*

a) a total P.A.D.S. score of 10 or better is obtained,
b) a minimum score of 1 is obtained in each P.A.D.S.
    assessment category,
c) a total P.A.D.S. score of less than 10 is accompanied by
    physician clearance
    (anesthesia or surgeon as indicated by individual case)
d) the patient is free of new medical complaints, signs, and
    symptoms
    (e.g. shortness of breath, chest pain, etc.)

DISCHARGE CHECKLIST

Post-Anesthesia Discharge Scale (P.A.D.S.) Score? _____

Evaluated by physician (anesthesia or surgery, as appropriate)? ☐
Adult escort present? ☐
Follow up appointments given? ☐
Post-operative instructions given and understood? ☐
Prescriptions given, if any? ☐

AMBULATORY SURGERY UNIT: POST - ANESTHESIA DISCHARGE SCALE			
ASSESSMENT	**POST-OP**	**DISCHARGE**	**DISCHARGE CRITERIA**
VITAL SIGNS	2 ☐ 1 ☐ 0 ☐	2 ☐ 1 ☐ 0 ☐	V.S. within 20% of baseline. V.S. within 20 to 40% of baseline. V.S. over 40% of baseline.
ACTIVITY	2 ☐ 1 ☐ 0 ☐	2 ☐ 1 ☐ 0 ☐	Ambulates at pre-operative level. Requires more assistance than pre-operatively. Unable or unwilling to ambulate.
ORIENTATION	2 ☐ 1 ☐ 0 ☐	2 ☐ 1 ☐ 0 ☐	Alert & oriented consistent with baseline. Sleepy, but alert and oriented when awake. Difficult to awaken and / or disoriented.
PAIN / NAUSEA / VOMITING	2 ☐ 1 ☐ 0 ☐	2 ☐ 1 ☐ 0 ☐	Complaint: None or minimal. Moderate complaints: Required medication(s). Severe complaints: Re-medication.
INTAKE	2 ☐ 1 ☐ 0 ☐	2 ☐ 1 ☐ 0 ☐	Tolerated food and fluids. Tolerated fluids only. Not taking food or fluids, or has I.V.
BLEEDING	2 ☐ 1 ☐ 0 ☐	2 ☐ 1 ☐ 0 ☐	Dressing dry or has scant bleeding. Moderate bleeding, dressing re-inforced. Severe bleeding, surgeon attended patient.
TOTALS			

FORM NO. AS2 Rev. 6/94

Figure 11–5. Sample of written policy used to facilitate patient flow through the ambulatory surgical unit. (IV = intravenous.)

SPECIAL SITUATIONS

Although most postophthalmic surgery anesthesia courses are smooth and uncomplicated, certain situations present with some frequency.

- Hypertension

As mentioned, patients routinely on antihypertensive medication should have taken it before their operation. They should also resume their usual regimen postoperatively as soon as possible.

The causes of hypertension must be considered. The most common sources in the recovery room setting are pain from the surgical site (more common after ophthalmic plastic cases than anterior chamber surgery), poor preoperative blood pressure control, a full bladder (especially when mannitol has been used), or a general manifestation of restlessness (remember that hypoxia can be a cause of restlessness). Treatment is appropriate to the cause. Short-acting medications or reductions in dose should be considered if the patient is ambulatory. For the patient who is hypertensive without complaints or without another identifiable cause, sublingual nifedipine will often be a satisfactory solution.

- Pain

Pain is usually minimal after anterior chamber surgery. It is somewhat greater after muscle and vitreoretinal surgery, and it can be significant after certain ophthalmic plastic procedures. Treatment options include oral analgesics, nonsteroidal anti-inflammatory agents, and narcotics. Pain referable to the eye itself, especially if accompanied with nausea, should prompt a consultation with the ophthalmologist in consideration of the possibility of increased intraocular pressure.

- Postoperative Nausea and Vomiting (PONV)

This problem presents more frequently after eye muscle and vitreoretinal surgery, and one should consider prophylaxis with metoclopramide, droperidol, or a phenothiazine. Ondansetron can be used for patients with a positive history of PONV or who fall into one of the high-risk populations (e.g., patients with a history of motion sickness or a history of irritable bowel).

Most patients should not be required to eat or drink postoperatively until they express a desire to do so. This practice, along with sensible first foods, will also serve to minimize this problem.

INDEX

Note: Page numbers in *italics* refer to figures; page numbers followed by t refer to tables.